Praise for *Practice & Leadership in Nursing Homes*

"As a nurse long involved in nursing home research, practice, education, and policy, as well as a contributor to the book Improving the Quality of Care in Nursing Homes, *I highly recommend this exceptional book. It's timely, comprehensive, and written by distinguished authors and interprofessional contributors who are among the very best in the field. Grounded in the 4 Ms framework, the 2022 NASEM report, and Moving Forward action plans, the text is organized to be maximally useful to nursing students and those who educate and employ them, including tips, practice essentials, and outstanding figures and tables that enhance the narrative."*

–Kathleen (Kitty) Buckwalter, PhD, RN, FAAN
Professor of Research & Distinguished Nurse Scientist in Aging
Donald W. Reynolds Center of Geriatric Nursing Excellence, College of Nursing
Oklahoma University Health Sciences Center
Professor Emerita, University of Iowa College of Nursing

"I commend the authors for an inspirational vision of both an environment that supports meaning and quality of life for older adults and a rewarding career in nursing homes. This in-depth, evidence-based roadmap to high-quality care in nursing homes is a powerful compilation of the expertise of leaders in our field, incorporating the socio-political context, theoretical frameworks, practice standards, and professional roles, action strategies, and case examples. This is a must-read!"

–Heather M. Young, PhD, RN, FAAN, FGSA
Professor, Betty Irene Moore School of Nursing, University of California, Davis

PRACTICE & LEADERSHIP IN NURSING HOMES

Building on Academic-Practice Partnerships

JoAnne Reifsnyder, PhD, MSN, MBA, RN, FAAN

Ann Kolanowski, PhD, RN, FAAN

Jacqueline Dunbar-Jacob, PhD, RN, FAAN

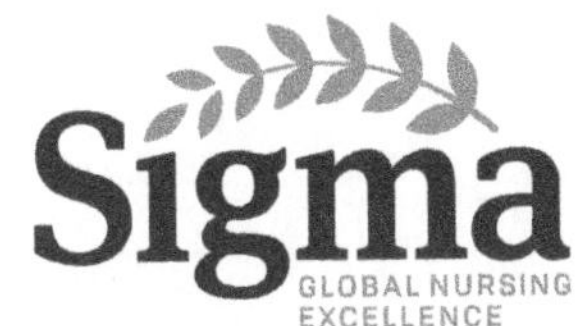

Sigma Theta Tau International Honor Society of Nursing (Sigma) is a nonprofit organization whose mission is developing nurse leaders anywhere to improve healthcare everywhere. Founded in 1922, Sigma has more than 135,000 active members in over 100 countries and territories. Members include practicing nurses, instructors, researchers, policymakers, entrepreneurs, and others. Sigma's more than 540 chapters are located at more than 700 institutions of higher education throughout Armenia, Australia, Botswana, Brazil, Canada, Colombia, Croatia, England, Eswatini, Finland, Ghana, Hong Kong, Ireland, Israel, Italy, Jamaica, Japan, Jordan, Kenya, Lebanon, Malawi, Mexico, the Netherlands, Nigeria, Pakistan, Philippines, Portugal, Puerto Rico, Scotland, Singapore, South Africa, South Korea, Sweden, Taiwan, Tanzania, Thailand, the United States, and Wales. Learn more at www.sigmanursing.org.

Sigma Theta Tau International
550 West North Street
Indianapolis, IN, USA 46202

To request a review copy for course adoption, order additional books, buy in bulk, or purchase for corporate use, contact Sigma Marketplace at 888.654.4968 (US/Canada toll-free), +1.317.687.2256 (International), or solutions@sigmamarketplace.org.

To request author information, or for speaker or other media requests, contact Sigma Marketing at 888.634.7575 (US/Canada toll-free) or +1.317.634.8171 (International).

ISBN: 9781646481255
EPUB ISBN: 9781646481262
PDF ISBN: 9781646481323
MOBI ISBN: 9781646481446

Library of Congress Control Number: 2023038680

Publisher: Dustin Sullivan
Acquisitions Editor: Emily Hatch
Cover Designer: Kim Scott/Bumpy Design
Interior Design/Page Layout: Kim Scott/Bumpy Design
Indexer: Larry Sweazy
Managing Editor: Carla Hall
Development Editor: Nicole Sholly
Project Editor: Todd Lothery
Copy Editor: Todd Lothery
Proofreader: Erin Geile

DEDICATIONS

This book is dedicated to the diverse women and men who comprise the nursing home careforce, providing expert, loving care to our nation's most vulnerable citizens. And to the memory of my mother, Anita, whose model as an endlessly compassionate and wise professional nurse inspired me to dedicate my life to caring for others.

–JoAnne Reifsnyder

To the memory of my husband, Kollie, and my son, Mark, whose lives gave me eternal love. And to Cindy and David, whose lives give me endless joy.

–Ann Kolanowski

In recognition of my husband, Rolf, whose personal experience in skilled nursing exemplified the benefits of post-acute care that nursing homes offer, and to my colleagues, Jacob Kariuki, Yurun Cai, and Beth Schwartz, whose enthusiastic teaching in the nursing home created nursing students interested in pursuing gerontology as a career.

–Jacqueline Dunbar-Jacob

ACKNOWLEDGMENTS

This book was created for our nation's future nurses by an interprofessional team of experts in the care of older adults. We want to thank Dr. Terry Fulmer for her persistent, visionary leadership that finds common ground and acts with haste and purpose to solve problems. As the pandemic entered year two, she convened a group of advisors with a commitment to improving the care of older adults and issued a challenge: We will propose an actionable, meaningful project by the end of a third meeting. Out of those three meetings emerged a consensus around partnering nursing schools with nursing homes to improve care and to excite new generations of nurses about caring for the elderly. Funded by the John A. Hartford Foundation, the Jewish Healthcare Foundation, and the Independence Foundation, a two-year demonstration titled *Revisiting the Teaching Nursing Home* (RTNH) kicked off in 2021. The work built on findings from the *Teaching Nursing Home* work in the 1980s led by Dr. Mathy Mezey and other nurse pioneers. As advisors to the 2021 demonstration, it became clear to us that a textbook was needed to support the education of undergraduate nursing students in nursing homes—a complex environment where most nursing students had little clinical experience beyond a nursing fundamentals course, if that. This book represents a collaboration across disciplines to bring to life the challenging and rewarding practice and leadership opportunities in nursing homes.

Many thanks to Nancy Zionts (RTNH Principal Investigator) and her team members, whose passion, creativity, and dedication have created a snowball of interest, support, and energy around the work. We also wish to thank the many members of the RTNH advisory teams, including:

Jewish Healthcare Foundation/Health Careers Futures
Nancy Zionts, MBA
Judith Black, MD, MHA
Stacie Bonenberger, MOT, OTR/L
Emily Franke, MSW, LSW
Lisa George, MPH, CHES
Anneliese Perry, MS, NHA
Maureen Saxon-Gioia, MSHSA, BSN, RN

Nursing Home Partners
UPMC Canterbury Place
Tracy Mason, RN, RNAC-CTA
Charles Rhodes, MD, MBA, MS, NHA
Presbyterian Senior Care, The Willows
Taylor McMahon, RN, CNDLTC
Centre Care Rehabilitation and Wellness
Andrew Naugle, BBA, NHA
Felicia Heaton, NHA
Wesley Enhanced Living MainLine
Dan Hood, MHA, LNHA
Kim Ratliff, BSN, RN, CNDLTC

School of Nursing Partners
University of Pittsburgh
Yurun Cai, PhD
Jackie Dunbar-Jacob, PhD, RN, FAAN
Pennsylvania State University Ross and Carol Nese College of Nursing
Marie Boltz, PhD, GNP-BC, FGSA, FAAN
Donna Fick, PhD, GCNS-BC, FAAN
University of Pennsylvania School of Nursing
Desiree Fleck, PhD, CRNP, CPNP-AC
Nancy Hodgson, PhD, RN, FAAN

The John A. Hartford Foundation
Terry Fulmer, PhD, RN, FAAN
Amy Berman, RN, LHD (hon), FAAN
Jane Carmody, DNP, MBA, RN, FAAN

Evaluation – University of Pittsburgh
Howard Degenholtz, PhD, FGSA
Chelsea Dickson, MPH

National and Statewide Advisory Board
Alice Bonner, PhD, RN, FAAN, Chair
Melissa Batchelor, PhD, RN, FNP, FGSA, FAAN

Erika Fricke
Ann Kolanowski, PhD, RN, FAAN
JoAnne Reifsnyder, PhD, MSN, MBA, RN, FAAN
Shari Ling, MD
Jennie Parker Martin, MPH
Susan Reinhard, PhD, RN
Eric Rodrieguez, MD
Susan Ryan, MA
Susan Sherman, MA, RN, FAAN
Ann Torregrossa, Esq
Deborah Trautman, PhD, RN, FAAN
Joan Weiss, PhD, RN, CRNP, FAAN
Heather Young, PhD, RN, FAAN

Working Group
Laurie Badzek, LLM, JD, MS, RN, FNAP, FAAN
Ellen Blackwell, MSW
Sophie Campbell, MSN, RN, CRRN, RAC-CT, CNDLTC
Mike De Stefon, BSOT, OTR/L, NHA
Sierra Funk, DNP, MSN, RN
Bobbi Gray, NHA, MPA
Aime Harrison, MPT
Christine Kasper, PhD, RN, FAAN, FACSM
Jacob Kariuki, PhD, AGNP-BC
Jenny Knecht, MSN, CRNP
Anne Mitchell, PhD, CRNP
Brianna Morgan, MSN, CRNP
Nicole Peterson, DNP, A/GPCNP-BC, CRNP
Brittney Sarnese, CTRS, CDP
Justine Sefchik, PhD, RN
Elizabeth A. Schlenk, PhD, RN, CNL, FAAN
Kim Strauch, MSN, RN, ANP-BC
Erin Vigne, MA, RN
Antonia Villarruel, PhD, RN, FAAN

Finally, we wish to acknowledge and thank the many contributors to this text, whose rich and diverse experience spanning nursing home operations, clinical care, nursing education, policy, regulatory affairs, technology, and finance have made the book not just possible but unmatched in quality of content. Our deepest gratitude to Abby Maglich, intern at the John A. Hartford Foundation, who provided invaluable administrative support. And a special thank you to our chapter leads Greg Alexander, Melissa Batchelor, Marie Boltz, Alice Bonner, Barbara Bowers, Julie Britton, Tara Cortes, Elizabeth Galik, Maureen Saxon-Gioia, Jennifer Sidelinker, Jasmine Travers, and Nancy Zionts.

ABOUT THE EDITORS

JoAnne Reifsnyder, PhD, MSN, MBA, RN, FAAN, is Professor, Health Services Leadership and Management, at the University of Maryland School of Nursing. She has held executive and leadership roles in hospice, hospice-related medication management, and skilled nursing. Her career clinical expertise is serious illness care for older adults. For 10 years, Reifsnyder served as the Chief Nursing Officer for Genesis HealthCare, the nation's largest skilled nursing provider. She is a fellow in the American Academy of Nursing, was appointed by former HHS Secretary Alex Azar to CDC's Healthcare Infection Control Practices Advisory Committee to bring expertise in long-term care, is a member of NASEM's Roundtable on Quality Care for People with Serious Illness, and is an advisor to the John A. Hartford Foundation and Jewish Healthcare Foundation-funded demonstration Revisiting the Teaching Nursing Home.

Ann Kolanowski, PhD, RN, FAAN, is Professor Emerita at the Penn State Ross and Carol Nese College of Nursing. She conducts research on nonpharmacological interventions for symptoms of distress and delirium in people living with dementia in nursing homes. Her research has been supported by grants from the National Institute of Nursing Research, the Alzheimer's Association, and the Hartford, Commonwealth, and Neuroscience Nursing Foundations. Kolanowski has published over 180 papers on dementia care in scientific journals and serves on many scientific advisory boards. She was the recipient of the 2012 Doris Schwartz Gerontological Nursing Research Award and is a fellow in the American Academy of Nursing and the Gerontological Society of America. Kolanowski was the founding Director of the Hartford Center of Geriatric Nursing Excellence at Penn State University.

Jacqueline Dunbar-Jacob, PhD, RN, FAAN, is Distinguished Service Professor and Dean Emeritus (Nursing) at the University of Pittsburgh. She was the founding Co-chair of the Implementation Steering Committee for the 2021 Essentials for the American Association of Colleges of Nursing and continues to serve on that committee. She was a participant in the NHLBI and NIA Working Conference on the Recognition and Management of Coronary Heart Disease and the Elderly (1985), National Academy of Sciences Workshop on Adaptive Aging (2003), and NIH Office of Medical Applications of Research State-of-the-Science Panel on Preventing Alzheimer's and

Cognitive Decline (2010). Dunbar-Jacob chaired the Scientific Advisory Board for the NIH Roadmap Initiatives for the Patient Reported Outcomes Measurement Information System from 2004–2011. She was PI and CO-PI of the NSF project on the development of Personal Robotic Assistants for the Elderly (2000–2005). A registered nurse and licensed psychologist, she is a fellow of the American Academy of Nursing, the American Psychological Association, the American Heart Association, the Society of Behavioral Medicine, and the Academy of Behavioral Medicine Research. She is Principal for Revisiting the Teaching Nursing Home at the University of Pittsburgh (2021–2023) and consultant on the project to the Jewish Healthcare Foundation.

AUTHORS

Katherine M. Abbott, PhD, MGS, FGSA, is Executive Director of the Scripps Gerontology Center and a Professor of Gerontology at Miami University in Oxford, Ohio. Abbott's research focuses on preference-based person-centered care and the social networks and health of older adults receiving long-term services and supports. She is the co-founder of Preference Based Living, whose mission is to conduct studies that build understanding of individual preferences and test innovative methods to honor preferences for people receiving long-term services and supports.

Gregory L. Alexander, PhD, RN, FAAN, FACMI, FIAHSI, is a nurse informaticist focused on improving quality of nursing home care. His scientific contributions were forged from nearly $40 million in research funding as Principal Investigator and Co-investigator on grants funded by the NIH, CMS, AHRQ, RAND, and others. His scholarly work includes over 300 peer-reviewed publications, proceedings, and presentations, including the first book for information technology implementation in long-term care: *An Introduction to Health Information Technology in LTPAC Settings* (2018). For the first time, he has shown that mean total HIT maturity in nursing homes has consistently increased over a seven-year longitudinal study. He identified structural disparities in HIT maturity in US nursing homes. He has shown that significant correlations exist between HIT maturity and 18 unique quality measures, which led to disparities in resident outcomes. He co-wrote the National Academies of Sciences, Engineering, and Medicine nursing home report on quality, released in 2022.

Melissa Batchelor, PhD, RN, FNP, FGSA, FAAN, is an Associate Professor at George Washington (GW) University's School of Nursing and Director of GW's interdisciplinary Center for Aging, Health and Humanities. Her research related to handfeeding residents with dementia (MelissaBPhD.com/NOSH) has been supported by the John A. Hartford Foundation, the Robert Wood Johnson Foundation Nurse Faculty Scholars program, and the National Institutes of Health/National Institute of Nursing Research. She is a fellow of the American Academy of Nursing and the Gerontological Society of America and served the US Senate Special Committee on Aging in the office of Senator Susan Collins (R-ME) as a Health and Aging Policy Fellow. She was the recipient of the 2022 NHCGNE Claudia J. Beverly Innovation Award and recognized as a Distinguished Gerontological Nurse Educator. Her weekly podcast, *This Is Getting Old: Moving Towards an Age-Friendly World*, is globally ranked (top 10%).

Liza L. Behrens, PhD, RN, is Assistant Professor at the Penn State Ross and Carol Nese College of Nursing. Behrens has more than 20 years of progressive experience providing nursing care to older adults in multiple care settings, including psychiatric and medical hospitals, outpatient clinics, nursing homes, and home-based care. She has held many leadership positions in nursing and in clinical research. She conducts research to develop and deliver individualized (person-centered) interventions to improve the quality of life and care for older adults living with dementia in nursing homes. Her recent work explores how risk perceptions of nursing home staff, family, and residents influence decision-making around honoring residents' preferences for activities of daily living and care. Behrens has published over 35 peer-reviewed papers on delivering person-centered dementia care in nursing homes.

Stacey E. Bergmann, MS, CTRS, ADC, CDP, has over 20 years of experience in the senior living industry providing recreation therapy and dementia care for older adults alongside a multidisciplinary team. She received her bachelor of psychology from the University of Delaware and attended Temple University to receive her education and training in therapeutic recreation. Bergmann received her master of health science degree from St. Francis University with a focus on health education and research in dementia care. As an advanced practice Certified Therapeutic Recreation Specialist and Dementia Consultant, she specializes in evidence-based, holistic care that promotes well-being for older adults. Bergmann was a Research Facilitator for Penn State Nursing's EIT-4-PBSD study. She is the owner of B-Enriched Living, focused on enriching lives for older adults by educating and empowering those who serve. She is also a Cognitive Care Coach and Community Consultant for AlzBetter and Wellness Coordinator for Friends Life Care. She is President of VOICE PA and is an advocate and champion for person-directed living.

Amy Berman, RN, LHD(hon), FAAN, is a Senior Program Officer with the John A. Hartford Foundation, where she works on the Foundation's development and dissemination of innovative, cost-effective models of care that improve health outcomes for older adults. Berman is the program officer overseeing the Age-Friendly Health Systems and Revisiting the Teaching Nursing Home initiatives funded by the Foundation, which both support the reliable delivery of evidence-based care in nursing homes. She also leads many of the Foundation's efforts focused on improving end-of-life and serious illness care. She is a member of the American Academy of Nursing, the Gerontological Society of America, the American Geriatrics Society, and the Sigma Theta Tau International Honor Society of Nursing. Berman has been the recipient of numerous honors for her advocacy on behalf of older adults and those facing serious illness, including the President's Award from the American Academy of Hospice and Palliative Medicine, the CAPC Innovation Award from the Center to Advance Palliative Care, and most recently, the Hospice and Palliative Nurses Association Champion Award.

Dawn Clayton Bieber, BS, OTR/L, has over 30 years of experience providing occupational therapy services to clients in skilled nursing facilities (SNF), assisted living facilities (AL), IRF, HH, and more. Bieber has served as an Advisory Council Member for the Geriatric Special Interest Section Listserv for AOTA (2007–2010) and has held several positions with the Pennsylvania Occupational Therapy Association, including Vice President, over the past 20 years. Bieber has clinical and operational experience and has worked to build and support collaborative relationships and integrated clinical programming that promotes aging in place and safety for residents and caregivers. She has presented at both the national and state level on the topics of dementia, falls management, and occupational therapy services in retirement communities.

Laura Block, BS, BSN, RN, is a doctoral student at the University of Wisconsin-Madison School of Nursing and an RN with experience in post-acute and long-term care settings. Block's research focuses on improving care for adults living with dementia who have complex biopsychosocial needs—and is inspired by her experiences working in nursing homes. She has contributed to research on transitional care for older adults living with dementia, behavioral and psychological symptoms of dementia, and person-centered care in nursing homes. Block is the recent recipient of a National Institute on Aging Ruth L. Kirschstein National Research Service Award (NRSA/F31) for her dissertation work, which will examine symptoms and treatment considerations for nursing home residents living with comorbid dementia and mental health conditions.

Marie Boltz, PhD, GNP-BC, FGSA, FAAN, is a geriatric nurse practitioner with extensive, cross-setting clinical and administrative experience. She has also taught at all university levels (undergraduate, master's, DNP, PhD). Boltz's areas of research include cross-setting interventions to promote functional health in older adults, support of informal and formal carers, and translational dementia research, funded by NIH and multiple foundations. She serves on editorial boards, as a reviewer for several academic journals, and as Editor of *Evidence-Based Geriatric Nursing Protocols for Best Practice* and *Dementia Care: An Evidence-Based Approach.* Boltz's expertise and commitment to gerontology have yielded numerous publications, national and international presentations, and invitations to serve on national research review panels, mentorship teams, and interdisciplinary research projects. Her scholarship has been recognized with the Doris Schwartz Gerontological Nursing Research Award (awarded by the Gerontological Society of America) and fellowship in the American Academy of Nursing and the Gerontological Society of America.

Alice Bonner, PhD, RN, FAAN, has been a nurse practitioner for over 30 years. She is currently Senior Advisor for Aging at the Institute for Healthcare Improvement and Chair of Moving Forward: Nursing Home Quality Coalition. She is also adjunct faculty at the Johns Hopkins University School of Nursing. From 2015 to 2019, Bonner served as Secretary of the Executive Office of Elder Affairs for the Commonwealth of Massachusetts. From 2011 to 2013, Bonner served as Director of the Division of Nursing Homes in the CMS in Baltimore, Maryland.

Barbara J. Bowers, PhD, RN, FAAN, is Professor Emerita at the University of Wisconsin-Madison, School of Nursing. Her research has focused on organizational models of care, particularly culture change models, staff development, and resident quality of life. Her work has been funded by the National Institutes of Health, the Commonwealth Fund, The Cargill Foundation, and the Robert Wood Johnson Foundation. Bowers has collaborated with researchers across many countries and served on local, state, and federal policy workgroups related to long-term care. She was the founding Director of the Center for Aging Research and Education at the University of Wisconsin-Madison, served as Director of Qualitative and Mixed Methods Education for the Institute for Clinical and Translational Research at the University of Wisconsin-Madison, and was Associate Editor of *The Gerontologist.* She has published widely on organizational models of long-term care and workforce development. Bowers received the Doris Schwartz Gerontological Nursing Research Award in 2022 and is a fellow in the American Academy of Nursing and in the Gerontological Society of America.

Julie Britton, DNP, MSN, RN-BC, GCNS-BC, FGNLA, has spent the last 35 years working in post-acute and long-term care settings. She began her career as a licensed practical nurse and returned to school to obtain her associate degree in nursing from Louisiana State University. She then earned her bachelor's degree in nursing from Temple University and obtained her master's degree and doctor of nursing practice from Gwynedd Mercy University, where she was awarded the Nurse Excellence

Award from Sigma Theta Tau International Honor Society of Nursing (Sigma). In 2011, Britton was one of 14 nurses selected nationwide to participate and complete the Sigma Theta Tau Geriatric Nursing Leadership Academy Fellowship program. She is board certified as a clinical nurse specialist in gerontology, is a fellow of the Geriatric Nurse Leadership Academy, and is certified as a Green Belt in Lean Six Sigma. Britton is Chair of the National Nurse Executive Council and is active in AHCA, where she serves on the Regulatory/Survey Committee. She also serves as an advisor for Moving Forward Nursing Home Quality Coalition and the National Senior Care Advisory Board. Britton is currently active in AONE, ANA, AADNS, NADONA, PADONA, Sigma, NJHCA, DNPA and PSNA. Her career path has been built on serving others in the delivery of care of the older adult, families, and communities to support healthy aging, maximum functioning, and quality of life. She promotes shared governance and believes in involving those at the front line/end users in shared decision-making.

Noll L. Campbell, PharmD, MS, is an Associate Professor in the Department of Pharmacy Practice at Purdue University, an Investigator at the Indiana University Center for Aging Research at the Regenstrief Institute, and a Scientist with the Indiana University Center for Health Innovation and Implementation Science. His research is focused on the measurement and management of adverse cognitive effects of medications in older adults with acute and chronic cognitive impairment. This work includes the use of behavioral economic principles to evaluate the impact of deprescribing interventions on clinical and operational outcomes in various care environments. His work has been funded by the National Institute of Health's National Institute on Aging, the Agency for Healthcare Research and Quality, and the pharmaceutical industry. He was awarded a New Investigator Award from the American Geriatrics Society in 2012, a Hulman Award for Achievement in Geriatrics from the Indiana Public Health Association in 2014, a Departmental Best Paper Award in 2019, and the Chaney Family Early Scholar Award from the Purdue University College of Pharmacy in 2021. Campbell also serves as the President-Elect of the American Delirium Society.

Sophie A. Campbell, MSN, RN, CRRN, RAC-CT, CNDLTC, is the Executive Director Educational Programming and Services for PADONA (Pennsylvania Association of Directors of Nursing Administration). In this position, she assesses the educational needs of Pennsylvania's long-term care nurse leaders and coordinates and schedules education with industry experts—while also providing information necessary for nurse leaders in their roles. Campbell provides nursing education, including education and mentoring for the directors of nursing in long-term care. She has a master's degree in nursing administration from the University of Pittsburgh. Prior to beginning her position with PADONA, she was the Director of Clinical Operations for the national accounting firm Baker Tilly and spent several years prior to that in operations in multiple positions, with the majority of her career in long-term care.

Joan G. Carpenter, PhD, CRNP, ACHPN, FPCN, is an Assistant Professor at the University of Maryland School of Nursing, a Health Scientist at the US Department of Veterans Affairs, and a nurse practitioner with Coastal Hospice and Palliative Care. Carpenter is an expert in geriatric palliative care, specializing in post-acute and long-term care settings. Her research focuses on the implementation and evaluation of nonpharmacologic palliative care interventions to improve the quality of life, reduce symptom burden, and enhance decision-making for people living with serious illness and their care partners.

Jeanne Copeland, MS, CCC-SLP, FNAP, RAC-CT, is a Clinical Director and speech-language pathologist for Powerback. She is a National Academies of Practice Distinguished Public Policy Fellow (FNAP) and a certified Resident Assessment Coordinator (RAC-CT). She specializes in utilizing interprofessional practice and evidence-based techniques to achieve patient-centered and clinically meaningful outcomes with the medically complex population. She enjoys presenting at state and national conventions on a range of topics including dementia and the SLP's role within an interprofessional collaborative model when working with medically complex patients. Copeland strives to educate and motivate others to embrace everyday opportunities for leadership, advocacy, and interprofessional collaborative practice when working with older adults.

Tara A. Cortes, PhD, RN, FAAN, FGSA, is the Executive Director of the Hartford Institute for Geriatric Nursing and a Professor at New York University Rory Meyers College of Nursing. Prior to joining the NYU College of Nursing, Cortes was President and CEO of Lighthouse International, a leading not-for-profit organization dedicated to fighting vision loss and helping people prevent vision impairment. Cortes spent the initial phase of her career in nursing education at Hunter College and then served as the Director of Nursing Research and Information Systems at Columbia Presbyterian Medical Center. She was the Chief Nursing Officer at Rockefeller University Hospital and continued her career in nursing leadership and hospital administration at Mount

Sinai Medical Center and at Bridgeport Hospital, before assuming the senior leadership role at Lighthouse International. Cortes was appointed as a Health and Aging Fellow (2013–2015) in the American Political Science Association Congressional Fellowship Program and served as a Senior Advisor at CMS in the Medicare-Medicaid Coordination Office. Cortes is a fellow of the American Academy of Nursing and of the New York Academy of Medicine. She is a past fellow of the Robert Wood Johnson Executive Nurse Fellows Program. She was appointed by the Secretary of Health and Human Services to the Advisory Committee for Primary Care Training in Medicine and Dentistry and served on an NIH expert panel to review the efficacy and safety of COVID-19 vaccine protocols for older adults.

Howard B. Degenholtz, PhD, FGSA, is Professor of Health Policy and Management and Faculty Affiliate of the Center for Bioethics and Health Law. He was the founding Director of the Doctoral Program in Health Services Research and Policy. Degenholtz is a health services researcher who focuses on long-term services supports and aging. He is currently the lead for a seven-year mixed method evaluation of the Commonwealth of Pennsylvania Community HealthChoices program. He has published on a wide range of topics including methods to measure and improve quality of life for people living in nursing homes. He is a member of AcademyHealth and a fellow in the Gerontological Society of America. He is the Social Media Editor of *The Gerontologist*, Associate Editor for LTSS of *Innovation in Aging*, and on the editorial board of the *Journal of Aging and Social Policy*.

Karen Eshraghi, MSW, received her bachelor's in social work from Spalding University and her master's in social work from Temple University. Currently, Eshraghi is the Director of Grants and Research for Abramson Senior Care in North Wales, Pennsylvania, and has extensive experience in providing quality improvement programming for residential senior care settings, including skilled nursing. She also is serving as a Project Director for NIH-level studies with Penn State College of Nursing to advance the science of person-centered care in nursing homes.

Sam Fazio, PhD, is Senior Director of Quality Care and Psychosocial Research at the Alzheimer's Association. Fazio has worked for the Alzheimer's Association since 1994 in a variety of areas, including education and training, program services, and medical and scientific relations. He currently works in the care and support area, where he oversees quality care standards and social/behavioral research initiatives. Fazio received his doctorate in developmental psychology from Loyola University Chicago.

Prior to working for the Alzheimer's Association, Fazio worked for Rush Presbyterian St. Luke's Medical Center at the Alzheimer's Family Care Center, an adult day center specifically designed for people with dementia. He has worked in the field of aging since 1987 and has a broad range of experience, including research, leadership and management, working with older adults and families, and direct care. Fazio has presented both nationally and internationally and published many journal articles and book chapters. He is the author of *The Enduring Self in People with Alzheimer's: Getting to the Heart of Individualized Care* and the co-author of *Rethinking Alzheimer's Care.*

Donna Fick, PhD, GCNS-BC, FAAN, is the Elouise Ross Eberly Endowed Professor of the Ross & Carol Nese College of Nursing at The Pennsylvania State University and Director of the Tressa Nese and Helen Diskevich Center of Geriatric Nursing Excellence. Fick is best known for her NIH-funded clinical research and implementation in mentation, delirium superimposed on dementia, and ultra-brief delirium detection at the bedside. Along with Edward R. Marcantonio, MD, and their team, she has transformed the way clinicians approach delirium and DSD. Their tools, the UB-2 and UB-CAM, are used in health systems across the world. The UB-CAM is available as a free app here: https://apps.apple.com/us/app/ub-cam-delirium-screen/id1591656740. She has been a member or Co-chair of the interdisciplinary panel for the American Geriatrics Society Beers Criteria for inappropriate medication use in older adults since 2002. She serves on the American Geriatrics Society Board as President-Elect, and as a member of the National Academy of Science Forum on Aging, Disability, and Independence. She also serves as a faculty and advisory member on Creating an Age Friendly Health System Initiative with the John A. Hartford Foundation and the Institute for Healthcare Improvement, and the Revisiting the Teaching Nursing Home Project. Fick has completed as PI & MPI three NIH-funded R01s on delirium in persons with dementia. She is board-certified in geriatrics, and her goal in her research and service is to improve the care of older adults, persons with disabilities, and their care partners. She lives in rural Pennsylvania near her three adult children and enjoys gardening and trail running in the mountains.

Emily K. Franke, MSW, LSW, is a licensed social worker who currently serves as a Program Specialist supporting the Jewish Healthcare Foundation's Aging Team and the foundation's behavioral health initiatives. With expertise in behavioral health, grief recovery, end-of-life choices, caregiving, and psychopharmacology, she brings a wealth of knowledge to her role. Franke's professional journey includes valuable experiences as a pre-licensed therapist at the Benedum Geriatric Center, therapist in private practice, and psychiatric social worker on the Integrated Health and Aging Program unit at Western Psychiatric Hospital. Her dedication lies in providing support to individuals grappling with symptoms of depression and anxiety in the context of medical diagnoses, as well as those facing caregiver or career-related burnout. Complementing her practical experience, Franke earned dual bachelor's degrees in psychology and gender, sexuality, and women's studies from the University of Pittsburgh, where she also achieved her master's degree in social work. During her master's program, she was recognized as a Hartford Fellow, focusing her efforts on developing specialized skills to serve the diverse older adult population, with a particular emphasis on LGBTQIA+ older adults.

Terry Fulmer, PhD, RN, FAAN, is President of the John A. Hartford Foundation in New York City, a national philanthropy dedicated to improving the care of older adults. She serves as the chief strategist for the Foundation, and her vision for better care of older adults is catalyzing the Age-Friendly Health Systems social movement. She is an elected member of the National Academy of Medicine and recently served on the independent Coronavirus Commission for Safety and Quality in Nursing Homes. She previously served as Dean of Health Sciences at Northeastern University and founding Dean of the New York University College of Nursing. Fulmer is nationally and internationally recognized as a leading expert in geriatrics and is also known for conceptualization and development of the national NICHE program and research on the topic of elder abuse and neglect. She is the first nurse to have served on the board of the American Geriatrics Society. She is also the first nurse to have served as President of the Gerontological Society of America, which awarded her the 2019 Donald P. Kent Award for exemplifying the highest standards for professional leadership in the field of aging.

Elizabeth Galik, PhD, CRNP, FAAN, FAANP, is a Professor and Chair of the Department of Organizational Systems and Adult Health at the University of Maryland School of Nursing and a nurse practitioner who specializes in the medical and neuropsychiatric care of older adults with dementia. She teaches in the Adult Gerontological Primary Care Nurse Practitioner program and has served as a Principal Investigator on externally funded research grants that have focused on improving care practices within post-acute and long-term care settings. Galik has practiced clinically as an RN and nurse practitioner in post-acute and long-term care settings for over 25 years. She is the Editor-in-Chief of *Caring for the Ages,* a Past President of the Gerontological Advanced Practice Nurses Association, and a fellow in the American Academy of Nursing, the American Association of Nurse Practitioners, and the Gerontological Society of America. She has served as an expert advisor for CMS to improve behavioral health in long-term care and acute care settings.

Andrea Gilmore-Bykovskyi, PhD, RN, is Associate Professor and Associate Vice Chair for Research in the BerbeeWalsh Department of Emergency Medicine at the University of Wisconsin School of Medicine and Public Health. A practicing geriatric nurse, Gilmore-Bykovskyi leads an active program of research focused on promoting effective, meaningful, and equitable care for people living with dementia—particularly during challenging points in the health and care continuum such as during acute illness and advanced disease. She is especially passionate about partnering directly with people living with dementia and caregivers to fully integrate their perspectives into the research process and results to strengthen attention and progress toward meaningful outcomes.

Laura N. Gitlin, PhD, FGSA, FAAN, an applied research sociologist, is Distinguished Professor, Dean Emerita of the College of Nursing and Health Professions at Drexel University and the inaugural Executive Director of its AgeWell Collaboratory. The AgeWell Collaboratory oversees Drexel's AgeFriendly University international designation and partners with over 80 community-based organizations serving racially, ethnically, and culturally diverse communities involving older adults and families. Gitlin is internationally recognized as an intervention scientist. Her research focuses on developing, evaluating, implementing, and disseminating novel home and community-based interventions that seek to improve quality of life indicators for older adults and/or their family members. She and her teams have developed interventions to address depressive symptoms (Get Busy Get Better), caregiving challenges (COPE, Skills2Care), functional challenges (ABLE, CAPABLE), dementia-related clinical symptoms (Tailored Activity Program) and caregiver support (Adult Day Service Plus, COPE). She applies a social ecological, health equity, and implementation lens to develop and evaluate person-centered and person-directed approaches to support individuals/families within their living contexts using nonpharmacological, behavioral, cognitive, and environmental strategies. Her interventions have resulted in improved physical and psychosocial outcomes, reduced mortality, and healthcare savings. Some of her interventions are being implemented globally and in agencies throughout the USA. She is a well-funded researcher with continuous research and training grant funding from federal agencies and private foundations for over 35 years. She and her teams have received numerous awards for their innovation and interventions.

Sherry A. Greenberg, PhD, RN, GNP-BC, FGSA, FNAP, FAANP, FAAN, is Professor and Hess Endowed Chair in Nursing Education at Monmouth University, Marjorie K. Unterberg School of Nursing and Health Studies. Greenberg is Past President of the Gerontological Advanced Practice Nurses Association. She is a fellow in the American Academy of Nursing, American Association of Nurse Practitioners, Gerontological Society of America, National Academies of Practice, and New York Academy of Medicine, as well as Distinguished Educator in Gerontological Nursing through the National Hartford Center of Gerontological Nursing Excellence. Greenberg earned her academic nursing degrees, baccalaureate, master's, and PhD from the University of Pennsylvania School of Nursing and was a Jonas Nurse Leaders Scholar. She has worked as a certified gerontological nurse practitioner in acute, long-term care, and outpatient primary care practices and has taught at undergraduate, graduate, and doctoral nursing levels.

Melodee Harris, PhD, RN, FAAN, is an Associate Professor at the University of Arkansas for Medical Sciences College of Nursing. Her leadership is reflected in her geropsychiatric practice in rural Arkansas nursing homes. She is Co-investigator on an Administration for Community Living grant and leads the Mission Day Break Award on Food Insecurity and Suicide Prevention program for older adults and veterans in Arkansas. Harris was Co-investigator on a $1.9 million Health Resources and Services Administration Advanced Nursing Education grant to train gerontological nurse practitioner students in rural primary care. Harris leads the Gerontological Advanced Practice Nursing Association Position Paper on Geropsychiatric Nursing. She serves on the National Hartford Center of Gerontological Nursing Excellence board of directors. Harris was a 2007–2009 John A. Hartford Scholar. Her research interests include dementia, sleep, massage, and geropsychiatric nursing.

Taylor McMahon, RN, CNDLTC, is the Director of Nursing at The Willows Presbyterian Senior Care Network in Oakmont, Pennsylvania, and is continuing her education at Chatham University. The Willows is part of the Pennsylvania-based "Revisiting the Teaching Nursing Home" initiative. As one of three regional areas implementing Age-Friendly Health Systems, The Willows is partnering with the University of Pittsburgh School of Nursing to establish a "teaching" environment where students, academics, and healthcare workers collaborate to improve care for residents and foster nursing careers in nursing homes and geriatrics. McMahon's love of geriatrics nursing began when she started her career at Presbyterian Senior Care Network in personal care at Westminster Place in 2014. She supported the nursing home team in quality improvement efforts to decrease hospital readmissions in the development and implementation of COPD/CHF clinical pathways, risk assessment tools, and education. McMahon recently received the American Hospital Association Next Generation Leadership Fellowship with a project focus of embedding the Age-Friendly Framework in the affordable housing sector and to aid in personal and professional development to better serve her team and residents.

Sheila L. Molony, PhD, APRN, FAAN, is a Professor of Nursing at Quinnipiac University, a fellow of the Gerontological Society of America, and a fellow of the American Academy of Nursing. Molony's research emphasizes the importance of individually tailored care, actively listening to the voices of older adults and families, and using these perspectives to shape healing environments in long-term care. Molony's work clarifies the concept of at-homeness, and she has developed a reliable and valid measure of this construct that has been used nationally and internationally. Molony's work includes the publication of Dementia Care Practice Guidelines for Assessment and Care Planning in a special issue of *The Gerontologist.* Molony is currently leading an NIH/NIA-funded project using human centered design to create positive psychosocial measures for individuals living with dementia.

Stefanie Mozgai, RN, is the Assistant Commissioner of Certificate of Need and Licensing at the New Jersey Department of Health, where she maintains oversight and accountability of the licensing process of all state-licensed healthcare facilities to ensure access to services and that those services meet the licensing standards. She also oversees the Office of Program Compliance, which is responsible for the administration of both state enforcement and federal penalties issued on behalf of the CMS. The nurse aide certification program and the licensed nursing home administrator board are also included within her division. Prior to assuming that role in January of 2022, Mozgai was the Assistant Commissioner of Health Facility Survey and Field Operations within NJDOH and had the responsibility for ensuring compliance with state and federal requirements and the overall management of the survey and certification process for over 2,000 licensed and certified healthcare facilities including hospitals, ambulatory care, and long-term care facilities. She spent one year at the CMS, functioning as Director of the Division of Continuing and Acute Care Providers, which developed survey policies and protocols for all acute care providers. She was the government liaison to the New Jersey Board of Nursing from 2019 to 2021 and was a member of the National Association for Health Facility Survey Agencies and served as the President from 2019 to 2020.

Christine Mueller, PhD, RN, FGSA, FAAN, is a Professor at the University of Minnesota School of Nursing. Her research career has focused on improving the care of elders living in nursing homes by addressing factors that can influence quality of nursing home care such as nurse staffing and care delivery models. She has provided national leadership on teaching geriatric nursing, with a particular emphasis on using the nursing home setting as a clinical learning laboratory for teaching geriatric nursing. As part of the Minnesota Hartford Center for Gerontological Nursing Excellence, she and her colleagues developed a nationally recognized program, *Faculty Learning About Geriatrics.* Mueller is a fellow in the American Academy of Nursing and the Gerontological Society of America. She served on the National Academy of Medicine Committee on Nursing Home Quality.

Nancy Munoz, DCN, MHA, RDN, FAND, is an instructor in the UMass, Amherst Nutrition Department. For 35 years, she functioned in a number of clinical nutrition and food service management leadership roles for Genesis Healthcare. Currently, Munoz serves as the Chief of Nutrition and Food Services for the VA Southern Nevada Healthcare System, overseeing the care provided to 72,000 veterans in the Las Vegas Valley. She serves on numerous committees, including the National Pressure Injury Advisory Panel, WoundSource, Dietetics in Healthcare Communities, the Healthy Aging Dietetics Practice Group of the Academy of Nutrition and Dietetics, and the Academy of Nutrition and Dietetics Positions Committee, among others.

Christine Pabico, PhD, RN, NE-BC, FAAN, Director of ANCC's Pathway to Excellence program, is a thought leader and expert in creating and sustaining high reliability organizations and positive practice environments. Her passion is to provide organizations around the globe strategies for success in creating work environments that support, engage, and empower staff to lead from the bedside. In addition, she is a recognized champion for safeguarding clinician well-being. Pabico has over 25 years of leadership experience, is ANCC board-certified as a Nurse Executive, and is a fellow of the American Academy of Nursing. Her passion for creating healthy work environments extended to her doctoral work, where she studied the relationships among nurse manager competency, the nursing practice environment, and frontline nurses' intent to stay. For her volunteer work, Pabico sits on the editorial board of the *American Nurse Journal* and the board of the Philippine Chamber of Commerce. She is a faculty for iLDP (PNAA's leadership development program) and President-elect for the Philippine Nurses Association in Metro DC.

Flora Petillo, MSN, CRNP, CWS, is a gerontological nurse practitioner with over 25 years of experience providing primary care in post-acute care. She is the Chief Operating Officer of GPS, a large multi-state, post-acute provider practice.

Marilyn Rantz, PhD, RN, FAAN, Curators' Professor Emerita, has a sustained career focused on improving quality of care for older people, particularly those living in nursing homes. She is a member of the National Academy of Medicine (formerly IOM) and a much sought-after leading researcher and expert in quality measurement and nursing home practice. Rantz recently completed the CMS-funded Missouri Quality Initiative (MOQI). She and her multidisciplinary research teams have a track record of over $103 million in funding to conduct cutting-edge research in long-term care, new delivery models of care for older adults, and technology development to enhance aging in place of community-dwelling elders. Rantz is the only individual to be twice named as an Edge Runner by the American Academy of Nursing for two different innovations: 2008 for Aging in Place and TigerPlace and 2012 for the Quality Improvement Program for Missouri (QIPMO). In 2020, she was named a Living Legend in Nursing by the American Academy of Nursing.

Kim Ratliff, BSN, RN, CNDLTC, is the Director of Nursing at Wesley Enhanced Living in Pennsylvania, which is is a part of Revisiting the Teaching Nursing Home, a program aimed at improving the quality of care in long-term care facilities and engagement in residents' care. Ratliff is a graduate of Messiah College and has worked in long-term care since 1984. She has held many positions including Nursing Assistant, Charge Nurse, Supervisor, Assistant Director of Nursing, and finally Director of Nursing.

Maureen Saxon-Gioia, MSHSA, BSN, RN, is a nurse project manager for aging initiatives with the Jewish Healthcare Foundation. In this role, she champions professional nursing education through Revisiting the Teaching Nursing Home, a pilot to foster academic relationships with schools of nursing and nursing homes, and the Pennsylvania Long-Term Care Learning Network for Nursing Facilities, with the goal of improving healthcare quality and safety and the strength of the careforce. Her career spans many years as a point-of-care nurse in an academic medical center. Saxon-Gioia also has experience in post-acute care for patients receiving home health services and led compliance and quality improvement activities to promote value-based care and professional nursing development through evidence-based care initiatives. Her combination of clinical and quality improvement experience fuels her passion for helping others promote change in healthcare.

Bethany Sewell, MSW, is a clinical social worker with a concentration in geriatrics and palliative care. She is currently a Project Manager at The PAIR (Palliative and Advanced Illness Research) Center at the University of Pennsylvania School of Medicine, where she supports grant-funded research projects aimed at improving the lives of all people affected by serious illness. Prior to that, Sewell worked at Genesis HealthCare as the Director of Clinical Research, but her commitment to improving the lives of the geriatric population started well before entering the realm of clinical research. The majority of Sewell's career has been spent as a clinical social worker in long-term care, where she has supported patients, residents, and families by navigating complex systems and exploring patients' care preferences to support goal-concordant care and ensure high-quality patient-centered care and improved outcomes.

Marianne Shaughnessy, PhD, AGPCNP-BC, GS-C, FAAN, is the Director, Geriatric Research, Education and Clinical Center Programs within the Office of Geriatrics and Extended Care (OGEC) at the Department of Veterans Affairs. Shaughnessy is responsible for oversight and activity of the 20 Geriatric Centers of Excellence nationwide. She has over 30 years of experience as a nurse and is certified as an adult-gerontological primary care nurse practitioner. She has worked in the VA since 1999. Prior to joining OGEC, Shaughnessy was the Associate Director for Education and Evaluation for the Baltimore Geriatric Research, Education, and Clinical Center (GRECC) and held an academic appointment as Associate Professor at the University of Maryland at Baltimore School of Nursing. She previously served as faculty in the schools of nursing at the University of Pennsylvania and the University of North Carolina at Greensboro. Her research interests include stroke rehabilitation and delirium identification and management. She has published more than 40 peer-reviewed journal articles and other publications. Shaughnessy earned her PhD, MSN, and BSN degrees from the School of Nursing at the University of Pennsylvania.

Jennifer C. Sidelinker, DPT, PT, is a Clinical Research Facilitator for Aegis Therapies. With over 30 years of clinical and clinical leadership experience in a variety of older adult care settings, Sidelinker has led the development and implementation of diverse, interprofessional clinical projects and programs (examples include implementation of an evidence-based rehab approach to fall risk identification and management and a SNF team-based Falls and Mobility System Review grounded in the Age-Friendly Health System 4M framework). She is a board-certified clinical specialist in geriatric physical therapy (GCS) and an active member of her state and national professional organization. She has written and presented at the state and national level on a variety of topics, including interprofessional practice, transitions in care, value-based care delivery, and evidence-based fall risk management and prevention. Sidelinker has a passion for excellence in evidence-informed clinical care delivery and summarizes her core personal and professional drivers with this statement: "I am an avid lifelong learner, and a thoughtful, practical, and collaborative problem-solver."

Elena O. Siegel, PhD, is Associate Professor Emeritus at Betty Irene Moore School of Nursing at UC Davis, Associate Director, National Office for the Betty Irene Moore Fellowship for Nurse Leaders and Innovators, and a member of the school's founding faculty. Her research in nursing home leadership and management teams focuses on building the capacity of directors of nursing and nursing home administrators to enhance quality and value, with emphasis on successful implementation of evidence-based quality improvement initiatives in day-to-day practice. Her research has been funded by Robert Wood Johnson Foundation, John A. Hartford Foundation, Foundation of National Association of Long Term Care Administrator Boards, National Council of State Boards of Nursing, Archstone Foundation, and California Association of Healthcare Facilities (California Department of Public Health – CMS Civil Money Penalty funds).

Brian D. Stever, BSN, RN, RAC-CT, is the owner of Stever Advisors, LLC, where he consults on Medicare/Medicaid matters in long-term care. He received his bachelor of science in nursing and nursing training from Messiah University in Mechanicsburg, Pennsylvania. He has been involved in the Resident Assessment Instrument process for over 25 years in a wide range of areas in long-term care. His focus has been in developing and educating staff on the correct capture of services provided and ensuring that residents receive the care they deserve. He has been involved in work groups with the Centers for Medicare & Medicaid Services (CMS) on the original Resident Assessment Protocols. He was also an educator for CMS, where he educated groups on the quality measures process as well as the original Nursing Home Compare website. He also worked with the Commonwealth of Pennsylvania on the development of the Pennsylvania Case Mix system for MDS 3.0. He is a Past Vice President of the board for the Pennsylvania Association of Nurse Assessment Coordinators, PANAC, and currently serves on the board. As a board member, he serves on the Advisory Committee for the Pennsylvania Office of Long-Term Living as well as on the Education Committee for the Pennsylvania Long-Term Learning Network.

Amy Stewart, MSN, RN, RAC-MT, RAC-MTA, DNS-MT, QCP-MT, is the Vice President of Education and Certification Strategy for the American Association of Post-Acute Care Nursing (AAPACN). Prior to this she was a curriculum development specialist for AADNS. Before joining the AAPACN staff, she was a legal nurse consultant for the law firm Hall, Prangle, & Schoonveld (HPS) in Chicago. She has over 25 years of experience in the post-acute healthcare industry, with expertise in the areas of the Resident Assessment Instrument (RAI), clinical reimbursement, quality, and regulatory change. Prior to joining HPS, Stewart was the Division Director of Reimbursement for 18 skilled nursing facilities in the Chicagoland area, part of a larger hospital system that participated in CMS innovative payment models. Previous roles include Director of Nursing, Pharmacy Quality Consultant, Wound Care Consultant, and MDS Coordinator. Steward is a Master Teacher for AAPACN's RAC-CT, RAC-CTA, DNS-CT and QCP programs and is a nationally recognized speaker and subject matter expert on a variety of post-acute care topics.

Robyn I. Stone, DrPH, is Senior Vice President for Research at LeadingAge and Co-director of the LeadingAge LTSS Center @UMass Boston, a research center with offices in Washington, DC, and Boston, Massachusetts. A noted researcher and internationally recognized authority on aging services, Stone has been engaged in policy development, program evaluation, large-scale demonstration projects, and other applied research activities for more than 40 years. She was a political appointee in the Clinton Administration, serving in the US Department of Health and Human Services as Deputy Assistant Secretary for Disability, Aging, and Long-Term Care Policy. She also served as Assistant Secretary for Aging. Her widely published work addresses long-term care policy and quality, chronic care for people with disabilities, the aging services workforce, affordable senior housing, and family caregiving. In addition, she is a fellow of the Gerontological Society of America and the National Academy of Social Insurance and was elected to the National Academy of Medicine in 2014. Stone received a master's degree in public policy from the University of Pittsburgh Graduate School of Public and International Affairs and a doctor of public health degree from the University of California, Berkeley. Her work bridges the worlds of research, policy, and practice to improve the care delivered to older adults—particularly lower-income populations—and to ensure the best quality of life for these individuals and their families.

Jasmine L. Travers, PhD, MHS, RN, AGPCNP-BC, is an Assistant Professor at NYU Rory Meyers College of Nursing. Her career is dedicated to designing and conducting research to improve health outcomes and reduce health disparities in vulnerable older adult groups using both quantitative and qualitative approaches. Her current work focuses on mitigating disparities in access and use of in-home and facility-based long-term care for older adults (i.e., home and community-based settings, nursing homes, and assisted living). Travers has published widely on the topics of aging, long-term care, health disparities and inequities, workforce diversity and workforce issues, vaccinations, and infections and has disseminated study findings in over 50 publications in high-impact aging and interdisciplinary policy, research, and clinical journals. These articles have been cited over 1,700 times and have a Google h-index of 20. Very recently, Travers served on the National Academies of Sciences, Engineering, and Medicine Committee on the Quality of Care in Nursing Homes, which, on April 6, 2022, released the widely anticipated report *The National Imperative to Improve Nursing Home Quality.*

Kimberly Van Haitsma, PhD, FGSA, is a clinical geropsychologist and Professor at Pennsylvania State University Ross and Carol Nese College of Nursing. At the college of nursing, she directs the Program for Person-Centered Living Systems of Care (PPCLSC) located in the Center of Geriatric Nursing Excellence and is an Adjunct Research Scientist at the Polisher Research Institute, Abramson Senior Care. She has served as a Principal Investigator or Co-principal Investigator on more than 35 grants awarded from federal, state, and foundation sources. Over her career, she has published more than 100 articles in peer-reviewed journals, many of which are co-published with former students. Van Haitsma's areas of research include development and testing of various mental health education and intervention approaches; innovative methodological and measurement development; and testing intervention and implementation strategies that facilitate the uptake of evidence-based, person-centered, preference-informed care practices targeting older adults with multiple chronic care conditions.

Joan Weiss, PhD, RN, CRNP, FAAN, is an adult and gerontological nurse practitioner who serves as the Deputy Director in the Division of Medicine and Dentistry at the Health Resources and Services Administration (HRSA). She oversees workforce development programming in geriatrics, primary care, graduate medical education, behavioral health, and oral health. Her experience in interprofessional practice and education spans 30 years. She is the Subject Matter Expert for the Federal Advisory

Committee on Interdisciplinary Community-Based Linkages. She is the HRSA representative on the US Department of Health and Human Services' (HHS) Advisory Council on Alzheimer's Disease Research, Care, and Services; the Family Caregiving Advisory Council; and the Grandparent Advisory Council. She is a recipient of the 2015 Secretary's Meritorious Group Award for taking important steps to find a cure and improve care for people with dementia. She is the recipient of the 2022 HRSA Administrator's Lifetime Achievement Award for extraordinary federal service dedicated to leadership, commitment, and expertise in the fields of interprofessional education, primary care, geriatrics, and dementia care.

Sheryl Zimmerman, PhD, is a University Distinguished Professor in the Schools of Social Work and Public Health and Co-director of the Program on Aging, Chronic Illness, and Long-Term Care in the Cecil G. Sheps Center for Health Services Research, University of North Carolina at Chapel Hill. She is nationally recognized as a leader in research and dissemination related to care for persons with dementia based on her work developing and evaluating measures, collecting data, and testing interventions in nursing homes and assisted living communities across the United States. In 1996, Zimmerman founded the Collaborative Studies of Long-Term Care, the largest ongoing national research consortium of long-term care settings across the country, which has participated in more than 70 projects with continuous funding from the National Institutes of Health, the Agency for Healthcare Research and Quality, and foundations. Zimmerman led two large projects on dementia care in long-term care that resulted in three special issues of peer-reviewed journals; in addition, she has written five books and more than 400 peer-reviewed manuscripts and is currently Editor-in-Chief Emeritus and Senior Associate Editor of *JAMDA – The Journal of Post-Acute and Long-Term Care Medicine.* Zimmerman worked closely with the national office of the Alzheimer's Association to develop its 2018 Dementia Care Practice Recommendations and co-authored two sets of the recommendations. Currently, she is co-leading a National Institute on Aging (NIA)-funded consortium to evaluate related outcome measures and care tools and promote their use and is Principal Investigator on two related NIA-funded projects—one evaluating new process and outcome measures and the other evaluating an online dementia training program.

Nancy D. Zionts, MBA, COO/Chief Program Officer for the Jewish Healthcare Foundation, is responsible for the grant agenda for the Foundation and its operating arms: Pittsburgh Regional Health Initiative and Health Careers Futures and WHAMglobal. Areas of focus include aging/long-term care and end of life, quality and safety, health careers, and women's health. She currently leads the Foundation's Revisiting the Teaching Nursing Home Initiative and the Statewide Long-Term Care Learning Network for Nursing Facilities and serves on the national Moving Forward Coalition for long-term care. She was the lead principal team member on federally funded projects including the CMS-funded RAVEN (Initiative to Reduce Avoidable Hospitalizations among Nursing Facility Residents). She has been active in many of the Foundation's initiatives including its Working Hearts, Women's Health Inequity in Older Age, Closure and Caregiver Champions Initiatives, the Fellowship On Death and Dying, Tomorrow's HealthCare, the Champions Programs, and Pennsylvania Health Funders Collaborative. She also was involved in the development of relevant publications including "Longer Lives Better Health: Helping Seniors Preserve their Physical, Mental and Social Well-being"; "Moderating the Effects of Aging: A Caregiver's Manual"; and "Closure Community Conversations Implementation Guide." Zionts is the 2020 Kelly Pruitt Age Friendly Leadership Award winner from the Southwestern Pennsylvania Partnership for Aging. Zionts, a native of Montreal, Canada, holds a bachelor's degree in chemistry and an MBA, both from Concordia University.

ADDITIONAL BOOK RESOURCES

To download a sample chapter and other free book resources, visit the Sigma Repository at https://sigma.nursingrepository.org/handle/10755/23523 or scan the QR code below.

SPECIAL NOTE TO READERS

Here at Sigma, we realize that language is constantly evolving. The meaning of a word often changes over time, some words become obsolete, and some terms that were once acceptable may become controversial or even offensive, depending on the context or circumstances. We have made every effort to make language choices that are inclusive and not offensive. Should you identify words in this book that you believe negatively impact a group or groups of people, please reach out to us at Publications@SigmaNursing.org.

TABLE OF CONTENTS

About the Editors ... xi
Authors ... xiii
Additional Book Resources ... xxxiii
Foreword ... xliii
Introduction ... xlvii

CHAPTER 1 The Journey to Improve Nursing Care ... 1

Introduction ... 1
A Brief History of Nursing Homes ... 2
- Federal Government Intervention ... 3
- Trending to For-Profit Status ... 4

Historical Efforts to Improve Quality of Care and Quality of Life in Nursing Homes ... 5
- Models of Care That Guide Nursing Home Practice ... 6
- The Good Life Model ... 8

Culture Change Models of Care ... 11
- The Neighborhood or Household Model ... 12
- The Eden Alternative ... 12
- Wellspring ... 13
- The Green House Nursing Home ... 13

Summary ... 13
References ... 14

CHAPTER 2 Creating a Culture of Care ... 19

Introduction ... 19
Descriptions of Organizational Culture ... 20
Just Culture vs. Punitive Culture ... 21
How Nursing Homes Become Age-Friendly Health Systems ... 22
- Key Drivers and Steps to Implementing the 4Ms ... 23
- Determining a Nursing Home's Baseline: What Policies and Practices Are in Place Now? ... 24
- Leadership and Teamwork ... 24
- Co-Designing Tools and Resources With Nursing Home Partners ... 24

Creating an Age-Friendly Ecosystem....25
Establishing a Baseline....26
Focusing on Mentation....26
Assessing and Acting on a Change in Condition: Consider Delirium....26
The 4Ms as a Set....28
Teaching Nursing Homes....29
Working Together to Integrate the 4Ms and Improve Organizational Culture....30
A Case Example....30
Positive Practice Environments and Shared Governance....31
Standard 1: Shared Decision-Making....32
Standard 2: Leadership....33
Standard 3: Safety....34
Standard 4: Quality....34
Standard 5: Well-Being....34
Standard 6: Professional Development....35
Summary....35
References....36

CHAPTER 3 Diversity, Equity, Inclusion: Staff and Residents....41
Introduction....41
Inequities Defined....42
Who Among the Nursing Home Workforce Experiences Inequities?....43
Overview of the Nursing Home Resident Population....44
Health Disparities Defined....45
Who Experiences Disparities and How?....45
Implications for Nursing Policy and Practice....48
Summary....54
References....55

CHAPTER 4 Person- and Family-Centered Care: Comprehensive Care Planning....61
Introduction....61
AACN Essentials....62
The 4Ms of Age-Friendly Care....63
Assessing Preferences for Care and Activities....64

Assessing and Cultivating At-Homeness....67
Approaches to Care....70
Function-Focused Care Approach....77
Assessment of Function....79
Function-Focused Care Planning and Interventions....80
Environmental Approaches....82
Policies That Support FFC....82
FFC Education....83
Negotiated Risk....83
Partnering With Family as Team Members....84
Summary....86
References....87
Resources....92

CHAPTER 5 Models of Nursing Care Delivery....95

Introduction....95
Nursing Care-Delivery Models....96
Care-Delivery Models Used in Today's Nursing Homes....97
Person-Centered Care Requires a Transformational Leader....99
Models of Palliative and End-of-Life Care....101
Palliative Care....101
Hospice Care....102
External Palliative Care Consultations....103
Primary Palliative Care....104
Resources for Palliative and Hospice Care....104
Models of Transitional Care....106
A Closer Look at Hospital Readmissions: Are They Avoidable?....107
Current Practice Gaps That Contribute to Poor Transitions....108
Transitional Care Interventions....109
Dementia Care Model....113
Care Needs of People Living With Dementia in Nursing Homes....114
Dementia-Specific Care Models and Interventions....115
The Key Essentials of Dementia Care....118
Summary....123
References....124

CHAPTER 6 Common Geriatric Syndromes 131

Introduction 131
A Holistic and Multifactorial Approach to Common Geriatric Syndromes 132
Screening for Geriatric Syndromes 133
Medications Associated With Geriatric Syndromes 133
Atypical Presentation of Illness Among Nursing Home Residents 134
Characteristics of Nursing Home Residents 135
Cognitive Impairment 135
Dementia 136
Delirium 138
Nursing Interventions for Cognitive Impairment 140
Malnutrition 141
Nursing Interventions for Malnutrition 143
Frailty 143
Geriatric Syndromes Related to the Case Study 146
Nursing Interventions Related to the Case Study 146
Falls 146
Assessment 148
Nursing Interventions for Fall Prevention 149
Urinary Incontinence 151
Assessment 152
Nursing Interventions for Urinary Incontinence in the Nursing Home 152
Summary 153
References 153

CHAPTER 7 Developing the Workforce of the Future 159

Introduction 159
Nursing Positions in Nursing Homes 160
Director of Nursing 160
Licensed Nursing Staff 164
Advanced Nursing Practice 168
Key Factors That Reflect the Nurse Practice Environment in Nursing Homes 170
Nursing Care-Delivery Models 171
NursingHome Compare 172

Nurse Staffing....173
Factors to Consider in Selecting a Nursing Home as a Place of Employment .173
Opportunities to Enhance the Role of RNs in the Nursing Home Setting 175
Summary 181
References....181

CHAPTER 8 Staff Development and Training 185

Introduction 185
Revisiting the Teaching Nursing Home 185
Professional Practice in Long-Term Care 187
Advanced Nursing Roles in Long-Term Care 190
Organizational Structure 190
Leadership, Management, and Mentorship....191
Performance Evaluation and Feedback.... 192
Competency-Based Education.... 192
Acuity as an Indicator of Education Needs 194
Certification 196
Benefits 196
Barriers 197
The Role of Educator 198
Methods of Training 199
Engaging Staff in Effective and Efficient Care Delivery 200
Avoiding Burnout and Practicing Self-Care 201
Burnout.... 202
Self-Care 202
Summary 205
References.... 205

CHAPTER 9 The Interprofessional Team and Collaborative Practice 209

Introduction 209
Why Nurses Need to Be Familiar With the Interprofessional Team....210
Nurse....211
Pharmacist.... 212
Central Pharmacy.... 212
Consultant Pharmacist 213

Medication Management and Legal Requirements .213
Rehabilitation Services .214
Physical Therapist .215
Occupational Therapist .219
Speech Therapist 223
Registered Dietitian/Nutritionist 228
RDN Education 228
RDN Role 229
RDN and Food Service Manager 230
Recreation Therapist 230
Education Requirements and Certification 230
Recreational Services .231
Social Worker .233
Resident Rights 234
Discharge Planning .235
Advance Care Planning 236
Putting It All Together – Case Example 238
Introduction 238
Case Details 239
Discussion 242
Conclusion 242
Summary 243
References 243

CHAPTER 10 Regulatory Context .247

Introduction 247
Nursing Home Survey and OBRA Background 248
The History of Nursing Home Regulations 248
Purpose/Intent .251
Types of Surveys .253
Standard and Life Safety Code Surveys 254
Focused Surveys .255
Abbreviated Standard Survey .257
Complaint .257

Special Focus Facilities. 258
CMS SOM Chapter 7 258
The Survey Process. 260
Ways LT/PAC Facilities Prepare for Survey. 260
How Surveyors Prepare for Survey. 262
What to Expect on Survey 262
How Survey Results Are Measured/The 2567 Statement of Deficiencies 264
Implications of Survey Results. 266
Five Star Rating Scoring Rules for Survey/Health Inspection Results 266
Survey Scoring Rules Summary 266
Rating Methodology for Facilities With Abuse Deficiencies 267
Summary 270
References. 271

CHAPTER 11 Financing Long-Term Care 275

Introduction 275
How Nurses Are Paid. 276
Why Learn About Nursing Home Financing? 276
How Financing and Your Role as Part of the Nursing Staff Intersect 277
The Financing System in Long-Term Care Is Complex 277
The Varied Payors for Nursing Homes: Who Pays for What? 278
What Services Can Be Billed for in Nursing Homes 280
Respite Care. 282
Hospice and Palliative Care 282
Consolidated Billing Under Medicare: What Is Excluded 283
The Reimbursement Bottom Line for Nursing Staff 285
Nursing Staff and Documentation: Where Financing and the Care You Provide Intersect. 285
The Payment Structures for Nursing Homes 286
Why Your Documentation Matters 290
Nonprofit Nursing Homes Versus For-Profit Nursing Homes. 293
Summary 293
References. 294

CHAPTER 12 Improving Quality in Nursing Homes 297

Introduction 297

Quality Measures 298

The Resident Assessment Instrument/Minimum Data Set 299

Long-Stay Versus Short-Stay Quality Measures 300

Shared Decision-Making to Increase Quality of Care 302

Safety Measures 303

Cultivating a Culture of Safety 303

Complying With Safety Protocols 304

Quality Improvement Programs and Processes in Nursing Homes 305

Models of Quality Care in Nursing Homes 306

The 4Ms Framework 309

Balancing Quality and Safety With What Matters to the Resident 311

Summary 314

References 314

CHAPTER 13 Nursing Home Health Information Technology 319

Introduction 319

Federal Policy Driving Technology Adoption in U.S. Nursing Homes 320

Inputs to Nursing Home Quality: The Case for Health Information Technology 320

Key Points of Failure for IT Adoption in Nursing Homes 320

Nursing Homes and the Technology Environment 323

Framework and Attributes for Nursing Home IT Maturity 323

Opportunities for IT Maturity Infrastructure Development and Testing 324

Recognizing IT Structural Disparities That Impact Quality of Nursing Home Care 325

Specialized Technologies for Nursing Home Systems 326

Interoperability and a Use Case for Evaluating Nursing Home Admissions 331

Current State and Evolution of Nursing Home Technology 333

Nursing Home Electronic Health Records 333

Telehealth 334

Summary 334

References 335

Index 339

FOREWORD

This book gives me great hope. The breadth and depth of the roster of authors, who are among our preeminent scientists and nurse leaders in the field of nursing home care, alerts us that we are in a different moment for evidence-based practice in nursing homes. The COVID-19 pandemic shocked all of us by exposing the incredible vulnerability of older adults and nursing home staff. How did we get to that place? The National Academies of Sciences, Engineering, and Medicine (NASEM) report *The National Imperative to Improve Nursing Home Quality* (2022) documented in painful detail the genesis and trajectory of the problems that were laid bare by the pandemic. As a nation, we are steeped in ageism, where older adults experience prejudice by virtue of the fact of their long lives. One need only look at our greeting cards, mandatory retirement in certain industries, national media, higher education, and the way in which we think about care delivery for the very old. Fortunately, a new coalition called Moving Forward is taking the NASEM report recommendations and moving them into action. The coalition is now more than 800 members strong, with Dr. Alice Bonner chairing the effort.

Further, we now have the evidence-based messaging recommendations to discuss issues related to nursing home care because of the excellent research reports produced by the Frameworks Institute, including "Communicating About Nursing Home Care: Findings and Emerging Recommendations" (Aassar & Volmert, 2022), funded by the John A. Hartford Foundation. This report reflects the urgency to improve the national conversation about nursing homes and nursing home care and underscores the need to communicate effectively about nursing homes by focusing on solutions and collective societal responsibility to garner public support for the deep reform needed to ensure the changes we make result in quality, safety, reliability, and appropriate payment reform for how nursing homes will exist and operate going forward.

Education and the strengthening of the nursing home workforce is another key area that must be addressed. Over 2,600 colleges or universities offer a nursing degree program in the United States, and over 900 are baccalaureate programs. Who is educating the nursing personnel who practice in our country's nursing homes? Look at any curricula and you will find very little didactic content and often an absence of clinical practicums in nursing homes. Herein lies one of the significant barriers to improving nursing home care. We are teaching future nurses that this area of practice is less important and that they need to know less in order to work in nursing homes.

Additionally, the salary inequity that registered nurses experience in nursing home practice versus acute care/hospital practice is another example of societal ageism that devalues those in nursing homes. It does not have to be this way. Can we reimagine the current state of our nursing education, clinical practice, and ultimately the staffing and salary that would be required for true equity for those who require skilled nursing home care? I have suggested that all nursing homes should be closed in order to force our hand as a country (Fulmer et al., 2020). Imagine the backup in emergency departments, surgical suites, and inpatient units. Further, imagine the dramatic increase in demand for quality home care this would create. Our nursing homes were largely built in the 1960s with a standard two-bed shared bathroom layout. It is little wonder that infection spread rampantly during COVID-19 as well as during any given flu season.

One approach to address education and workforce issues can be found in the Revisiting the Teaching Nursing Home initiative, now underway in the state of Pennsylvania. This effort implements a contemporary version of the Teaching Nursing Home model envisioned by the Robert Wood Johnson Foundation in the 1980s (Mezey, 1989). In the three regions of Pennsylvania, faculty and nursing home leaders and staff are demonstrating how enhanced partnerships between academic nursing schools and skilled nursing facilities can improve quality and cost outcomes. The partnership draws upon existing resources from the Age-Friendly Health Systems initiative while integrating lessons learned and partnerships created through the COVID-19 pandemic and the original Teaching Nursing Home model implementation. The Pennsylvania State University College of Nursing, University of Pennsylvania School of Nursing (Penn Nursing), and University of Pittsburgh School of Nursing provide faculty and educational support. The John A Hartford Foundation, Jewish Healthcare Foundation, Independence Foundation, and Henry L. Hillman Foundation co-fund this important initiative. The goal is to engage every nursing school and every nursing home in Pennsylvania in this vital work. Having completed phase 1 of the program, we now move into phase 2 and have rebranded the effort to be named the Teaching Nursing Home Collaborative (TNHC) to more fully reflect the incredible momentum and uptake of this model for nursing home–academic partnerships across Pennsylvania. Our TNHC intersects with the broader ongoing Age-Friendly Health System movement under the leadership of the Institute of Healthcare Improvement. It further intersects with the Moving Forward Coalition in a powerful way.

Pennsylvania is a highly useful testing ground, and I am grateful to the National Advisory Board and to all the faculty and staff who are willing to reexamine our academic practice partnerships and opportunities for improvement. I am also grateful to Senior Program Officers Amy Berman and Jane Carmody, my friends, and experts in gerontological nursing, who lead this work for the John A. Hartford Foundation. Let me also acknowledge the expert team at the Jewish Health Foundation, including Chief Operating Officer and Chief Program Officer Nancy Zionts; Nurse Project Manager of Aging Initiatives Maureen Saxon-Gioia; Program Associate Emily Franke; and Program Manager of Aging Initiatives Anneliese Perry; along with the many members of that team who contribute on any given day. Our Teaching Nursing Home national advisory board of stellar experts in the field have been priceless.

Our editors have crafted an outstanding textbook that provides the opportunity for all of us to address the care we all want in nursing homes with a focus on creating a culture of care that is person- and family-centered, based on science, and respectful of the workforce. The person who brings your breakfast tray is an important sentinel person to observe if something is changing for the resident. The authors describe excellence in teamwork, the family's role on the team, and how we can elevate an exciting and compelling model for all staff considering working in the nursing home environment. It starts with appropriate education and exciting clinical experiences with expert faculty who can bring the science alive and provide experiential learning to the students. These faculty are key role models and have a powerful influence over how the experience is shaped and the students respond. I am grateful to Drs. JoAnne Reifsnyder, Ann Kolanowski, and Jackie Dunbar-Jacob for editing this exceptional textbook that should be required for every nursing student and every nursing faculty member.

–Terry Fulmer, PhD, RN, FAAN
President, The John A. Hartford Foundation

REFERENCES

Aassar, M., & Volmert, A. (2022, April 11). *Communicating about nursing home care: Findings and emerging recommendations.* Frameworks Institute. https://www.frameworksinstitute.org/publication/communicating-about-nursing-home-care-findings-and-emerging-recommendations/

Fulmer, T. T., Koller, C. F., & Rowe, J. W. (2020, Sept. 21). Reimagining nursing homes in the wake of COVID-19. *NAM Perspectives.* National Academy of Medicine. https://nam.edu/reimagining-nursing-homes-in-the-wake-of-covid-19/

Mezey, M. (1989). The Teaching Nursing Home program: Outcomes of care. *Nursing Clinics of North America, 24*(3), 769–780.

National Academies of Sciences, Engineering, and Medicine. (2022). *The national imperative to improve nursing home quality: Honoring our commitment to residents, families, and staff.* National Academies Press. https://nap.nationalacademies.org/catalog/26526/the-national-imperative-to-improve-nursing-home-quality-honoring-our

INTRODUCTION

JoAnne Reifsnyder, PhD, MSN, MBA, RN, FAAN
Ann Kolanowski, PhD, RN, FAAN
Melodee Harris, PhD, RN, FAAN
Sherry Greenberg, PhD, RN, GNP-BC, FGSA, FNAP, FAANP, FAAN

WHY WE WROTE THIS BOOK

The many contributors to this textbook represent some of the best researchers, clinicians, and educators in geriatrics and, in particular, the specialized care of patients who return home after rehabilitation in nursing homes and those who live there long term. As an outgrowth of a Pennsylvania-based demonstration project funded by the John A. Hartford Foundation (JAHF), the Jewish Healthcare Foundation, and the Independence Foundation titled "Revisiting the Teaching Nursing Home" (RTNH; JAHF, n.d.), this book has been created as a resource to support more meaningful and productive collaboration between schools of nursing and their neighboring nursing homes.

The RTNH demonstration aims to address the long-term care (LTC) workforce shortage by introducing nursing students to geriatric nursing, better preparing the health workforce, and improving quality of care within nursing homes (JAHF, n.d.). The project is a renewal of the Teaching Nursing Home model that was pioneered in the 1980s (Mezey et al., 1984), which found that creating partnerships between nursing schools and nursing homes improved clinical outcomes within the homes, mainly by reducing hospitalizations. As advisors to the RTNH demonstration, the editors of this book quickly recognized that there was no nursing textbook for undergraduate nursing students that provided a singular focus on the challenges and opportunities of nursing practice in this complex environment.

The term "nursing home" may evoke images both positive and negative depending on one's experience and frame of reference. Nursing homes have existed in the United States as convalescent centers for older adults for many decades. Chapter 1 of this book provides an in-depth historical perspective on the evolution of nursing homes from almshouses for the poor in the 17th century to modern day facilities that provide both short-term, post-acute rehabilitation and long-term skilled nursing for older adults who require more care than can be provided at home.

Nursing homes are places of residence primarily for older adults, although the LTC nursing home population may include adults as young as 18 who meet criteria for nursing home care. The majority of children with special needs are cared for at home, although an estimated 5,000 children live in facilities that specialize in their care (Friedman et al., 2014). This textbook focuses on the care of older adults in nursing homes, both as short-term patients receiving rehabilitation after a hospital stay and long-term residents.

In February 2020, a nursing home in Kirkland, Washington, was the "initial US epicenter" of the novel coronavirus SARS-CoV-2 outbreak that would come to be known as COVID-19 (White, 2021). In early March of 2020, the World Health Organization declared COVID-19 a pandemic (Cucinotta & Vanelli, 2020). Early in the pandemic, testing supplies were limited, available to nursing homes only through departments of health and only in small quantities, making it difficult to detect COVID-19 and isolate residents other than those with symptoms. Nursing homes reported widespread shortages of personal protective equipment, and as staff developed symptoms and needed to be excluded from work, staffing challenges that existed pre-pandemic intensified.

Precautions taken to slow the spread of COVID-19 from the community into nursing homes as well as within nursing homes included closing facilities to visitors and eliminating congregate meals, activities, and rehabilitation. Confined to their rooms for months on end, many residents experienced anxiety, depression, and functional and cognitive decline (Levere et al., 2021). By January 2022, COVID-19 had accounted for more than 200,000 deaths among nursing home residents and staff and more than 23% of all COVID-19-related deaths in the US (Chidambaram, 2022). The impact of illness and death was disproportionately borne by patients and residents of ethnic and racial minorities (Weech-Maldonado et al., 2021).

The devastating effects of the COVID-19 pandemic in nursing homes will be the subject of research and commentary for many years to come. The crisis laid bare the many deficiencies in the US system of care for its most vulnerable citizens. Constructed primarily in the 1960s–1990s, nursing homes typically have small, shared living quarters (two, three, or even four beds in a single room) and shared toilets, which made isolation of residents who tested positive, those with symptoms, and those who were exposed to an infected roommate extremely difficult.

Nurse staffing levels were already lower than standards set by the Centers for Medicare & Medicaid Services in half of all US nursing homes (Harrington et al., 2016). One study found that there were significant declines in staffing levels during severe COVID-19 outbreaks that had not recovered nearly four months after an outbreak (Shen et al., 2022). At this writing, staffing levels in nursing homes still remain 12% below pre-pandemic levels (Altarum, 2023), which, as already stated, were lower than required in a large proportion of facilities before the pandemic.

The many staff who did remain at the bedside through the pandemic have also suffered. Nursing home staff reported somatic problems, worries, and stress that significantly impacted their mental health (Palosky, 2021). Direct-care staff faced impossible choices during the pandemic, putting their own lives and their families' lives at risk while at the same time experiencing burnout and demoralization from the negative media coverage of nursing homes (Espinoza, 2022).

A MAJOR CALL FOR REFORM

In response to the pandemic, the National Academies of Sciences, Engineering, and Medicine (NASEM) formed a committee to address long-standing issues that have impacted quality of care in nursing homes. The committee, composed of 17 members and chaired by a nurse, Betty Ferrell, issued their report in 2022 following a year-long study. That report, *The National Imperative to Improve Nursing Home Quality: Honoring Our Commitment to Residents, Families, and Staff*, included strong recommendations toward the goal of promoting person-centered care in our nation's nursing homes (NASEM, 2022).

Importantly, the committee concluded that the goals they established should not be approached in a piecemeal manner but rather must be addressed as an integrated set to make real progress. These are the seven broad goals for a comprehensive approach to person-centered care:

Goal one: Deliver comprehensive, person-centered, equitable care that ensures the health, quality of life, and safety of nursing home residents; promotes resident autonomy; and manages risks

Goal two: Ensure a well-prepared, empowered, and appropriately compensated workforce

Goal three: Increase transparency and accountability of finances, operations, and ownership

Goal four: Create a more rational and robust financing system

Goal five: Design a more effective and responsive system of quality assurance

Goal six: Expand and enhance quality measurement and continuous quality improvement

Goal seven: Adopt health information technology in all nursing homes

The following table is a guide to finding content in the textbook related to each of the reform goals specified in the NASEM report.

NASEM REPORT	CONTENT LOCATION IN THE TEXTBOOK
Goal one	Chapters 1, 2, 3, 4, 5, 6
Goal two	Chapters 3, 5, 7, 8, 9
Goal three	Chapters 1, 11
Goal four	Chapters 1, 11
Goal five	Chapters 10, 12
Goal six	Chapters 10, 12
Goal seven	Chapter 13

Across these goals, the role of the professional nurse was viewed as central to realizing improvements in settings that bear our discipline's name.

Funded by the John A. Hartford Foundation, the Moving Forward Coalition was established as a two-year initiative to define near and long-term actionable plans (JAHF, 2022) to realize the goals outlined in the landmark NASEM report. The coalition is organized into subgroups, each accountable for one of the seven major goals. Considerable structural and policy change is unquestionably needed to make progress on the goals. Nevertheless, the coalition has attracted and emboldened a large and diverse set of stakeholders who intend to do just that.

As you will read throughout this text, there is reason for optimism about nursing practice in the nursing home sector. There are exemplary nursing homes throughout the country providing engaged, compassionate, person-centered, and wellness-focused care to older adults across the spectrum of disease and disability. Highly skilled and committed nurses lead teams of RNs, LPNs, and certified nursing assistants (CNAs) to practice at the top of their skill sets, offering advanced training in specialties such as memory care, cardiac care, wound care, and palliative care. For the nursing student interested in honing comprehensive assessment and care management skills, there is no better environment in which to learn about complex chronic illness. Chapter 8 covers staff development, training, and performance evaluation.

Importantly, the integration of technology including electronic health records in nursing homes has lagged behind such development in other care settings. Chapter 13 addresses the current state and future opportunities surrounding the use of technology to document key data elements about care and to enhance clinical decision support.

The addition of advanced practice (registered) nurses (APNs/APRNs)—nurses with graduate degrees in nursing specialties—has brought medical care closer to the point of care. These APNs collaborate with all members of the interprofessional team to assure quality of care. As part of advocacy and policy efforts, the Gerontological Advanced Practice Nurses Association (GAPNA) has adopted position statements related to LTC, available on the GAPNA website at https://www.gapna.org/advocacy/policies-position-statements.

The GAPNA position statements are applicable to all nurses caring for older adults and working in nursing home settings, as knowledge of roles and expectations is crucial. One example is the position statement "Eliminating Practice Barriers of the Gerontological APRN in the Long-Term Care Setting," which delineates the critical role of the gerontological APRN in LTC, highlights barriers to APRN practice, and suggests recommendations for continued advancement of the role of the APN in nursing homes.

Finally, and most importantly, older adults have lived rich, full, complicated lives—and they have stories to tell and wisdom to impart. As most geriatric-trained nurses will tell you, they can't imagine caring for any other population. But nursing homes are complicated, and many changes are needed.

This textbook aims to reduce the negative attitudes that surround nursing practice in nursing homes by illustrating how high-quality nursing care and positive resident outcomes can be achieved when nurses practice at the top of their licenses. This book will challenge you to think about where you could fit in and how you might lead the changes that will advance care for older adults who receive care and live in the nursing homes of tomorrow.

OVERVIEW OF NURSING HOMES AND THE PROFESSIONAL NURSE IN THESE SETTINGS

In the US, the post-acute and LTC delivery system includes a broad range of health, personal care, and support services that meet the needs of older people and other adults whose capacity for self-care is limited because of chronic diseases or disabilities and other health-related conditions (Administration for Community Living, 2021). Services provided in these settings include social work, mental health and counseling, therapies (physical, occupational, respiratory [in some locations], and speech), therapeutic recreation, skilled nursing care, pharmacy, hospice, and dietary and nutrition.

Settings that deliver these services are quite varied and include adult day care centers, home health agencies, hospices, assisted living and other residential care communities, inpatient rehabilitation facilities, LTC hospitals, and nursing homes. While the post-acute and LTC delivery system has changed substantially over the last 30 years, nursing homes continue to be a major provider of post-acute and LTC. In fact, the use of nursing homes for short-term post-acute care and rehabilitation has steadily increased over the last decade.

Nursing homes (also called skilled nursing facilities) are among the most challenging and rewarding places for professional nurses to practice. Arguably, it is here, more than any other healthcare setting, that nurses can apply their competencies and leadership skills that are essential to the needs of older adults who reside there. Within nursing homes, professional nurses deliver a broad range of services and supports including promotion of health and well-being/disease prevention, chronic disease care, regenerative or restorative care, and hospice/palliative/supportive care (American Association of Colleges of Nursing [AACN], 2021).

Because older adults reside in these settings over long periods of time, nurses have a unique opportunity to develop a deep understanding of each resident's needs, values, and preferences for everyday living. Professional nurses also experience the positive effect of their clinical leadership on improving the quality of care delivered by staff and the quality of life enjoyed by residents.

Nursing homes are quite different from acute-care settings, where much of clinical nursing education occurred in the past. To deliver quality care in the nursing home, it is essential that nurses first understand the population that is served in these settings and the characteristics that define their care needs.

Characteristics of People Residing in Nursing Homes

In 2018, an estimated 1,321,200 people were residents in nursing homes. The vast majority were over the age of 65 (81.1% of short-stay residents and 84.6% of long-stay residents), and most were women (59.0% of short-stay residents and 66.6% of long-stay residents). Non-Hispanic white residents comprised 73.9% of the total population, while 14.9% of residents were non-Hispanic Black service users (Sengupta et al., 2022). See Chapter 3 for a discussion of diversity, equity, and inclusion in the nursing home setting. Sixty-two percent of all residents used Medicaid as their payor source (see Chapter 11 for an in-depth discussion of LTC finance).

The care needs of nursing residents are complex due to their functional limitations and high disease burden. Over 87% of residents need assistance with bathing, dressing, toileting, walking or locomotion, transferring in and out of a chair or bed, and eating. This care needs to be delivered in a manner that maintains and/or restores function and is consistent with the resident's goals, preferences, and priorities. Chapter 4 introduces you to person-/family-centered care, function-focused care, and assessing preferences for care; Chapter 2 describes Age-Friendly care, where what matters to the resident is one of four pillars.

Residents of nursing homes also have a high disease burden, many with multiple co-morbidities including arthritis (27.6%), diabetes (34.8%), heart disease (20.1%), hypertension (76.9%), and osteoporosis (11.4%). Importantly, almost half of older adults in these settings have a dementia diagnosis (49.1%), and 48.8% have depression (Sengupta et al., 2022). Finely tuned assessment skills are needed to make sense of atypical symptoms that older adults often present with.

Chapter 6 introduces you to the concept of chronic disease management and evidence-based interventions that can modify and reduce frailty and common geriatric syndromes (i.e., falls, delirium, incontinence) that result from the interaction of multiple physical, cognitive, and psychological comorbidities. Chapter 9 describes how the interprofessional team in a nursing home collaborates on a single plan of care to address a patient/resident's chronic conditions, goals and preferences, functional status, and quality of life. Quality and safety regulations are covered in Chapter 10, while Chapter 12 provides information on the quality and safety measures used in nursing homes and how to improve in those areas.

This brief description of the characteristics of nursing home residents will help nurses appreciate the complexity of residents' needs and the concomitant need for highly skilled professional nurses who can lead teams of direct caregivers in the delivery of person-centered care.

Professional Nurse Roles in Nursing Homes

The professional nurse is the onsite provider in LTC and often the first line in communication and care coordination with residents, families, primary care providers, and other specialists. Because the care delivery model in nursing homes (covered at length in Chapter 5) is one in which the professional nurse functions as a team leader and supervises/mentors the staff (LPNs, CNAs) at the point of care, higher level nursing skills such as critical thinking, teamwork, decision-making, integration of evidence-based practice, and therapeutic communication are critical (Mueller et al., 2018). However, foundational clinical skills—such as physical assessment, medication administration and management, and the use and care of medical devices including feeding tubes or ventilators—are equally important.

APRNS are key team members in addressing issues related to the care of older adults in LTC, including the following:

- Providing high-quality, evidence-based care to medically and socially complex older adults

- Assessing and managing acute and chronic conditions, including infectious illnesses, such as COVID-19, influenza, and others
- Managing mental health problems
- Coordinating transitional care needs
- Educating and advocating for older adults, families, and caregivers
- Working with care partners to address caregiving needs

Chapter 7 presents and discusses the role of APRNs in nursing homes.

COMPETENCIES NEEDED FOR PROFESSIONAL NURSING PRACTICE IN NURSING HOMES

Professional nurses who work in LTC are expected to maintain a level of competence to promote positive outcomes for the population they serve. A number of organizations have identified competencies needed by nurses who practice in all settings, including the unique specialty of geriatric/gerontological nursing.

The AACN developed *The Essentials: Core Competencies for Professional Nursing Education* as a compass to guide the accountability of nursing graduates for mastering basic skills. Ten domains are included in the Essentials (AACN, 2021):

- Knowledge for Nursing Practice
- Person-Centered Care
- Population Health
- Scholarship for Nursing Discipline
- Quality and Safety
- Interprofessional Partnerships
- Systems-Based Practice
- Informatics and Healthcare Technologies
- Professionalism
- Personal, Professional, and Leadership Development

Knowledge, skills, and attitudes are integrated across the domains (AACN, 2021). All 10 competency domains are relevant to LTC. Each chapter in this textbook includes a table that illustrates which domains and competencies from the Essentials are covered in that chapter.

The Quality and Safety Education for Nurses (QSEN) Competencies were developed to prepare RNs with basic practices on patient-centered care, teamwork and collaboration, evidence-based practice, quality improvement, safety, and informatics (Cronenwett et al., 2007). Similar to the AACN Essentials, knowledge, skills, and attitudes are associated with each competency domain (Cronenwett et al., 2007). The QSEN Competencies align with nursing home goals for quality care.

The Geropsychiatric Competency Enhancements for Entry-Level Professional Nurses are meant to deepen the AACN Essentials and other competencies. Specific competency enhancements for RNs in LTC are:

- Identifying mental health and cognitive disorders
- Recognizing age-related change
- Supporting and advocating for older adults with cognitive, affective, or behavioral symptoms and issues related to decisional capacity
- Guardianship and power of attorney
- Ensuring safe and effective transitions of care between other environments and LTC

As leaders of the interprofessional team in LTC, RNs are also subject to Interprofessional Collaborative Practice Competencies, including Values and Ethics, Roles/Responsibilities, Interprofessional Communication, and Teams/Teamwork (Interprofessional Education Collaborative, 2011). Interprofessional collaboration is especially important in memory care (Harris et al., 2013; Jackson et al., 2016).

Perhaps there is no more vulnerable population than older adults living in LTC. RNs who work in LTC represent a unique specialty and are expected to maintain a professional level of competence to promote positive outcomes for the population served.

ORGANIZATIONS THAT SUPPORT PROFESSIONAL PRACTICE IN NURSING HOMES

A number of organizations provide networking, professional development, mentoring, and support for the professional nurse who practices in the nursing home. The following table provides a brief overview of key organizations involved in the nursing and interprofessional care of older adults. In addition to the noted national organizations, there are multiple centers of geriatric/gerontological nursing excellence around the country, mainly based at academic institutions, committed to implementing innovative educational, practice, research, and policy endeavors related to the preparation of the next generation of nursing leaders who will care for older adults, including those residing in nursing homes. Many of these centers can be found on the National Hartford Centers of Gerontological Nursing Excellence website listed in the table.

Nursing Organizations Involved in Long-Term Care of Older Adults

ORGANIZATION	BRIEF DESCRIPTION	WEBSITE
American Geriatrics Society (AGS)	Society of geriatrics healthcare professionals dedicated to improving the health, independence, and quality of life of older people. Members include geriatricians, geriatrics nurse practitioners, social workers, family practitioners, physician assistants, pharmacists, and internists who are pioneers in advanced-illness care for older individuals, with a focus on championing interprofessional teams, eliciting personal care goals, and treating older people as whole persons. Mission: To improve the health, independence, and quality of life for older people.	https://www.americangeriatrics.org

(continues)

Nursing Organizations Involved in Long-Term Care of Older Adults *(continued)*

ORGANIZATION	BRIEF DESCRIPTION	WEBSITE
Center to Advance Palliative Care (CAPC)	National organization dedicated to increasing the availability of quality, equitable healthcare for people living with serious illness and their family caregivers. As the nation's leading resource in its field, CAPC provides healthcare professionals and organizations—health systems, hospitals, hospices, home health agencies, LTC facilities, medical groups, health plans, and other entities—with the training, tools, and technical assistance necessary to effectively meet this need. It is part of the Icahn School of Medicine at Mount Sinai, in New York City.	https://www.capc.org
Gerontological Advanced Practice Nurses Association (GAPNA)	Premier professional organization that represents the interests of APNs, RNs, clinicians, educators, and researchers involved in the practice or advancement of caring for older adults. Members are active in academia, research, and a variety of clinical practice settings across the healthcare continuum—including primary care, acute care, post-acute care, home care, and LTC. Across this broad spectrum, GAPNA provides opportunities for education, leadership, research, advocacy, networking, and the advancement of evidence-based care. Mission: Promoting excellence in advanced practice nursing for the well-being of older adults. Gerontological Nursing Certification Commission (GNCC), the certification arm of GAPNA, offers an APRN specialty certification in gerontology, the APRN Gerontological Specialist-Certified (GS-C) to distinguish APRNs who possess expert knowledge, experience, and skill in managing the complex health needs of older adults.	https://www.gapna.org GNCC certification information: https://www.gapna.org/certification

ORGANIZATION	BRIEF DESCRIPTION	WEBSITE
Gerontological Society of America (GSA)	Fosters collaboration among behavioral and social scientists, physicians, nurses, biologists, psychologists, social workers, educators, economists, policy experts, practice leaders, those who study the humanities and the arts, and other scholars and researchers in aging. Mission: Cultivate excellence in interdisciplinary aging research and education to advance innovations in practice and policy.	https://www.geron.org
HIGN—Hartford Institute for Geriatric Nursing	Since its start in 1996, HIGN has sought to shape the quality of healthcare of older adults. HIGN is the geriatric arm of the NYU Rory Meyers College of Nursing and has become, over the years, a beacon for all those who wish to advance geriatric care through nursing leadership and interprofessional team care. Has notable e-learning resources, ConsultGeri nursing protocols and resources, and *Try This:* Series on Best Practices in Nursing Care to Older Adults. Mission: To advance age-sensitive and equitable healthcare for all older adults.	https://hign.org HIGN e-learning resources available at: https://hign.org/consultgeri-resources/elearning
National Association of Directors of Nursing Administration in Long Term Care (Nadona LTC)	Leading advocate, mentor, and educational organization for directors of nursing, assistant directors of nursing, RNs, and nurse leaders in long-term and post-acute care. Mission: Leading professional organization for current and aspiring nursing leaders through professional development, board certification, and clinical expertise related to the promotion of health and wellness of individuals in the LTC and post-acute care continuum.	https://nadona.org Multiple certifications and certificate programs available at: https://nadona.org/exams

(continues)

Nursing Organizations Involved in Long-Term Care of Older Adults *(continued)*

ORGANIZATION	BRIEF DESCRIPTION	WEBSITE
National Association of Health Care Assistants (NAHCA)	National professional association of and for certified nursing assistants (CNAs). Intent is to enhance quality of life and care for frail, older, disabled people; enhance the professional standing of CNAs and other similarly credentialed caregivers through recognition, education, advocacy, and motivation; and form strong relationships with the other professionals within the LTC system. Mission: Elevate the professional standing and performance of CNAs and other caregivers through recognition, advocacy, education, and empowerment while building a strong alliance with healthcare providers to maximize success and quality patient care.	https://www.nahcacna.org
National Hartford Center of Gerontological Nursing Excellence (NHCGNE)	Collaboration of national and international nursing schools and institutions demonstrating commitment to gerontological nursing. Certificate of Recognition for Excellence as a Distinguished Educator in Gerontological Nursing available to those eligible. Mission: Enhance and sustain the capacity and competency of nurses to provide quality care to older adults.	https://www.nhcgne.org Information about the Distinguished Educator in Gerontological Nursing Program available at: https://www.nhcgne.org/leadership-development/distinguished-educator-in-gerontological-nursing-program
National Hospice and Palliative Care Organization (NHPCO)	Largest nonprofit membership organization representing hospice and palliative care programs, providers, and professionals who care for people affected by life-limiting illness. Committed to improving end-of-life care and expanding access to hospice care with the goal of enhancing quality of life. Mission: To lead and mobilize the transformation of care delivery to ensure equitable access to high-quality, interdisciplinary, person-centered care for those living with serious illness.	https://www.nhpco.org

The nursing profession has an extraordinary and historic opportunity to improve care in settings that bear its name. The starting point is nursing education and you, the next generation of professional nurses. Traditionally, nursing students have not been prepared to lead teams for the delivery of high-quality LTC. There have been many misconceptions about practice in nursing homes and the role of the professional nurse. This textbook, written by experts in the field, will dispel many of these misconceptions and provide a foundation for clinical practice in a unique and exciting setting. It is a beginning step toward helping you implement the NASEM recommendations for person-centered care in the nursing home.

REFERENCES

Administration for Community Living. (2021). *Understanding long-term care.* https://acl.gov/ltc/basic-needs/

Altarum. (2023, Feb. 23). *Health care adds 58,000 jobs amid strong economywide job growth.* https://altarum.org/sites/default/files/uploaded-publication-files/Altarum-HSEI-Labor-Brief_Feb_2023.pdf

American Association of Colleges of Nursing. (2021). *The essentials: Core competencies for professional nursing education.* https://www.aacnnursing.org/Portals/42/AcademicNursing/pdf/Essentials-2021.pdf

Chidambaram, P. (2022). *Over 200,000 residents and staff in long-term care facilities have died from COVID-19.* Kaiser Family Foundation. https://www.kff.org/policy-watch/over-200000-residents-and-staff-in-long-term-care-facilities-have-died-from-covid-19/

Cronenwett, L., Sherwood, G., Barnsteiner, J., Disch, J., Johnson, J., Mitchell, P., Sullivan, D. T., & Warren, J. (2007). Quality and safety education for nurses. *Nursing Outlook, 55*(3), 122–131. https://doi.org/10.1016/j.outlook.2007.02.006

Cucinotta, D., & Vanelli, M. (2020, March 19). WHO declares COVID-19 a pandemic. *Acta Biomedica, 91*(1), 157–160. https://doi.org/10.23750/abm.v91i1.9397

Espinoza, R. (2022). The impact of COVID-19 on direct care workers. *Generations Journal* (Spring). https://generations.asaging.org/impact-covid-19-direct-care-workers

Friedman, S. L., Kalichman, M. A., Council on Children with Disabilities, Norwood Jr., K. W., Adams, R. C., Brei, T., Burke, R. T., Davis, B. E., Houtrow, A. J., Kuo, D. Z., Levy, S. E., Turchi, R. M., Wiley, S. E., & Murphy, N. A. (2014, October). Out-of-home placement for children and adolescents with disabilities. *Pediatrics, 134*(4), 836–846. https://doi.org/10.1542/peds.2014-2279

Harrington, C., Schnelle, J. F., McGregor, M., & Simmons, S. F. (2016). The need for higher minimum staffing standards in U.S. nursing homes. *Health Services Insights, 9,* 13–19. https://doi.org/10.4137/HSI.S38994

Harris, M., Mayo, A., Balas, M. C., Aaron, C. S., & Buron, B. (2013, June). Trends and opportunities in geropsychiatric nursing: Enhancing practice through specialization and interprofessional education. *Journal of Nursing Education, 52*(6), 317–321. https://doi.org/10.3928/01484834-20130509-03

Interprofessional Education Collaborative. (2011). *Core competencies for interprofessional collaborative practice.* https://ipec.memberclicks.net/assets/2011 Original.pdf

Jackson, M., Pelone, F., Reeves, S., Hassenkamp, A. M., Emery, C., Titmarsh, K., & Greenwood, N. (2016, Aug. 16). Interprofessional education in the care of people diagnosed with dementia and their carers: A systematic review. *BMJ Open, 6*(8), e010948. https://doi.org/10.1136/bmjopen-2015-010948

John A. Hartford Foundation. (n.d.). *Revisiting the Teaching Nursing Home.* https://www.johnahartford.org/grants-strategy/revisiting-the-teaching-nursing-home

John A. Hartford Foundation. (2022, Sept. 12). *Moving forward: Nursing Home Quality Coalition.* https://www.johnahartford.org/dissemination-center/view/moving-forward-nursing-home-quality-coalition

Levere, M., Rowan, P., & Wysocki, A. (2021, May). The adverse effects of the COVID-19 pandemic on nursing home resident well-being. *Journal of Post-Acute and Long-Term Care Medicine, 22*(5), 948–954. https://doi.org/10.1016/j.jamda.2021.03.010

Mezey, M., Lynaugh, J., & Cherry, J. (1984). The Teaching Nursing Home program. *Nursing Outlook, 32*(3).

Mueller, C., Duan, Y., Vogelsmeier, A., Anderson, R., McConnell, E., & Corazzini, K. (2018, November). Interchangeability of licensed nurses in nursing homes: Perspectives of directors of nursing. *Nursing Outlook, 66*(6), 560–569. https://doi.org/10.1016/j.outlook.2018.09.004

National Academies of Sciences, Engineering, and Medicine. (2022). *The national imperative to improve nursing home quality: Honoring our commitment to residents, families, and staff.* National Academies Press. https://doi.org/doi:10.17226/26526

Palosky, C. (2021, April 6). *KFF/post survey reveals the serious mental health challenges facing frontline health care workers a year into the COVID-19 pandemic.* Kaiser Family Foundation. https://www.kff.org/coronavirus-covid-19/press-release/kff-post-survey-reveals-the-serious-mental-health-challenges-facing-frontline-health-care-workers-a-year-into-the-covid-19-pandemic/

Sengupta, M., Lendon, J. P., Caffrey, C., Melekin, A., & Singh, P. (2022, May). Post-acute and long-term care providers and services users in the United States, 2017–2018. *Vital and Health Statistics, 3*(47), 1–93. https://www.ncbi.nlm.nih.gov/pubmed/35604771

Shen, K., McGarry, B. E., Grabowski, D. C., Gruber, J., & Gandhi, A. D. (2022, July). Staffing patterns in US nursing homes during COVID-19 outbreaks. *JAMA Health Forum, 3*(7), e222151. https://doi.org/10.1001/jamahealthforum.2022.2151

Weech-Maldonado, R., Lord, J., Davlyatov, G., Ghiasi, A., & Orewa, G. (2021). High-minority nursing homes disproportionately affected by COVID-19 deaths. *Frontiers in Public Health, 9,* 606364. https://doi.org/10.3389/fpubh.2021.606364

White, E. M. (2021, Sept. 1). Underreporting of early nursing home COVID-19 cases and deaths in federal data. *JAMA Network Open, 4*(9), e2123696. https://doi.org/10.1001/jamanetworkopen.2021.23696

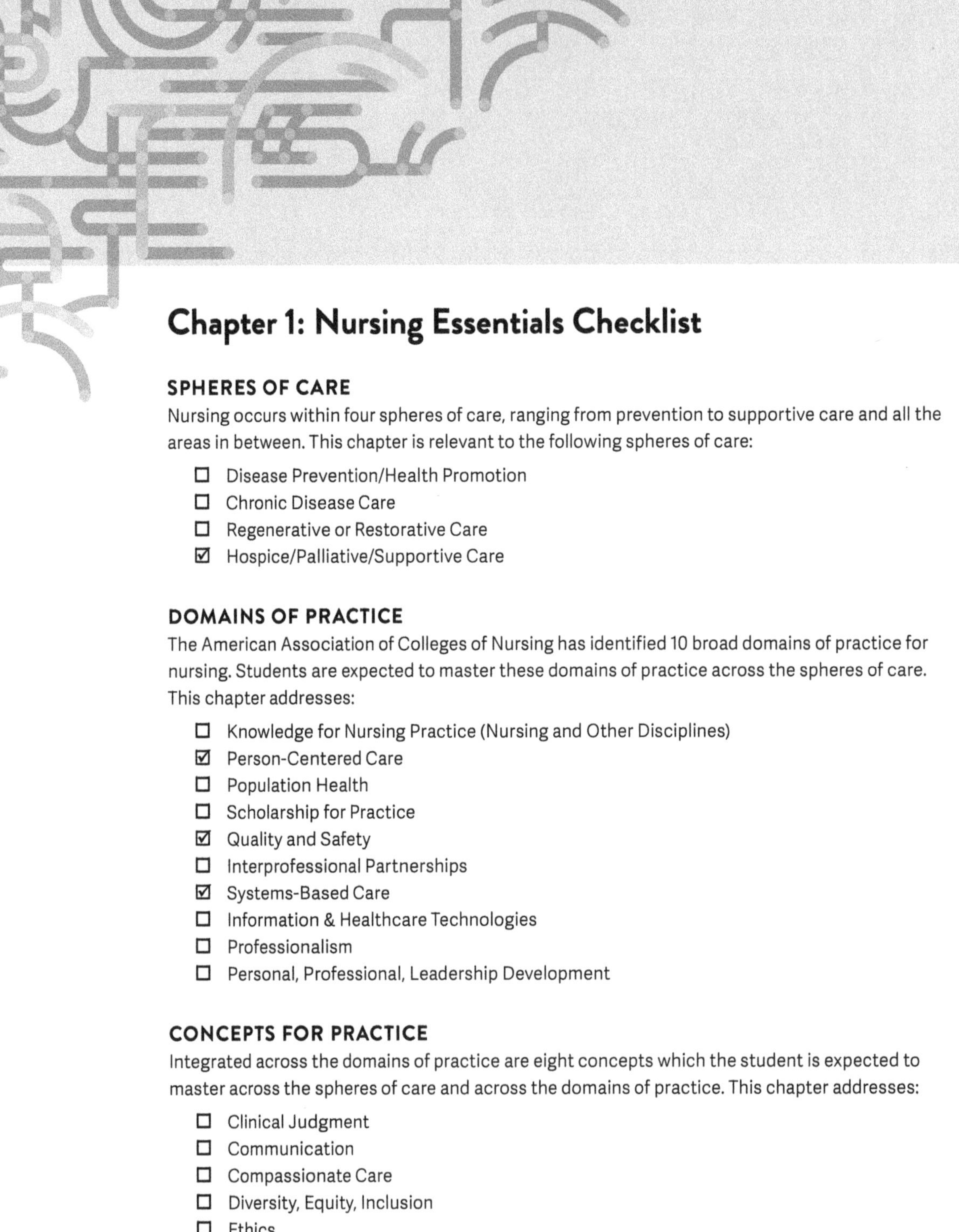

Chapter 1: Nursing Essentials Checklist

SPHERES OF CARE

Nursing occurs within four spheres of care, ranging from prevention to supportive care and all the areas in between. This chapter is relevant to the following spheres of care:

- ☐ Disease Prevention/Health Promotion
- ☐ Chronic Disease Care
- ☐ Regenerative or Restorative Care
- ☑ Hospice/Palliative/Supportive Care

DOMAINS OF PRACTICE

The American Association of Colleges of Nursing has identified 10 broad domains of practice for nursing. Students are expected to master these domains of practice across the spheres of care. This chapter addresses:

- ☐ Knowledge for Nursing Practice (Nursing and Other Disciplines)
- ☑ Person-Centered Care
- ☐ Population Health
- ☐ Scholarship for Practice
- ☑ Quality and Safety
- ☐ Interprofessional Partnerships
- ☑ Systems-Based Care
- ☐ Information & Healthcare Technologies
- ☐ Professionalism
- ☐ Personal, Professional, Leadership Development

CONCEPTS FOR PRACTICE

Integrated across the domains of practice are eight concepts which the student is expected to master across the spheres of care and across the domains of practice. This chapter addresses:

- ☐ Clinical Judgment
- ☐ Communication
- ☐ Compassionate Care
- ☐ Diversity, Equity, Inclusion
- ☐ Ethics
- ☐ Evidence-Based Practice
- ☑ Health Policy
- ☐ Social Determinants of Health

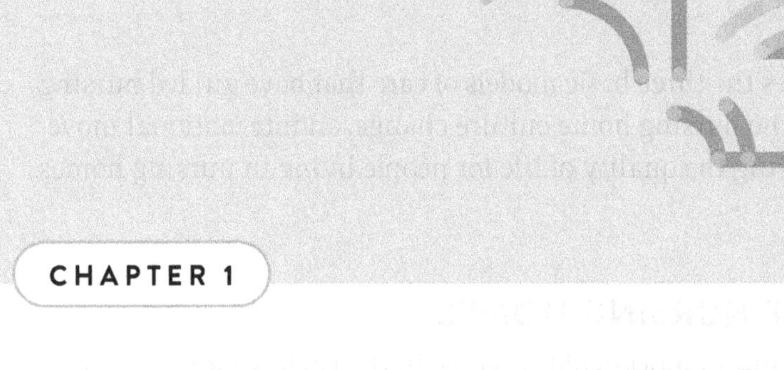

CHAPTER 1

THE JOURNEY TO IMPROVE NURSING CARE

Barbara J. Bowers, PhD, RN, FAAN
Robyn I. Stone, DrPH
Laura N. Gitlin, PhD, FGSA, FAAN

OBJECTIVES

1. **Trace the historical evolution of nursing homes.**
2. **Understand the "home" function of nursing homes and its relationship to quality of care and quality of life.**
3. **Describe models of care and the nursing home culture change movement.**

INTRODUCTION

In America's early years, elder care was the responsibility of the person's family. Eventually, almshouses or poorhouses were established to care for older persons but provided only the most basic needs—shelter, food, and a bed—with little concern for the safety and cleanliness of that shelter. These establishments provided no services to meet the social or healthcare needs of the individuals who resided there. Over time, religious and fraternal organizations began to offer an alternative to almshouses and provided a clean and safe place to live, social support, and a decent quality of life. The nursing home as we know it today didn't exist until the 1940s. Models of care have been developed in the decades since, becoming increasingly focused on the person as a whole instead of solely on what their medical and clinical needs might be. This chapter briefly explores the history of the care and support of older people in the

United States and introduces the three basic models of care that have guided nursing home practices, as well as the nursing home culture change, an international movement committed to improving the quality of life for people living in nursing homes that began in the 1980s.

A BRIEF HISTORY OF NURSING HOMES

Responsibility for the care and support of older people in the US has a long and complex history. Early settlers brought with them many practices from their countries of origin. For example, in the 1700s, all 13 of the US colonies had enacted filial obligation laws that mandated family responsibility for indigent older adults and required families to pay for any care and services provided by the state to support their older relatives (Gillick, 2017). While these laws are no longer widely used, they are still on the books in many states.

European colonists also brought the concept of almshouses or poorhouses with them to the US. *Almshouses*, common as early as the 1600s, were public institutions established to house poor individuals, people with disabilities, orphans, and older adults who had no family or neighbors to support them (Haber, 1993). Rooted in the Elizabethan Poor Laws, this "indoor relief" was the only form of public welfare. Poverty, disability, and illness were viewed as moral failures, and almshouses were meant to reform through order and structure (Watson, 2010). They were also intended to protect society from the corrupting influences of the poor and feeble.

Almshouses were locally run by a county, village, or other governmental entity and were based on the principles of basic hospitality and shelter (Wagner, 2005). These environments simply provided a roof, a bed, and a daily meal for vulnerable individuals who had no resources. The buildings were designed as warehouses with little, if any, attention given to providing a clean and safe space for vulnerable older adults and others to live. People were cramped into wards, and no services were provided to meet the social or healthcare needs of individuals who were in poor health, frail, and at risk for further deterioration. Buildings tended to have poor ventilation and were cold in the winter and unbearably hot in the summer. Poor older adults and younger persons with disabilities who had to rely on public assistance to survive, including living in almshouses, were viewed as "undeserving" and stigmatized; consequently, there was no public interest in improving the living conditions in these institutions (National Academies of Sciences, Engineering, and Medicine [NASEM], 2022).

During the 1800s and early 1900s, distinctions were increasingly made between those considered "deserving" and those considered "undeserving." Almshouses were increasingly viewed as unacceptable housing for the "deserving poor"—those destitute individuals who were in these circumstances through no fault of their own, but rather had no access to resources because they had lost their primary source of family support (Watson, 2010). The worthy poor included orphaned children who had lost breadwinning parents, widows whose husbands had died leaving them without the skills to work, and older people who were no longer able to work and who had no family to care for them.

In response, many religious and fraternal organizations began to establish orphanages and old age homes in their communities. These organizations transformed existing houses into congregate living residences or purposefully built structures that were designed to be more homelike and to provide a clean and safe place to live, social support, and a decent quality of life for older residents (Katz, 1984). The specialty of geriatric nursing grew out of nurses' concerns for the poor conditions experienced by older people living in almshouses (Schell, 1993).

As almshouses disappeared, many people received room, board, and some level of services from the homes run by these charitable religious or fraternal institutions. Social workers who did not want to place older adults in almshouses, which they considered unsafe and unsanitary, sought alternative placements in either religious or fraternally supported homes or proprietary homes where room and board and minimal supports could be purchased for a small fee (Watson, 2010).

Federal Government Intervention

In 1935, the Social Security Act established the first government-sponsored pension for older people, providing funds for them to remain in the community, reducing the number of older people relying on charitable homes for the aged (Haber, 1993), and catalyzing a boom in proprietary "rest homes" and "convalescent homes" for older adults (Vladeck, 1980). Over time, these community-based residential facilities became known as *boarding homes,* housing sicker and frailer older adults and ushering in the era of the modern nursing home (Watson, 2010).

In 1946, Congress passed the Hill-Burton Act, which provided funds for nursing homes to be built in conjunction with hospitals and gave the federal government control over building and regulating these entities. Nursing home buildings were modeled after hospitals, and although they had no physicians, the physical environment helped to transform homes for older people from a primarily social service/welfare model with home-like attributes that were found in the charitable homes for the aged to a medical model.

The passage of Medicaid as an amendment to the Social Security Act in 1965 was a watershed for the modern nursing home (Vladeck, 1980). The legislation included coverage of residential care in nursing homes for low-income older adults and created significant opportunities for many in the private sector to build and operate private sector nursing homes. With a stable payment source for nursing home care through the Medicaid program, the number of nursing homes grew by 140% by the mid-1970s (Birnstengel, 2021). Today, Medicaid is the largest payor of nursing home care, providing over 60% of the funding for long-term nursing home residents (NASEM, 2022). Medicare is the primary payor for post-acute care, covering up to 100 days for care intended to rehabilitate individuals, with the aim of returning home to the community. Private pay accounts for approximately 26% of nursing home payments.

Trending to For-Profit Status

Initially, nursing homes were mostly nonprofit entities, run primarily by religious and philanthropic organizations or small, family-owned proprietary homes. Today, the majority of nursing homes (almost 70%) are for-profit, with nearly one-quarter nonprofit and 7% government-owned (Harris-Kojetin et al., 2019). Nearly 60% of all nursing homes are affiliated with a *chain*, defined as corporations that own or run two or more such facilities (Harris-Kojetin et al., 2019). Research documents that for-profit nursing homes consistently demonstrate lower levels of care quality, including satisfaction with care and clinical outcomes, than nonprofit nursing homes (Harrington et al., 2012; Stevenson & Grabowski, 2008; You et al., 2016). This relationship has also been observed when nonprofit homes convert to for-profit status, frequently showing a subsequent decline in performance (Stevenson & Grabowski, 2008).

One trend in for-profit ownership status is the growth in nursing homes owned by real estate investment trusts (REITs) or private equity firms. Approximately 12% of nursing homes are owned by REITs, and 5% of nursing homes have private equity ownership (Braun et al., 2023). *REITs* are for-profit public or private corporations that invest in income-producing properties; over the past two decades, nursing homes have been an attractive option because of the high value of the real estate and the steady patient/resident volume in the facilities. As of 2021, REITs held investments in 1,806 of the more than 15,000 nursing homes in the US.

Although a small part of the sector right now, private equity firms have generated considerable concern by consumer advocates, and more recently the federal government, due to the lack of transparency about how much profit is generated and where the profits are going. These nursing homes are under great pressure to generate high short-term profits, and recent research suggests that this type of ownership leads to poorer quality due to reduced staffing and services related to the need to generate profits quickly (Harrington et al., 2012). Declines in quality have also been seen when chains are purchased by private equity firms (Stevenson et al., 2013). There is also concern that these firms have little or no experience in the long-term care sector and are more likely to admit the highly lucrative post-acute patients covered by Medicare rather than the long-stay nursing home residents, many of whom are covered by Medicaid—a much less lucrative public payor.

HISTORICAL EFFORTS TO IMPROVE QUALITY OF CARE AND QUALITY OF LIFE IN NURSING HOMES

As a residential setting, nursing homes provide round-the-clock nursing care that is primary delivered by certified nursing assistants (CNAs), although facilities vary widely as to their organization, internal structure, service portfolios, and staffing.

As the name "nursing *home*" implies, these settings are also and perhaps foremost a "home"—the domicile or residence for real people, individuals who need special care or oversight but who nonetheless reside in a setting that becomes their home. A home is personal, highly individuated, variegated, and imbued with historical and present-day meanings and experiences for the person who resides there (Gitlin, 2003; Wahl, 2003). A home provides physical and emotional familiarity that helps to maintain a person's quality of life and ability to effectively function every day. This is particularly the case for individuals with chronic illnesses and frailties (Wahl et al., 2009), who are especially vulnerable to the influence of their living environment, supporting or serving as a barrier to a quality of life (Lawton, 1983; Wahl, 2019).

When people transition from their home (community place of residence) to a nursing home, many of these environmental supports for overall function may not be available to them. For nursing home residents, who typically have cognitive and/or physical frailties, environmental factors such as unfamiliar noises and lack of familiar sources of comfort, security, and accessibility to family and things they value can directly impact everyday moods, behaviors, physical and cognitive functioning, clinical outcomes, and overall quality of life. That is why nursing homes that are homelike in structure and function are increasingly gaining recognition and popularity. This approach entails the complex task of balancing allowance for personalization of rooms, spaces, and daily routines with constraints imposed by legal and regulatory features dictating nursing home practices (see Chapter 10).

The "home" function of nursing homes is increasingly recognized as equally significant as their healthcare and medical functions. Thus, the importance of a nursing home as a "home" should not be underappreciated. Understanding that as a home, the quality of life provided is as essential as medical care is core to nursing care. Nursing home as home requires a holistic understanding of residents, including their preferences, values and goals, and whatever contributes to quality of life. This holistic perspective is foundational to nursing practice in nursing homes, informing practices, interactions, and models of care that reflect respect and dignity afforded individuals residing in their homes and that go beyond the medical or clinical purpose.

A prime successful example of a nursing care facility built on these understandings is the Hogeweyk Dementia Village (https://hogeweyk.dementiavillage.com/), originally constructed in the Netherlands and being replicated in select locations around the world. Dementia villages are designed to enable residents with significant cognitive impairments to safely live in a community-like facility replete with easily accessible stores and coffeehouses where items can be purchased, music venues, gardening and workshop spaces, and daily craft and other activities.

Models of Care That Guide Nursing Home Practice

So, what is a "nursing home"? Is it a medical facility? Is it a home? Is it both? Nursing homes are at once *medical facilities,* highly regulated to reduce risk and attend to medical goals, and a person's *home,* with the goal of preserving quality of life. How these goals are implemented and the balance between them reflect different models of care that guide operations. These two goals can sometimes be in conflict, with the former approach emphasizing pathology and the latter approach reflecting a holistic, wellness, quality-of-life perspective. The model of care, in turn, shapes the scope and type of supports and treatments that are provided and guides the responsibilities and practices of nursing, with consequences for staff and residents alike.

As illustrated in Figure 1.1, conceptually, there are three basic *models of care* that have guided nursing home practices. The prevailing model of care in nursing homes has been the *traditional medical model* (Farre & Rapley, 2017). Due to its medical focus, this model has led to common overprescribing of medications to address a range of clinical symptoms and behaviors and unnecessary hospitalizations of residents to aggressively treat or manage conditions when palliative care is more consistent with resident wishes (Kales et al., in press). For example, let's say a resident develops urinary incontinence. This is a common and disruptive health problem among nursing home residents (Leung & Schnelle, 2008). The medical model perspective suggests the need for a diagnostic assessment including obtaining a medical history and urinalysis and ruling out possible reversible underlying conditions, including medication side effects. Treatments that might be considered are drug therapies and surgery. While this is appropriate in the case where incontinence is the result of an infection, the medical model often overlooks other causes and potential treatments for incontinence.

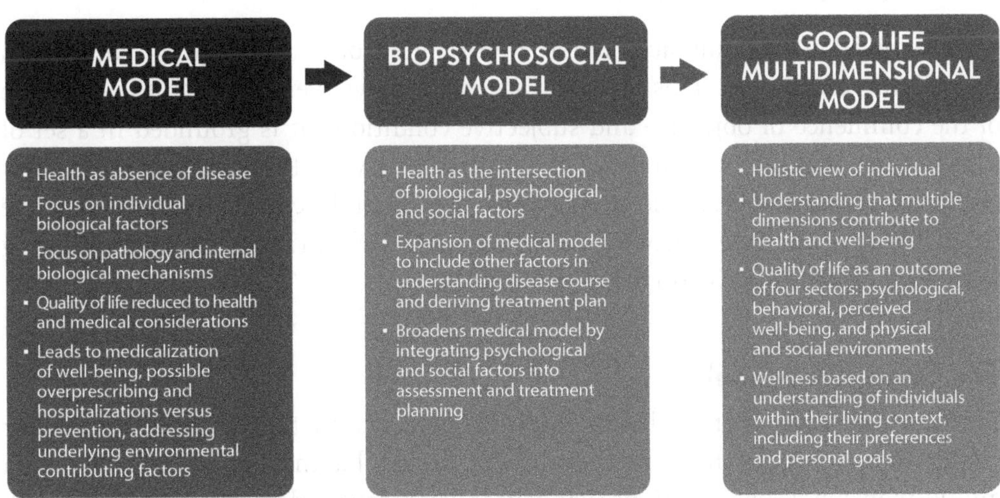

FIGURE 1.1 Models of care and key assumptions.

The medical model has been widely critiqued, even in the field of medicine, for being myopic and ignoring factors other than biology that may influence disease and illness processes. To broaden healthcare (which includes medical practice), starting in the late 1970s and early 1980s an adaptation of the medical model was posited and referred to as the *biopsychosocial model* (Engel, 1977). This model sought to preserve the biological foundation of healthcare medicine but expanded its focus to account for social, psychological, and behavioral factors that may influence symptomatology and illness processes. The biopsychosocial approach is an advancement as it seeks to understand different social and psychological dimensions to inform a treatment plan (Kusnanto et al., 2018). Nevertheless, the approach still defines health narrowly as the absence of disease and centers care around pathophysiology and biological conditions as root causes. However, it can help healthcare providers understand the psychosocial aspects of illness and promote a positive therapeutic relationship.

A shortcoming of this model is the failure to consider environmental conditions that can influence health and quality of life. In the example of the resident with urinary incontinence, this model would similarly have a health provider start with a diagnostic assessment and rule out possible underlying and reversible conditions such as infection. Other treatment considerations would include monitoring fluid intake, introducing a toileting schedule including prompted voiding techniques, and addressing the psychological impact of incontinence on the resident.

A third model of care embraces a more holistic view of understanding clinical and daily living challenges. This *quality-of-life model* views well-being as the outcome of the confluence of objective and subjective conditions. It is grounded in a set of assumptions that differ from other models, starting with the premise that quality of life is possible and desirable at every life stage. First developed and labeled as the "good life" by Dr. M. Powell Lawton in 1983, it has since been adapted for people living with dementia in 2018 (Gitlin & Hodgson, 2018).

The Good Life Model

The *Good Life model* is grounded in empirical evidence that older adults view their quality of life as more than just their health. Rather, having a good life is based on multidimensional considerations that have independent and joint effects. These multidimensional considerations can be grouped into four quadrants or sectors, with each having in turn multiple domains, as illustrated in Figure 1.2:

- The *behavioral competency* quadrant encompasses various health and functional states, including executive function, physical function, physical health, ability to do things one chooses, time use, cognitive status, and behavioral and psychological symptoms.
- The *psychological well-being* sector covers subjective experiences, including positive affect (joy, pleasure, happiness) and negative affect (depressed mood).
- The third sector, *perceived valuation*, refers to an individual's appraisal of their life and its quality, their perceived sense of well-being and purpose, and their sense of control, agency, and connectedness.
- Finally, the fourth quadrant, the *objective environment*, comprises both physical and social characteristics of factors external to an individual, such as the living environment, including its safety, comfort, layout, and availability of social supports (Wahl, 2007).

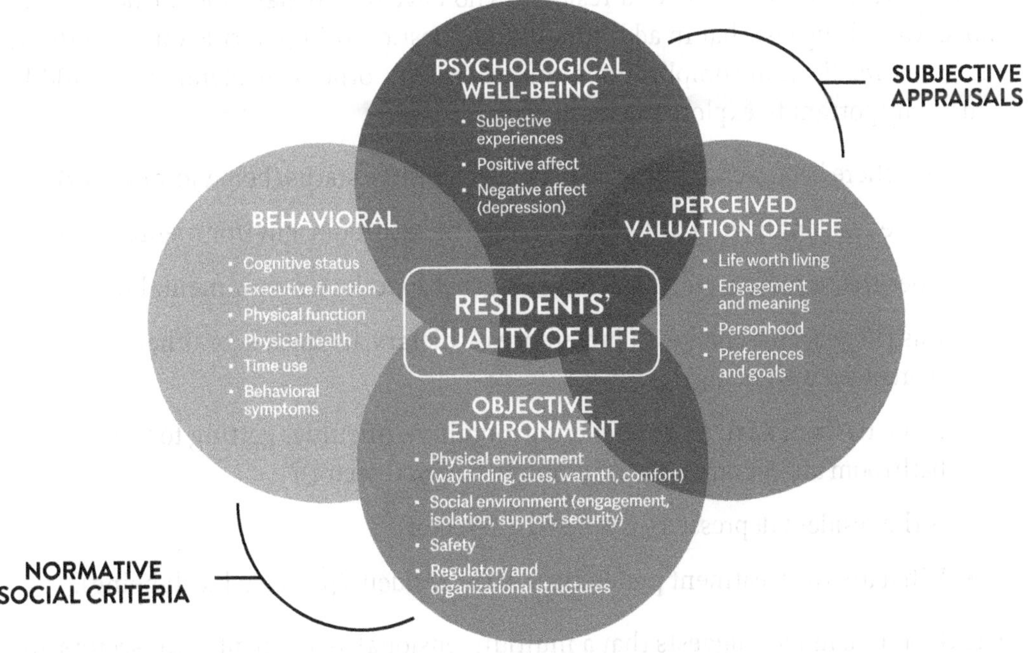

FIGURE 1.2 Good Life model of care. *Adapted from Gitlin and Hodgson (2019)*

Thus, the Good Life model considers individuals in the context of these combined influences of the biological, psychological personal appraisals and objective conditions. These sectors can be further grouped as representing subjective appraisals (perceived valuation of life and psychological well-being) and normative criteria (competencies and the objective environment). Several assumptions of this model are noteworthy:

- A good life is highly individuated and reflects the combination of normative, objective, and psychological elements and personal valuations (what matters to the person).
- To understand quality of life, each sector and their domains need to be assessed and apprehended.
- For any clinical challenge, a treatment plan needs to potentially consider all four quadrants.

Let's return to our example of a resident who develops urinary incontinence. This model would suggest that in addition to a diagnostic workup to rule out underlying infection, medication complications, and pathology, other considerations would be equally important to explore, such as:

- Has there been a change in the person's cognitive status (behavioral sector)?
- Is the resident having difficulty finding the bathroom (environmental sector)?
- Does the resident need visual or verbal cues to toilet (environmental sector)?
- Has there been a change in preferences—dietary, hydration, or other (perceived well-being)?
- Is the resident a fall risk and having mobility difficulties getting to the bathroom and/or on or off the toilet (behavioral sector)?
- Is the resident depressed (psychological sector)?
- What are the treatment preferences of the resident (perceived well-being)?

The Good Life model suggests that a multidimensional assessment of all sectors and their respective domains should guide treatment decision-making.

In summary, models of care are important to consider, as they inform the type of treatments developed for nursing home residents. Consideration of quality-of-life indicators for residents—including examining and understanding the role of normative factors (e.g., the objective environment) and subjective appraisals (e.g., perceived valuation of life)—changes the dynamical treatment processes from a medically dominated worldview to one that considers the person as a whole and encompasses psychological, social, environmental, behavioral, and personal valuations. The culture change movement, described in the next section, operationalizes this general model of care.

CULTURE CHANGE MODELS OF CARE

Nursing home culture change is an international movement committed to improving the quality of life for people living in nursing homes, particularly long-stay residents. It is an example of the Good Life model described above. The aim of nursing home culture change is to ensure general well-being, including a meaningful life for nursing home residents. The culture change movement began in the early 1980s as the result of some important discoveries (Koren, 2010). For example, in 1985 the National Citizens' Coalition for Nursing Home Reform (NCCNHR) published the findings from interviews with nursing home residents (NCCNHR, 1985). Nursing home residents from across the US identified their most common desires as:

- A pleasing, home-like environment
- Choice in daily activities (e.g., bath or shower, waking and sleeping times, etc.)
- Roommate selection
- Ongoing, varied, preferred activities
- Tasty and varied foods to select from
- Well-trained, well-supervised, consistent staff
- Respectful relationships with staff

In 1986, the Institute of Medicine (IOM) published a comprehensive review, *Improving the Quality of Care in Nursing Homes* (IOM, 1986), echoing many of the findings and recommendations in the NCCNHR project. In the early 1990s, practice leaders from nursing homes across the US created the Pioneer Network (Fagan, 2003) to transform nursing home life through promoting self-determination, meaningful engagement in life, individual choice, dignity, respect, and a home-like environment, also known as *person-centered care.* Each of these initiatives also emphasized the importance of resident relationships with staff, particularly direct-care staff (CNAs). This explains the almost universal emphasis of culture change programs on consistently assigning staff to the same residents and their efforts to decrease turnover. *Person-centered care* differs from *patient-centered care* in its focus on the whole person, not just a person's clinical or health needs.

Many nursing homes have implemented at least some culture change practices (ordering from a menu, resident choice of waking and sleeping times, consistent assignment of staff, etc.). However, there are a few comprehensive culture change models that integrate several culture change strategies in a structured and consistent way. Each of these comprehensive models, described in the following sections, also supports and empowers direct-care staff to reduce turnover and preserve the resident/staff relationships that are vital to resident quality of life.

The Neighborhood or Household Model

The household model creates small communities or households of residents and staff within a larger organization (Espinoza, 2018). Members of each household dine together at a communal table within their household. Food is often cooked in the household kitchen, releasing aromas that enhance pleasure and appetite (Chaudhury et al., 2017). The stable staff working with a small group of residents enhances the development of relationships between residents and staff, increases staff familiarity with resident preferences, and promotes resident/resident relationships (Hermer et al., 2017).

The Eden Alternative

The Eden Alternative model focuses on quality of life by eliminating resident boredom, loneliness, and helplessness (Thomas, 2003). Eden shares the values of the culture change movement but is distinguished by its emphasis on resident "care for living things." Eden homes are filled with live plants, host continual visits from animals (Hermer et al., 2017), and often integrate children from the community into home activities.

Wellspring

Wellspring differs from the other culture change models in its focus on clinical outcomes and staff development. The stated goals of the model are to enhance the quality of care and improve the quality of work life for nursing home staff. Resident quality of life is approached through a focus on empowering and retaining highly skilled staff. To achieve this, the Wellspring model has created a collaborative learning network that brings several nursing homes together to address resident care and resident life issues. Direct-care staff are empowered to identify issues and lead initiatives to address them. Nurse practitioners and clinical nurse specialists are shared across nursing homes as teachers, coaches, and consultants to staff on improving resident care. There is a strong focus on team-building among staff and continual learning (Stone et al., 2002).

The Green House Nursing Home

The Green House model is the most comprehensive of culture change models, including a transformation of the physical environment and a staffing structure that alters lines of authority, empowers direct-care staff, and ensures consistent staff assignment (Rabig et al., 2006). Green House nursing homes are comfortable, home-like environments. All residents have private rooms and bathrooms. Residents dine together at a common table, often including staff and family members of residents as well. Caregivers are assigned to each home and do not rotate. Residents and staff confer on recreational activities and daily care (Reinhard, 2022). Residents rise in the morning at their leisure and order the breakfast of their choice. Family members, including children, are generally quite comfortable and feel welcomed in Green House homes (Lum et al., 2008). Most Green House homes have open access to outdoor areas, something often desired but generally unavailable to nursing home residents.

SUMMARY

Nursing homes are struggling to emerge from the stigma and medically dominated focus of the past. Continuing their commitment to provide high-quality clinical care, nursing homes have increasingly been focused on the quality of residents' lives, particularly long-term residents for whom the nursing home has become "home." This is not a quick or easy transformation, and much work needs still to be done. New models have been proposed and tried in an effort to improve the lives of residents. These new person-centered models, described in this chapter, are intended to acknowledge the humanity of nursing home residents, to avoid reducing people to their disabilities and clinical diagnoses, and to acknowledge that for many, there is still the possibility of living a meaningful life. Real transformation will require shifting the education and attitudes of providers, altering organizational structures, significantly modifying state and federal regulations, and realigning funding mechanisms to support more humane models of care. Nurses will play a central role in this transformation.

REFERENCES

Birnstengel, G. (2021, March 5). *How'd we get here? The history of nursing homes.* Next Avenue. https://www.nextavenue.org/history-of-nursing-homes/

Braun, R. T., Williams, D., Stevenson, D. G., Casalino, L. P., Jung, H. Y., Fernandez, R., & Unruh, M. A. (2023, February). The role of real estate investment trusts in staffing US nursing homes. *HealthAffairs, 42*(2), 207–216. https://doi.org/10.1377/hlthaff.2022.00278

Chaudhury, H., Hung, L., Rust, T., & Wu, S. (2017, October). Do physical environmental changes make a difference? Supporting person-centered care at mealtimes in nursing homes. *Dementia, 16*(7), 878–896. https://doi.org/10.1177/1471301215622839

Engel, G. L. (1977, April 8). The need for a new medical model: A challenge for biomedicine. *Science, 196*(4286), 129–136. https://doi.org/10.1126/science.847460

Espinoza, R. (2018). *The household model: Creating a 'home' in nursing homes.* https://www.phinational.org/household-model-creates-real-home-people-living-nursing-homes/

Fagan, R. (2003). Pioneer Network: Changing the culture of aging in America. *Journal of Social Work in Long-Term Care, 2*(1–2), 125–140. doi: 10.1300/J181v02n01_09

Farre, A., & Rapley, T. (2017, Nov. 18). The new old (and old new) medical model: Four decades navigating the biomedical and psychosocial understandings of health and illness. *Healthcare, 5*(4). https://doi.org/10.3390/healthcare5040088

Gillick, M. R. (2017). *Old & sick in America: The journey through the health care system.* University of North Carolina Press.

Gitlin, L. N. (2003, October). Conducting research on home environments: Lessons learned and new directions. *Gerontologist, 43*(5), 628–637. https://doi.org/10.1093/geront/43.5.628

Gitlin, L. N., & Hodgson, N. A. (2018). *Better living with dementia: Implications for individuals, families, communities, and societies.* Elsevier/Academic Press

Haber, C. (1993). And the fear of the poorhouse: Perceptions of old age and impoverishment in early twentieth-century America. *Generations, 17*(2), 46–60.

Harrington, C., Olney, B., Carrillo, H., & Kang, T. (2012, February). Nurse staffing and deficiencies in the largest for-profit nursing home chains and chains owned by private equity companies. *Health Services Research, 47*(1 Pt 1), 106–128. https://doi.org/10.1111/j.1475-6773.2011.01311.x

Harris-Kojetin, L. D., Sengupta, M., Lendon, J. P., Rome, V., Valverde, R., & Caffrey, C. (2019). Long-term care providers and services users in the United States, 2015–2016. *Vital and Health Statistics, 3*(43). https://stacks.cdc.gov/view/cdc/76253

Hermer, L., Bryant, N. S., Pucciarello, M., Mlynarczyk, C., & Zhong, B. (2017). Does comprehensive culture change adoption via the household model enhance nursing home residents' psychosocial well-being? *Innovation in Aging, 1*(2). https://doi.org/10.1093/geroni/igx033

Institute of Medicine. (1986). *Improving the quality of care in nursing homes.* https://www.ncbi.nlm.nih.gov/books/NBK217556/

Kales, H., Maust, D., & Gitlin, L. N. (in press). Addressing dementia-related behavioral symptoms before, during and after the pandemic – Disrupting the behavior-prescribing reflex. *JAMA Psychiatry.*

Katz, M. B. (1984, Winter). Poorhouses and the origins of the public old age home. *Milbank Memorial Fund Quarterly Health and Society, 62*(1), 110–140.

Koren, M. J. (2010, February). Person-centered care for nursing home residents: The culture-change movement. *HealthAffairs, 29*(2), 312–317. https://doi.org/10.1377/hlthaff.2009.0966

Kusnanto, H., Agustian, D., & Hilmanto, D. (2018, May–June). Biopsychosocial model of illnesses in primary care: A hermeneutic literature review. *Journal of Family Medicine and Primary Care, 7*(3), 497–500. https://doi.org/10.4103/jfmpc.jfmpc_145_17

Lawton, M. P. (1983, August). Environment and other determinants of well-being in older people. *Gerontologist, 23*(4), 349–357. https://doi.org/10.1093/geront/23.4.349

Leung, F. W., & Schnelle, J. F. (2008, September). Urinary and fecal incontinence in nursing home residents. *Gastroenterology Clinics of North America, 37*(3), 697–707. https://doi.org/10.1016/j.gtc.2008.06.005

Lum, T. Y., Kane, R. A., Cutler, L. J., & Yu, T. C. (2008, Winter). Effects of Green House nursing homes on residents' families. *Health Care Financial Review, 30*(2), 35–51.

National Academies of Sciences, Engineering, and Medicine. (2022). *The national imperative to improve nursing home quality: Honoring our commitment to residents, families, and staff.* The National Academies Press. https://doi.org/doi:10.17226/26526

National Citizens' Coalition for Nursing Home Reform. (1985). *A consumer perspective on quality care: The residents' point of view.* https://theconsumervoice.org/uploads/files/issues/resident_pers.pdf

Rabig, J., Thomas, W., Kane, R. A., Cutler, L. J., & McAlilly, S. (2006, August). Radical redesign of nursing homes: Applying the Green House concept in Tupelo, Mississippi. *The Gerontologist, 46*(4), 533–539. https://doi.org/10.1093/geront/46.4.533

Reinhard, S. C., Hado, E., Bowers, B., Ryan, S., & DeVries, M. (2022). *Empowered direct care worker: Lessons from the Green House staffing model.* AARP Public Policy Institute. https://doi.org/https://doi.org/10.26419/ppi.00159.001

Schell, E. (1993). The origins of geriatric nursing. The chronically ill elderly in almshouses and nursing homes, 1900–1950. *Nursing History Review, 1*, 203–216.

Stevenson, D. G., Bramson, J. S., & Grabowski, D. C. (2013). Nursing home ownership trends and their impacts on quality of care: A study using detailed ownership data from Texas. *Journal of Aging & Social Policy, 25*(1), 30–47. https://doi.org/10.1080/08959420.2012.705702

Stevenson, D. G., & Grabowski, D. C. (2008, September–October). Private equity investment and nursing home care: Is it a big deal? *HealthAffairs, 27*(5), 1399–1408. https://doi.org/10.1377/hlthaff.27.5.1399

Stone, R. I., Reinhard, S. C., Bowers, B., Zimmerman, D., Phillips, C. D., Hawes, C., Fielding, J. A., & Jacobson, N. (2002). *Evaluation of the Wellspring model for improving nursing home quality* (Vol. 550). Commonwealth Fund New York.

Thomas, W. H. (2003). Evolution of Eden. *Journal of Social Work in Long-Term Care, 2*(1–2), 141–157. https://doi.org/10.1300/J181v02n01_10

Vladeck, B. C. (1980). *Unloving care: The nursing home tragedy*. Perseus Books Group.

Wagner, D. (2005). *The poorhouse: America's forgotten institution*. Rowman-Littlefield Publishers.

Wahl, H. W. (2003). Future developments in living environments for older people in the U.S. and Germany: Potential and constraints. In K. W. Schaie, H. W. Wahl, H. Mollenkopf, & F. Oswald (Eds.), *Aging independently: Living arrangements and mobility* (pp. 281–301). Springer Publications.

Wahl, H. W. (2007). Environmental gerontology. In J. E. Birren (Ed.), *Encyclopedia of gerontology* (2nd ed.). Elsevier.

Wahl, H. W. (2019). Linking the socio-physical environment to successful aging: From basic research to intervention to implementation science considerations. In R. Fernandez-Ballesteros, A. Benetos, & J. Robine (Eds.), *The Cambridge handbook of successful aging*. Cambridge Press.

Wahl, H. W., Fange, A., Oswald, F., Gitlin, L. N., & Iwarsson, S. (2009, June). The home environment and disability-related outcomes in aging individuals: What is the empirical evidence? *The Gerontologist, 49*(3), 355–367. https://doi.org/10.1093/geront/gnp056

Watson, S. D. (2010). From almshouses to nursing homes and community care: Lessons from Medicaid's history. *Georgia State University Law Review, 26*(3), 937–969.

You, K., Li, Y., Intrator, O., Stevenson, D. G., Hirth, R., Grabowski, D. C., & Banasszak-Holl, J. (2016). Do nursing home chain size and proprietary status affect experiences with care? *Medical Care, 54*(3), 229–234.

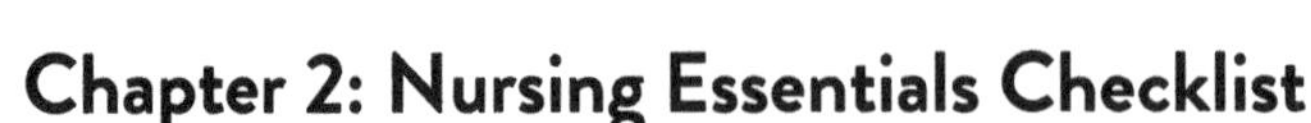

Chapter 2: Nursing Essentials Checklist

SPHERES OF CARE

Nursing occurs within four spheres of care, ranging from prevention to supportive care and all the areas in between. This chapter is relevant to the following spheres of care:

- ☑ Disease Prevention/Health Promotion
- ☑ Chronic Disease Care
- ☑ Regenerative or Restorative Care
- ☑ Hospice/Palliative/Supportive Care

DOMAINS OF PRACTICE

The American Association of Colleges of Nursing has identified 10 broad domains of practice for nursing. Students are expected to master these domains of practice across the spheres of care. This chapter addresses:

- ☑ Knowledge for Nursing Practice (Nursing and Other Disciplines)
- ☑ Person-Centered Care
- ☑ Population Health
- ☐ Scholarship for Practice
- ☑ Quality and Safety
- ☑ Interprofessional Partnerships
- ☑ Systems-Based Care
- ☑ Information & Healthcare Technologies
- ☑ Professionalism
- ☑ Personal, Professional, Leadership Development

CONCEPTS FOR PRACTICE

Integrated across the domains of practice are eight concepts which the student is expected to master across the spheres of care and across the domains of practice. This chapter addresses:

- ☐ Clinical Judgment
- ☑ Communication
- ☐ Compassionate Care
- ☑ Diversity, Equity, Inclusion
- ☐ Ethics
- ☑ Evidence-Based Practice
- ☐ Health Policy
- ☑ Social Determinants of Health

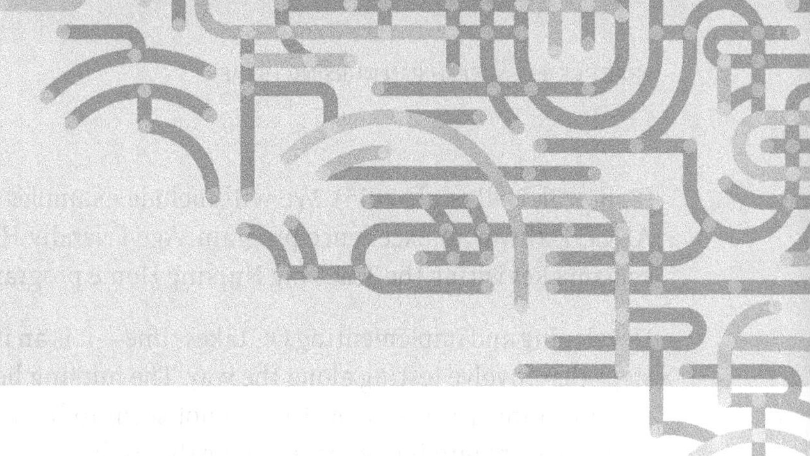

CHAPTER 2

CREATING A CULTURE OF CARE

Alice Bonner, PhD, RN, FAAN
Donna Fick, PhD, GCNS-BC, FAAN
Christine Pabico, PhD, RN, NE-BC, FAAN

OBJECTIVES

1. Define organizational culture.
2. Describe initiatives (Age-Friendly Health Systems, Revisiting the Teaching Nursing Home, Pathways to Excellence) that promote an organizational culture of care.
3. Understand how a culture of care affects the delivery of quality care, resident quality of life, and quality of the work environment.

INTRODUCTION

Organizational culture (OC) is a term that is often used to describe how an organization does things/gets work done. OC is about how leaders and everyone in the organization manage and support teams and workers through daily activities and also how they manage through change. Despite those elements being part of many OC definitions or descriptions, there is little consensus around what OC actually is in nursing homes (Doll et al., 2017).

This chapter discusses principles of OC, including related topics such as culture change and person-centered or resident-directed care. Our goal is for readers to think about how to describe OC and how OC can positively (or negatively) influence care practices, nursing home resident quality of life, staff joy in work, and intent to stay

(Banaszak-Holl et al., 2015). We will include examples that address OC, such as the ANCC Pathway to Excellence program, Age-Friendly Health Systems, and the Pennsylvania Revisiting the Teaching Nursing Home program.

Developing and implementing OC takes time—it is an iterative process, with interim steps that involve testing along the way. The nursing home team needs to be flexible in rethinking aspects of OC that do not seem to be working, particularly based on feedback from nursing home residents themselves.

DESCRIPTIONS OF ORGANIZATIONAL CULTURE

A fundamental principle of OC is that there are multiple ways to create and develop a positive and productive OC over time. Healthy OC involves brainstorming and coordinating with nursing home residents and with all staff members (all roles, not just senior leaders). Many nursing homes have a multicultural staff, so taking those different cultural beliefs into consideration is important (Debesay et al., 2022). The process often includes external partners (e.g., family members or care partners, advocates, quality advisors, and others) as well. Below are some elements of OC descriptions outlined by Michael D. Watkins in a 2013 issue of the *Harvard Business Review* (Watkins, 2013):

- Culture can be powerfully shaped by either positive or negative incentives, which may include financial rewards, recognition and advancement, or sanctions.
- Culture is consistent, observable patterns of behavior in organizations. Ideally, the organization (in this case, the nursing home) is designed so that the easier/easiest practice approach is the safest/best approach to achieve desired outcomes and meet residents' needs.
- It may also be a process of "sense-making," finding jointly held beliefs and ways to align purpose and shared actions.
- Cultures are multiple, overlapping, and dynamic. OC is shaped by and can overlap with other cultures, such as the broader societal culture in which the nursing home operates.

JUST CULTURE VS. PUNITIVE CULTURE

The concept of *Just Culture* is described by the Brigham and Women's Hospital (BWH) administration in Boston, Massachusetts, as: "A system of shared accountability in which organizations are accountable for the systems they have designed and for responding to the behaviors of their employees in a fair and just manner" (BWH, n.d., para. 1). Staff at BWH do not always feel comfortable speaking up when they see something that threatens patient safety and/or they feel blamed when errors occur.

The system's goal in implementing Just Culture is to create a strong culture of safety where staff are managed fairly when involved in an error, mistake, or adverse event. Just Culture involves looking for risk, not fault. The goal is to increase staff's comfort level in reporting and being open about errors. Another definition of *Just Culture* is "a learning culture that is constantly improving and oriented toward patient safety" (Boysen, 2013, p. 2). Common themes include avoiding blame, promoting comfort with identifying potential risks, continuous learning, and collaboration.

In contrast, a *punitive culture* is one in which individuals or teams are blamed when an error occurs (finding fault), and negative consequences are imposed. In this type of culture, those in authority (staff structure is often hierarchical) believe that the process will reduce the chance of that type of error in the future. There are often impediments to effective interprofessional communication around care processes (Xue et al., 2022).

Survey agencies are often perceived as having a punitive culture, meaning that when surveyors inspect nursing homes, they are looking for noncompliance with federal or state regulations that might require enforcement (e.g., a plan of correction, payment of fines, or a ban on new admissions). Researchers and clinicians familiar with nursing home models have advocated for more of a Just Culture within the survey system so that, in addition to nursing homes with infractions or compliance issues being identified, those that demonstrate positive quality outcomes and improvement are highlighted and positively recognized as well.

Nursing home teams should strive for an OC that recognizes best or better practices in Age-Friendly care and encourages transparency around reporting *near misses* (potential errors) and/or actual failures of care. The team must continuously review its own policies and practices and must ensure that the voices of nursing home residents and direct-care staff are always heard and that their recommendations and ideas are integrated into Age-Friendly care practices and daily routines as much as possible. In the next section we describe what an Age-Friendly Health System is and how it contributes to a positive OC.

Tips to Remember

- Describe or define OC. Talk about OC with new hires and make it a part of annual training with existing staff.
- Post a definition or description of OC on a whiteboard or bulletin board and place markers/pens nearby to encourage people to write their own comments.
- Be flexible and review OC at least annually—make updates or changes based on feedback, particularly from nursing home residents.
- Discuss recent OC examples that demonstrate a meaningful impact on resident outcomes and staff workflow/joy in work.

HOW NURSING HOMES BECOME AGE-FRIENDLY HEALTH SYSTEMS

The US older adult population is growing rapidly and has increasingly complex healthcare needs (Emery-Tiburcio et al., 2021). In 2016, the John A. Hartford Foundation began collaborating with the Institute for Healthcare Improvement (IHI), the American Hospital Association, the Catholic Health Association, and other healthcare organizations and government agencies to design, develop, implement, and test Age-Friendly Health Systems (AFHS; Fulmer et al., 2018). The bold vision is that together, we will build a social movement so that all care with older adults is Age-Friendly care.

The definition of *Age-Friendly care* is that it:

- Follows an essential set of evidence-based practices
- Causes no harm
- Aligns with What Matters to the older adults and their care partners

To be recognized as an AFHS, healthcare settings such as nursing homes must reliably provide a set of four evidence-based elements of high-quality care known as the *4Ms—What Matters, Medication, Mentation, Mobility*—to all eligible older adults with each encounter (see Figure 2.1).

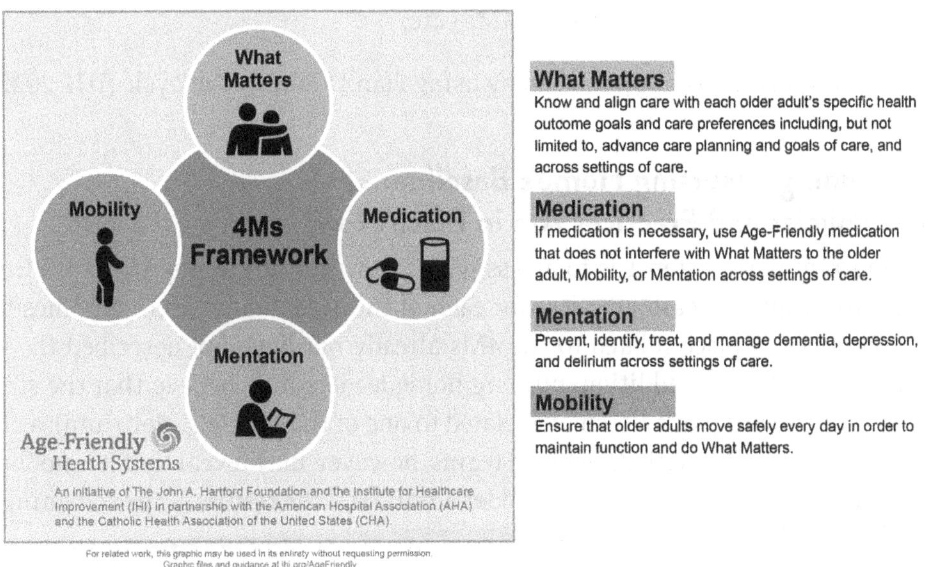

FIGURE 2.1 The 4 Ms framework of an Age-Friendly Health System.

Key Drivers and Steps to Implementing the 4Ms

There are two key drivers of Age-Friendly care:

- Assess: knowing about the 4Ms for each older adult
- Act on: incorporating the 4Ms into care delivery and care plan documentation

Both must be addressed by all relevant disciplines, and the information must be made accessible to each person on the healthcare team.

There are five basic steps to implementing the 4Ms in nursing home practice:

1. Assemble and prepare the team; begin to outline an approach.
2. Review, discuss, and understand current 4Ms goals, practices, and workflows on the unit; design or adapt workflows.

3. Provide care consistent with the 4Ms; sequence the process starting with one resident and one 'M,' then test the remaining three 'Ms.'
4. Integrate the 4Ms as a set for each resident and for the unit as a whole; study and measure performance.
5. Next steps: improve and sustain 4Ms care.

The five steps can also be approached by using Plan-Do-Study-Act cycle (IHI, 2022).

Determining a Nursing Home's Baseline: What Policies and Practices Are in Place Now?

An important part of step 1 is to assess what your unit or nursing home is already doing with respect to care practices for each of the 4Ms. Many nursing homes have some practices in place related to the 4Ms already but have not described the 4Ms as an integrated set. In addition, nursing home leaders may believe that the staff is conducting screening or assessment related to one of the 4Ms (e.g., delirium); a chart review and discussion with direct-care teams, however, may reveal that it is not being done consistently or reliably with all older adults, and the results of the screening are not being acted on.

Leadership and Teamwork

The Age-Friendly approach presents an opportunity for each nursing home to develop a positive OC and to demonstrate leadership and teamwork, valuing each person on the team and identifying champions to lead small groups in promoting Age-Friendly care. Senior leaders, managers, and direct-care teams will strengthen existing and/or future quality improvement efforts and work to prevent adverse events, enhance resident outcomes, and enhance quality of life for everyone.

Co-Designing Tools and Resources With Nursing Home Partners

Many in the management of nursing homes believe that because they serve primarily older adults, they are automatically an AFHS. Prototyping work done by IHI with nursing homes in 2021 and 2022 indicates that by carefully reviewing specific cases and scenarios, consistent and reliable implementation of the 4Ms as a set with each older adult is often not being done or documented at baseline (Bonner & Portale, 2022).

This is an opportunity to focus more reliably and consistently on key components of care that drive positive clinical and workforce outcomes, integrating each of the 4Ms and the 4Ms *as a set* in nursing home practice (IHI, 2023).

There are free tools and resources for nursing homes that wish to pursue becoming recognized as an AFHS as one way to promote a positive OC. For example, the IHI website has a publication called *Age-Friendly Health Systems: Guide to Care of Older Adults in Nursing Homes* and a companion workbook, *A Workbook for Nursing Home Teams* (IHI, 2022). Those resources are designed to be used together, as the guide has more content for leaders and senior staff members, whereas the workbook is designed for direct-care staff (nurses, CNAs, social workers, etc.) to use in their daily work with residents.

The workbook includes printable worksheets to guide teams through each step of the process for each of the 4Ms, as well as examples of evidence-based tools and processes that nursing homes may consider and test. It also includes a case study to demonstrate how a nursing home team completed the worksheet related to 4Ms implementation on one resident and the outcomes for that resident. Finally, it includes ways to measure how well Age-Friendly care is being implemented and evaluated.

CREATING AN AGE-FRIENDLY ECOSYSTEM

Nursing homes have traditionally been seen as separate from the rest of the healthcare and community-based care systems. However, that should not be our approach. People who reside in nursing homes for some period of time often return to their own homes or other less clinical residential settings such as assisted living or group homes. They may also have chronic health conditions that require frequent re-hospitalizations. In short, older adults often cycle through healthcare and community systems, leading to increased risks during multiple care transitions and across ecosystems unless we get away from practicing in silos (Britton et al., 2017; Dash et al., 2022).

A priority of the AFHS movement is to implement Age-Friendly care across settings, so that providers, professionals, older adults, family members/care partners, and policymakers are all speaking a common language with shared understanding of each older adult's goals, preferences, and priorities. This system needs to be sustainable and flexible enough to meet the needs of nursing home residents and staff members that may change over time. We need to create that Age-Friendly ecosystem to truly deliver Age-Friendly care in every encounter with every older person. Age-Friendly care is comprehensive and can form the foundation for a positive OC in a nursing home.

Establishing a Baseline

As previously stated, an important initial step in implementing Age-Friendly care is establishing a baseline—i.e., determining what the nursing home is currently doing to assess and act on the 4Ms and support the team integrating the 4Ms into their workflow. Many (or most) nursing homes may already focus on Mobility, Mentation, and Medication use but they may not be assessing and acting on them as a set and integrating them into plans of care. For instance, they may be surveying residents about their preferences for care or may be reviewing Medications, but they often lack a framework to bring this together and to use What Matters and preferences for care when thinking about and acting on Mobility, Mentation, and Medication use. The AFHS framework provides a reliable and equitable way to assure that the 4Ms are assessed in every older adult and acted upon for the resident in a way that improves the lives of older adults (Fulmer et al., 2022).

Focusing on Mentation

Diving more deeply into Mentation is a way to see how the 4Ms work together in a complementary and synergistic way. Mentation includes dementia, delirium, and depression. In the nursing home setting, Mentation is often assessed using the Minimum Data Set (MDS). Dementia and depression should be screened for on admission and should also be assessed annually and anytime there is a change such as a hospitalization, change in function, or acute illness.

Many residents in nursing homes have some degree of cognitive impairment. Even if a resident has an existing diagnosis of dementia, they should continue to be assessed annually and with any change. A staging tool for dementia should also be considered so that care, interventions, and caregiver support (both formal and informal) can be aligned with their stage of dementia. Assessment should always be paired with acting on Mentation to prevent or minimize adverse events and complications such as falls or a decrease in Mobility.

Assessing and Acting on a Change in Condition: Consider Delirium

In the nursing home setting, a change in condition may include a resident who has a change in function or who is suddenly sleeping more, eating less, or engaging less with others; this person could be developing delirium or delirium superimposed on dementia (DSD). Acting on the assessment should always entail looking for the underlying cause of the delirium; preventing complications of delirium such as falls, aspiration, or skin breakdown; understanding, maintaining, and restoring function; and managing expressions of behavior (Fick & Shrestha, 2022; Gitlin et al., 2010).

Delirium assessment is part of the MDS but should also be assessed when a resident has a change in function or acute change in Mentation is suspected. Delirium in the AFHS framework is assessed more frequently in the skilled or post-acute setting than in long-term care (LTC). DSD is the most common type of delirium in the nursing home setting and occurs in as many as 70% of nursing home residents (Komici et al., 2022).

When choosing tools for assessing DSD in the nursing home, consider tools that fit into the staff's workload and that have been tested in persons with dementia such as the DSD-4, the FAM-CAM, and the UB-CAM (Fick & Shrestha, 2022; Morandi et al., 2021). The American Delirium Society has delirium screening and prevention tips on its website. The UB-CAM delirium tool uses a two-step detection process, and the first step involves asking two questions called the *UB-2* that a nursing assistant can do:

1. "Please tell me the day of the week."
2. "Please tell me the months of the year backward, starting with December as your first month."

An incorrect answer on either question is a positive screen for delirium, and the nurse leader or other clinician should complete the rest of the questions on the UB-CAM. If they get both correct (meaning they do not screen positive for delirium), staff should document it as a vital sign and in their plan of care to show the resident's baseline. The nurse leader and staff should continue to implement delirium prevention such as daily activity and hydration (Fick et al., 2018; Fick & Shrestha, 2022; Marcantonio et al., 2022).

To our knowledge, this is the only delirium screen that has been tested on a large scale with nursing assistants completing the UB-2 step of the protocol. A free app for the UB-CAM is available for Apple and Android through their app stores; search for UB-CAM to find it.

Another tool that is very useful in the nursing home setting to pick up a worsening of function which may help in triggering the need for a delirium screen is the Stop and Watch tool. This early warning tool can be used by staff along with the UB-2. This tool watches for and reports changes such as communicating less, needing more help overall, no bowel movements in three days, eating or drinking less, increased sleepiness, and changes in Mobility. These can be signs of delirium in nursing home residents (Lapp et al., 2022).

Prevention of delirium in the nursing home setting includes evidence-based approaches targeting well-known delirium risk factors such as cognitive impairment, sleep deprivation, immobility, vision impairment, hearing impairment, and dehydration (Inouye et al., 2007). Studies have also shown that infection and fecal impaction are factors associated with delirium in the nursing home, and many cases are multi-causal (Komici et al., 2022).

Behaviors related to dementia should be acted on with recreational therapy activities, best practices for communication and touch, and best practice such as the Describe, Investigate, Create, and Evaluate or DICE approach that was developed by Helen Kales and colleagues (Gitlin et al., 2012). This approach involves working with staff to *describe* the behavior, *investigate* the causes (pain, delirium, fear, etc.), *create* interventions, and then *evaluate* if they are working to create a positive team culture.

THE 4MS AS A SET

To become recognized as an AFHS, the 4Ms must all be provided to each older adult *as a set*, and the relationships between all 4Ms should be considered. Implementation of the 4Ms and Age-Friendly care also requires systems and societal changes. This is addressed in the National Academies of Sciences, Engineering, and Medicine (NASEM, 2022) report on the quality of care in nursing homes.

As outlined in the previous section, *Mentation* in the nursing home setting may impact and be impacted by each of the other three Ms. For example, *What Matters* in a resident with dementia is about knowing the resident and including what makes them feel calm and communicating that with other staff, including agency staff (Rosgen, 2018).

Knowing older adults improves the detection of delirium and the management of behaviors in persons with dementia. We must provide the leadership and toolkits at the bedside to make it easier for nurses to understand and intervene *in the moment* for behavior and provide adequate staffing, infrastructure, and best practices for communication to address delirium causes, prevention, discharge teaching, and recovery (Fick, 2022; Fick & Shrestha, 2022)

Avoiding high-risk *Medications*, especially antipsychotics and anticholinergics, optimizes delirium prevention and management. Inappropriate Medication use has been shown to lead to harm in older adults, and there are evidence-based tools and lists of Medications to avoid in older adults that are updated regularly (American Geriatrics Society, 2019). Being willing to deprescribe across all settings of care is critical to quality of life and Age-Friendly care. Studies have shown that the failure to discontinue high-risk or inappropriate Medications is associated with increased all-cause mortality and harm (Coupland et al., 2019; Fick, 2020).

Mobility or movement has both an immediate and long-term benefit to Mentation and is a core intervention in the care of delirium, dementia, and depression. Daily movement in the nursing home and making daily Mobility goals with residents is more effective than thinking you're going to do it two or three times a week or in an activity. Mobility in the nursing home is everyone's responsibility—for example, helping residents walk to the dining room and encouraging movements in everyday activities of daily living. Some nursing home residents may mobilize using a wheelchair—they do not need to walk or run to be mobile. Those residents may do sit to stand exercises, leg exercises, simple chair stretches, arm exercises with small weights (2 lbs.), cardio drumming while sitting in a chair (*drumming* is using short pool noodles on an exercise ball that sits in a bucket), and other musical stretches and activities while sitting in the wheelchair. Integrating daily Mobility into each resident's day is vital. This daily movement will have an immediate impact on mood, Mentation, and behaviors that indicate distress (Basso & Suzuki, 2017; Fick, 2022).

TEACHING NURSING HOMES

Another program that addresses nursing home care of older adults and has the potential to promote a positive OC (a culture of care) is Teaching Nursing Homes (TNH). The TNH program began in the 1980s and sought to understand if a practice/academic partnership and geriatric nursing leadership could improve nursing home care (Huey, 1985). In addition to the wider Age-Friendly care movement, the Revisiting the Teaching Nursing Home project is also infusing Age-Friendly care and the 4Ms into the nursing home (Jewish Healthcare Foundation, 2021).

The relationships and partnerships between colleges of nursing and nursing homes are key to the Teaching Nursing Home program and to keeping the model sustainable beyond project funding. The Teaching Nursing Home project aims to be a true partnership between academic units and nursing homes with an "all teach all learn" model that brings geriatric education to nursing home staff and graduate and undergraduate nurses. Like the original program in the 1980s, it focuses on "What can nursing homes teach us?" (Huey, 1985). Part of that process involves connecting academic leadership principles with interprofessional team implementation in real-world settings such as nursing homes.

Working Together to Integrate the 4Ms and Improve Organizational Culture

One of the goals of the 4Ms is to have future nursing home leaders that are skilled in clinical care of older adults and also know, respect, and understand nursing home residents and culture. The Geriatric Workforce Enhancement Program, funded by the Health Resources and Services Administration and IHI, have educational modules, videos, and Age-Friendly care worksheets specific to Age-Friendly care in the nursing home setting for nursing assistants and all staff (Pennsylvania State University Ross and Carol Nese College of Nursing, n.d.). The RN leader in the nursing home can use materials like these to lead staff in rounds to improve care.

A Case Example

Many nursing homes struggle with severe workforce and "care force" shortages. They are also struggling with a shortage of individuals in the nursing home with leadership and geriatric certification, education, and training (Siegel et al., 2023). An example of this is from a nursing home that reached out saying they needed help with combative residents. The staff member who reached out expressed that he loved working with older adults but did not have a background in geriatrics. He was put into a leadership and education position with one year's experience as a registered nurse and no specialized training in geriatrics or LTC.

The nursing home was also facing high agency staff use and a shortage of nursing and recreational therapy staff. The nurses and nursing assistants were suddenly having a surge of challenging behaviors in their residents and were not trained or equipped in the moment to manage behavior in persons with dementia with best practices. This nursing home was a wonderful place and wanted to provide the best care, but it lacked a system to make it successful.

Through their work with academic nursing programs, the nursing home management strengthened the pipeline for recruiting nurses and also promoted positive relationships with managers to improve retention. They engaged with academic partners with expertise in the area of behavior management and empowered the frontline staff. The nurse leader in this situation can work with staff to address the language used to describe behavior, increase staff knowledge of the meaning of behavior, work to better understand what problems staff are encountering with behavior, and help them anticipate how they can prevent distressing behaviors with non-drug approaches.

A key implementation and quality improvement strategy is to engage frontline staff to problem-solve together, allowing them to help the educator or RN leader present the content so that they have real ownership in the problem and pride in the solutions. They may utilize tools such as DICE, defined earlier in this chapter (Gitlin et al., 2012).

POSITIVE PRACTICE ENVIRONMENTS AND SHARED GOVERNANCE

Nurses provide care and coordination in nursing homes, while certified nursing assistants (CNAs) provide vital support for delivering direct resident care. Extensive evidence demonstrates the correlation between nursing staff's (nurses and CNAs) ability to provide safe and effective care and a strong OC in the environment in which they practice (Dans & Lundmark, 2019). In addition, supportive practice environments that engage and inspire staff have a direct, positive impact on several outcomes including job satisfaction, employee retention, resident experience, care quality, and safety. For this reason, it is essential to create positive practice environments where nursing staff feel supported, valued, and empowered to optimize the role of RNs, CNAs, and other professionals.

To create a positive practice environment, a core set of organizational traits that support professional nursing practice must be present and enculturated. The American Nurses Credentialing Center's (ANCC) Pathway to Excellence Framework for Positive Practice Environments (Pathway Framework), an evidence-based blueprint that has been used across a variety of healthcare settings including acute care and LTC, identifies six standards to be essential (see Figure 2.2).

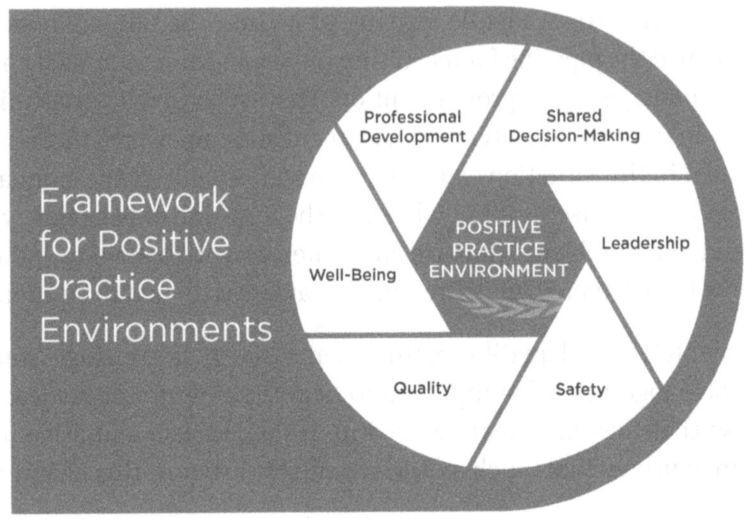

FIGURE 2.2 ANCC Pathway to Excellence Framework for Positive Practice Environments (ANCC, n.d.).

Pathway-LTC, launched in 2010, recognizes LTC organizations that substantiate the presence of essential elements necessary for creating and sustaining positive practice environments (ANCC, n.d.). What originally started as 12 standards has been streamlined to the six, highlighted in Figure 2.2. Pathway-LTC's mission underscores the program's position that every nurse and CNA deserves to work in an environment that gives them a voice, values their contribution, and safeguards their well-being. Living the six evidence-based standards that comprise the Pathway Framework leads to resident-centric, collaborative, safe, and healthy workplaces.

As team members receive support to further enhance their knowledge and skills, participate in shared governance councils, and care for their physical and mental health, they feel valued and become more loyal to the organization. Studies show that creating positive practice environments also has financial implications for organizations in the form of reduced turnover and improved quality and safety (Cadmus & Mastrocola, 2021; Cronshaw et al., 2021; Gensimore et al., 2020).

Standard 1: Shared Decision-Making

The cornerstone of the framework is shared decision-making. Giving the direct-care nursing staff a voice increases their engagement and makes them feel valued. Hardwiring this culture requires organizational structures and a professional practice model that supports shared governance. *Shared governance*, originally introduced in the 1970s, has become a widely used evidence-based structural model in acute-care settings to enable nurses to take an active participatory role in decisions that impact their practice, giving them a higher level of professional autonomy. Despite its well-documented benefits (improvement in nurse and resident or patient outcomes), shared governance is still rarely seen in nursing homes (ANCC, n.d.).

The critical concept of shared governance is *shared decision-making* between the direct-care staff and leaders. By fostering ownership and accountability, shared decision-making empowers frontline staff and positions them as their leaders' partners. When nursing staff feel heard and have input in decisions that impact their practice, their job satisfaction increases, they become more engaged, they fully own their work, and they feel fulfilled. Creating such an environment enables the nursing staff to function at their best and contributes to the organization's success.

Standard 2: Leadership

It is equally important to have leadership both at the organization (director of nursing, or DON) and unit (nurse managers, or NMs) levels that supports shared decision-making and the other essential elements of a positive practice environment. Successful transformation of an OC requires alignment of vision, mission, and goals throughout the organization and leaders to inspire this alignment. The NMs play an essential role in bringing the DON's vision to where the frontline staff are. They help the frontline staff recognize that what they do at the bedside influences the resident experience, outcomes, and the organization's success. NMs also play a critical role in creating the local culture since they are responsible for the 24-hour operation of the unit. They have firsthand knowledge of the issues faced by the team, and, more important, they have the best opportunity to remove barriers and address things that frustrate nurses.

Considering the essential role NMs play in supporting their teams, it is equally critical for them to be supported. This standard ensures that the organization provides role-specific orientation and ongoing leadership development opportunities for NMs to set them up for success. In addition, because of the long-standing challenges with leadership turnover, a plan must be in place for retaining the DON and NMs. Finally, this standard requires organizations to conduct succession planning and to have a strategy in place for planned or unplanned leadership turnover.

Standard 3: Safety

This standard prioritizes both residents and nursing staff safety. It is important for the organization to have policies and processes that protect their safety and well-being. In addition, nursing staff are engaged as active participants in improving safety. They participate in reviewing safety events and have a voice in identifying potential solutions or necessary changes to existing policies and procedures. Nursing staff also have input on daily staffing decisions and feel safe to communicate concerns about staffing plans. Most important, this standard highlights the significance of creating a respectful workplace culture free of incivility, bullying, and violence, which includes protection from verbal and physical abuse from residents and families. A Just Culture is fostered so that employees feel safe reporting concerns.

Standard 4: Quality

Quality is central to an organization's mission, vision, goals, and values. A culture of continuous quality improvement in the delivery of person-centered care and efforts to improve population health is promoted. Policies and processes are (1) developed or revised with the interprofessional team's input, (2) focused on improving resident outcomes, and (3) based on evidence and external benchmarks.

Standard 5: Well-Being

It is important to safeguard the well-being of clinicians because studies have shown that there is a direct correlation between clinician well-being and resident safety and outcomes (Elliott & Fry, 2021; Jun et al., 2021). NASEM also recognizes the practice environment to be fundamental in ensuring clinician well-being and patient/resident safety (Fahrenkopf et al., 2008; Grant & Pabico, 2022; National Academy of Medicine, 2022).

This standard requires leaders to assess workforce well-being proactively and periodically. They are expected to integrate employee well-being and resilience into strategic planning to ensure that it is at the forefront and always remains a priority. Having the nursing staff actively participate in the selection, planning, and evaluation of those well-being initiatives ensures that they will be meaningful and highly utilized.

Organizations must also have support processes in place to foster staff resilience and psychological safety and mitigate physical, psychological, and compassion fatigue. In addition to clinician burnout, compassion fatigue results in feelings of hopelessness, emptiness, lack of motivation, disengagement, disconnectedness, and eventually decreased sense of fulfillment. This standard requires organizations to have support processes that equip healthcare providers to recognize and effectively manage compassion fatigue and burnout.

Finally, leaders hardwire a culture of recognition. Meaningful recognition contributes to reduced stress and positive relationships and increases employees' sense of meaning in their work. It is an effective way to emotionally recharge nurses and support their well-being.

Standard 6: Professional Development

Professional development ensures that nurses and CNAs are competent to provide care and provides them with mentoring, support, and opportunities for lifelong learning. Developing competent staff begins with an individualized orientation that addresses specific learning needs to ensure a smooth transition to practice. To further meet the team's self-identified needs, staff must have input into the selection of nonmandatory educational offerings. A culture of lifelong learning is embraced; thus, opportunities for continued professional development such as conference attendance, participation in professional organizations, pursuit of certifications, or support for higher formal education are offered.

SUMMARY

It is up to us. In the nursing home (and other settings), it's not as simple as just educating staff, giving residents a worksheet, or putting it into the care plan. We must address underlying issues to provide nursing home teams with the staffing, tools, leadership, and training needed; to be able to understand expressions of behavior in persons with dementia; and to understand behavior as an unmet need or possible delirium.

Developing, promoting, and sustaining an organizational culture of care is vital to nursing home resident quality of life and quality of work life for direct-care workers and other nursing home staff. Education alone is not enough. While teaching about Age-Friendly care, we must also advocate for societal, system, financial, and policy changes and be active in helping implement the recommendations of the NASEM nursing quality report. This is our responsibility as a society. We can and must do better for older people and ourselves.

REFERENCES

American Geriatrics Society. (2019). 2019 updated AGS Beers Criteria® for potentially inappropriate medication use in older adults. *Journal of the American Geriatrics Society, 67*(4), 674–694. https://doi.org/10.1111/jgs.15767

American Nurses Credentialing Center. (n.d.). *About Pathway.* https://www.nursingworld.org/organizational-programs/pathway/overview/

Banaszak-Holl, J., Castle, N. G., Lin, M. K., Shrivastwa, N., & Spreitzer, G. (2015, June). The role of organizational culture in retaining nursing workforce. *The Gerontologist, 55*(3), 462–471. https://doi.org/10.1093/geront/gnt129

Basso, J. C., & Suzuki, W. A. (2017, March 28). The effects of acute exercise on mood, cognition, neurophysiology, and neurochemical pathways: A review. *Brain Plasticity, 2*(2), 127–152. https://doi.org/10.3233/BPL-160040

Bonner, A., & Portale, J. (2022, Dec. 6). *Promoting Age-Friendly care in nursing homes: Prototypes and implementation with nursing home teams.* IHI Forum, Orlando, Florida.

Boysen 2nd, P. G. (2013, Fall). Just Culture: A foundation for balanced accountability and patient safety. *Ochsner Journal, 13*(3), 400–406. https://www.ncbi.nlm.nih.gov/pubmed/24052772

Brigham and Women's Hospital. (n.d.). *What is Just Culture? Changing the way we think about errors to improve patient safety and staff satisfaction.* https://www.brighamandwomensfaulkner.org/about-bwfh/news/what-is-just-culture-changing-the-way-we-think-about-errors-to-improve-patient-safety-and-staff-satisfaction

Britton, M. C., Ouellet, G. M., Minges, K. E., Gawel, M., Hodshon, B., & Chaudhry, S. I. (2017, November). Care transitions between hospitals and skilled nursing facilities: Perspectives of sending and receiving providers. *The Joint Commission Journal on Quality and Patient Safety, 43*(11), 565–572. https://doi.org/10.1016/j.jcjq.2017.06.004

Cadmus, E., & Mastrocola, J. R. (2021, Jan. 12). Pathway to Excellence in long-term care organizations. *American Nurse Journal, 16*(1), 38–41. https://www.myamericannurse.com/pathway-to-excellence-in-long-term-care-organizations/

Coupland, C. A. C., Hill, T., Dening, T., Morriss, R., Moore, M., & Hippisley-Cox, J. (2019, Aug. 1). Anticholinergic drug exposure and the risk of dementia: A nested case-control study. *JAMA Internal Medicine, 179*(8), 1084–1093. https://doi.org/10.1001/jamainternmed.2019.0677

Cronshaw, A., Boddye, E., Reilly, L., Boardman, R., Portas, L., Hagan, J., Griffiths, S., Donovan, H., Clark, D., Collins, L., Linley, B., Salt, S., Sheahan-Parry, M., Cooper, J., Jones, K., Sunderland, M., Manning, J. C., & Marufu, T. C. (2021). Engaging nurses to achieve a culture of excellence: A children's hospital journey towards Pathway to Excellence accreditation. *Nursing Management, 28*(6).

Dans, M., & Lundmark, V. (2019). The effects of positive practice environments: Leadership must-knows. *Nursing Management, 50*(10), 7–10.

Dash, K., Shue, J., Driver, T., Bonner, A., Pelton, L., Snyder, R., Diep, A., Espinosa, S., & Fulmer, T. (2022). Developing a shared language to describe the age-friendly ecosystem: Technical meeting report. *International Journal of Geriatrics and Gerontology, 6*, 134.

Debesay, J., Arora, S., & Fougner, M. (2022, June 30). Organisational culture and ethnic diversity in nursing homes: A qualitative study of healthcare workers' and ward nurses' experiences. *BMC Health Services Research, 22*(1), 843. https://doi.org/10.1186/s12913-022-08184-y

Doll, G. A., Cornelison, L. J., Rath, H., & Syme, M. L. (2017, August). Actualizing culture change: The Promoting Excellent Alternatives in Kansas Nursing Homes (PEAK 2.0) program. *Psychological Services, 14*(3), 307–315. https://doi.org/10.1037/ser0000142

Elliott, R., & Fry, M. (2021). Psychological capital, well-being, and patient safety attitudes of nurses and midwives: A cross-sectional survey. *Nursing & Health Sciences, 23*(1), 237–244. https://doi.org/10.1111/nhs.12808

Emery-Tiburcio, E. E., Berg-Weger, M., Husser, E. K., Tumosa, N., Golden, R. L., Newman, M. H., Morley, J. E., Knecht-Fredo, J. M., Hupcey, J. E., & Fick, D. M. (2021, December). The geriatrics education and care revolution: Diverse implementation of Age-Friendly Health Systems. *Journal of the American Geriatrics Society, 69*(12), E31–E33. https://doi.org/10.1111/jgs.17497

Fahrenkopf, A. M., Sectish, T. C., Barger, L. K., Sharek, P. J., Lewin, D., Chiang, V. W., Edwards, S., Wiedermann, B. L., & Landrigan, C. P. (2008). Rates of medication errors among depressed and burnt out residents: Prospective cohort study. *BMJ, 336*(7642), 488–491. https://doi.org/10.1136/bmj.39469.763218.BE

Fick, D. M. (2020). Less really is more in inappropriate medication use in older adults: How can we improve prescribing and deprescribing in older adults? *The American Journal of Geriatric Psychiatry, 68*(8), 1175–1176. https://doi.org/10.1111/jgs.16485

Fick, D. M. (2022). Knowing the older adult with delirium superimposed on dementia. *The American Journal of Geriatric Psychiatry, 30*(10), 1079–1082. https://doi.org/10.1016/j.jagp.2022.06.003

Fick, D. M., Inouye, S. K., McDermott, C., Zhou, W., Ngo, L., Gallagher, J., McDowell, J., Penrod, J., Siuta, J., Covaleski, T., & Marcantonio, E. R. (2018). Pilot study of a two-step delirium detection protocol administered by certified nursing assistants, physicians, and registered nurses. *Journal of Gerontological Nursing, 44*(5), 18–24. https://doi.org/10.3928/00989134-20180302-01

Fick, D. M., & Shrestha, P. (2022). Delirium in persons with dementia: Integrating the 4Ms of Age-Friendly care as a set into the care of older people. *Journal of Gerontological Nursing, 48*(10), 3–6. https://doi.org/10.3928/00989134-20220909-01

Fulmer, T., Mate, K. S., & Berman, A. (2018, January). The Age-Friendly Health System imperative. *Journal of the American Geriatrics Society, 66*(1), 22–24. https://doi.org/10.1111/jgs.15076

Fulmer, T., Pelton, L., Zhang, J., & Huang, W. (2022). *Age-Friendly Health Systems: A guide to using the 4Ms while caring for older adults.* Institute for Healthcare Improvement.

Gensimore, M. M., Maduro, R. S., Morgan, M. K., McGee, G. W., & Zimbro, K. S. (2020). The effect of nurse practice environment on retention and quality of care via burnout, work characteristics, and resilience: A moderated mediation model. *The Journal of Nursing Administration, 50*(10), 546–553.

Gitlin, L. N., Kales, H. C., & Lyketsos, C. G. (2012, Nov. 21). Nonpharmacologic management of behavioral symptoms in dementia. *JAMA, 308*(19), 2020–2029. https://doi.org/10.1001/jama.2012.36918

Gitlin, L. N., Winter, L., Dennis, M. P., Hodgson, N., & Hauck, W. W. (2010, August). Targeting and managing behavioral symptoms in individuals with dementia: A randomized trial of a nonpharmacological intervention. *Journal of the American Geriatrics Society, 58*(8), 1465–1474. https://doi.org/10.1111/j.1532-5415.2010.02971.x

Grant, E. J., & Pabico, C. (2022). A framework for achieving the National Plan for Health Workforce Well-Being recommendations. *Nursing Management, 53*(10), 9–15. https://doi.org/10.1097/01.NUMA.0000874432.64403.fb

Huey, F. L. (1985). What teaching nursing homes are teaching us. *American Journal of Nursing, 85*(6), 678–683.

Inouye, S. K., Zhang, Y., Jones, R. N., Kiely, D. K., Yang, F., & Marcantonio, E. R. (2007). Risk factors for delirium at discharge. *Archives of Internal Medicine, 167*(13), 1406. https://doi.org/10.1001/archinte.167.13.1406

Institute for Healthcare Improvement. (2022). *Age-Friendly Health Systems: Guide to care of older adults in nursing homes.* https://241684.fs1.hubspotusercontent-na1.net/hubfs/241684/IHI-Age-Friendly-Guide-Nursing-Homes_March28-2022.pdf

Institute for Healthcare Improvement. (2023). *What is an Age-Friendly Health System?* https://www.ihi.org/Engage/Initiatives/Age-Friendly-Health-Systems/Pages/default.aspx

Jewish Healthcare Foundation. (2021, June 29). *Pennsylvania Teaching Nursing Home pilot aims to transform model care.* https://www.jhf.org/news-blog-menu/entry/pennsylvania-teaching-nursing-home-pilot-aims-to-transform-care-model-1

Jun, J., Ojemeni, M. M., Kalamani, R., Tong, J., & Crecelius, M. L. (2021). Relationship between nurse burnout, patient and organizational outcomes: Systematic review. *International Journal of Nursing Studies, 119*, 103933. https://doi.org/10.1016/j.ijnurstu.2021.103933

Komici, K., Guerra, G., Addona, F., & Fantini, C. (2022, Aug. 15). Delirium in nursing home residents: A narrative review. *Healthcare, 10*(8). https://doi.org/10.3390/healthcare10081544

Lapp, L., Egan, K., McCann, L., Mackenzie, M., Wales, A., & Maguire, R. (2022). Decision support tools in adult long-term care facilities: Scoping review. *Journal of Medical Internet Research, 24*(9), e39681. https://doi.org/10.2196/39681

Marcantonio, E. R., Fick, D. M., Jung, Y., Inouye, S. K., Boltz, M., Leslie, D. L., Husser, E. K., Shrestha, P., Moore, A., Sulmonte, K., Siuta, J., Boustani, M., & Ngo, L. H. (2022). Comparative implementation of a brief app-directed protocol for delirium identification by hospitalists, nurses, and nursing assistants. *Annals of Internal Medicine, 175*(1), 65–73. https://doi.org/10.7326/m21-1687

Morandi, A., Grossi, E., Lucchi, E., Zambon, A., Faraci, B., Severgnini, J., MacLullich, A., Smith, H., Pandharipande, P., Rizzini, A., Galeazzi, M., Massariello, F., Corradi, S., Raccichini, A., Scrimieri, A., Morichi, V., Gentile, S., Lucchini, F., Pecorella, L., Mossello, E., Cherubini, A., & Bellelli, G. (2021, July). The 4-DSD: A new tool to assess delirium superimposed on moderate to severe dementia. The *Journal of Post-Acute and Long-Term Care Medicine, 22*(7), 1535–1542.E3. https://doi.org/10.1016/j.jamda.2021.02.029

National Academies of Sciences, Engineering, and Medicine. (2022). *The national imperative to improve nursing home quality: Honoring our commitment to residents, families, and staff.* The National Academies Press. https://doi.org/10.17226/26526

National Academy of Medicine. (2022). *National Plan for Health Workforce Well-Being.* https://nam.edu/initiatives/clinicianresilience-and-well-being/national-planfor-health-workforce-well-being

Pennsylvania State University Ross and Carol Nese College of Nursing. (n.d.). *Nursing homes.* https://www.agefriendlycare.psu.edu/nursing-home

Rosgen, B., Krewulak, K., Demiantschuk, D., Ely, E. W., Davidson, J. E., Stelfox, H. T., & Fiest, K. M. (2018). Validation of caregiver-centered delirium detection tools: A systematic review. *Journal of the American Geriatrics Society, 66*(6), 1218–1225. https://doi.org/10.1111/jgs.15362

Siegel, E. O., Kolanowski, A. M., & Bowers, B. J. (2023, January–February). A fresh look at the nursing home workforce crisis: Transforming nursing care delivery models. *Research in Gerontological Nursing, 16*(1), 5–13. https://doi.org/10.3928/19404921-20230104-01

Watkins, M. D. (2013, May 15). What is organizational culture? And why should we care? *Harvard Business Review.* https://hbr.org/2013/05/what-is-organizational-culture

Xue, T. M., Colon-Emeric, C. S., Herndon, L., Hecker, E. J., Berry, S. D., Little, M. O., & McConnell, E. S. (2022, Sept. 7). Strengthening resident, proxy, and staff engagement in injury prevention in skilled nursing facilities. *The Gerontologist, 62*(8), 1112–1123. https://doi.org/10.1093/geront/gnab193

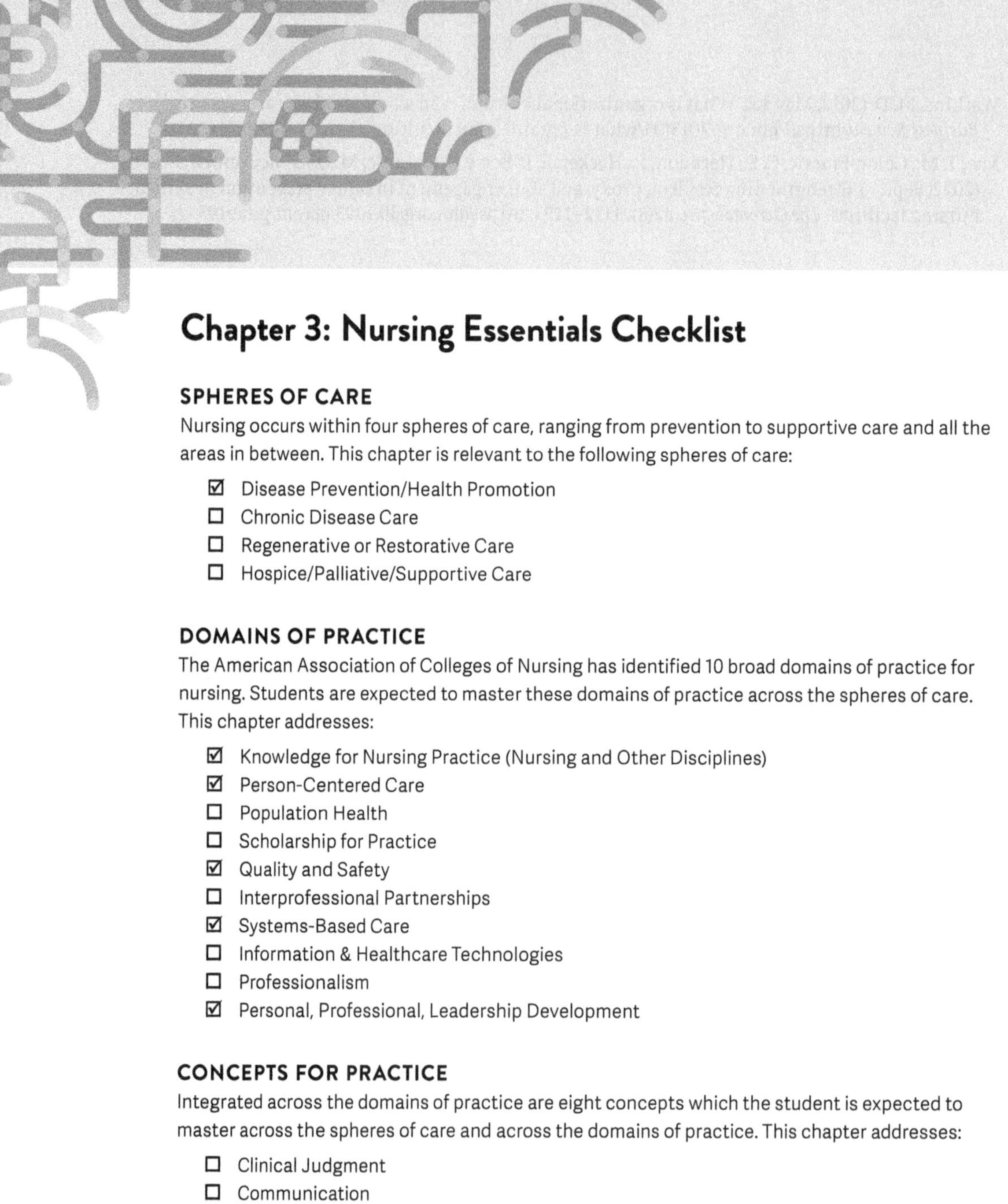

Chapter 3: Nursing Essentials Checklist

SPHERES OF CARE

Nursing occurs within four spheres of care, ranging from prevention to supportive care and all the areas in between. This chapter is relevant to the following spheres of care:

- ☑ Disease Prevention/Health Promotion
- ☐ Chronic Disease Care
- ☐ Regenerative or Restorative Care
- ☐ Hospice/Palliative/Supportive Care

DOMAINS OF PRACTICE

The American Association of Colleges of Nursing has identified 10 broad domains of practice for nursing. Students are expected to master these domains of practice across the spheres of care. This chapter addresses:

- ☑ Knowledge for Nursing Practice (Nursing and Other Disciplines)
- ☑ Person-Centered Care
- ☐ Population Health
- ☐ Scholarship for Practice
- ☑ Quality and Safety
- ☐ Interprofessional Partnerships
- ☑ Systems-Based Care
- ☐ Information & Healthcare Technologies
- ☐ Professionalism
- ☑ Personal, Professional, Leadership Development

CONCEPTS FOR PRACTICE

Integrated across the domains of practice are eight concepts which the student is expected to master across the spheres of care and across the domains of practice. This chapter addresses:

- ☐ Clinical Judgment
- ☐ Communication
- ☐ Compassionate Care
- ☑ Diversity, Equity, Inclusion
- ☑ Ethics
- ☐ Evidence-Based Practice
- ☐ Health Policy
- ☐ Social Determinants of Health

CHAPTER 3

DIVERSITY, EQUITY, INCLUSION: STAFF AND RESIDENTS

Jasmine L. Travers, PhD, MHS, RN, AGPCNP-BC

OBJECTIVES

1. Define inequities, health disparities, and diversity, equity, and inclusion (DEI).
2. Understand staff and resident issues related to DEI.
3. Propose ways to improve the nursing home environment so that it supports DEI.

INTRODUCTION

The nursing home workforce comprises nearly 1.6 million individuals who work across several positions in the nursing home (Centers for Disease Control and Prevention [CDC], 2022). These workers occupy recreational, occupational, speech language, physical therapy, housekeeping, environmental services, administrative, director, physician, advanced practice nursing, physician assistant, social work, and direct care roles (CDC, 2022; US Bureau of Labor Statistics [BLS], 2019). Direct-care workers, who make up the majority of the nursing home workforce and spend the most time with residents, include registered nurses (RNs), licensed practical nurses (LPNs), and certified nursing assistants (CNAs; CDC, 2022; BLS, 2019).

While the nursing home workforce in general is quite diverse in racial and ethnic makeup, immigration status, age, and gender, this diversity tends to be most concentrated in specific roles, leading to stark inequities experienced by a large proportion of the workforce. In this chapter, we define inequities, explore who experiences inequities in the nursing home environment, and discuss how a focus on diversity, equity, and inclusion (DEI) is necessary to reduce the inequities that both staff and residents experience in nursing homes.

INEQUITIES DEFINED

An *inequity* is defined as an instance of injustice or unfairness and is typically experienced by people with racial and ethnic minoritized backgrounds and/or those who identify as a sexual or gender minority, female, older adult, person living with disabilities, or immigrant (Merriam-Webster Dictionary, n.d.). Drivers of inequities include ignorance, bias, poor governance, culture, and racist policies, practices, and laws (National Academies of Sciences, Engineering, and Medicine [NASEM] et al., 2017).

Inequities have been commonly mistaken for *inequalities*, which occur when not everyone is given the exact same resources and do not include a measurement of actual needs or extant opportunities or resources. Importantly, inequities are avoidable and reflect a measurement of actual needs or extant opportunities or resources, making them different from inequalities (see Figure 3.1).

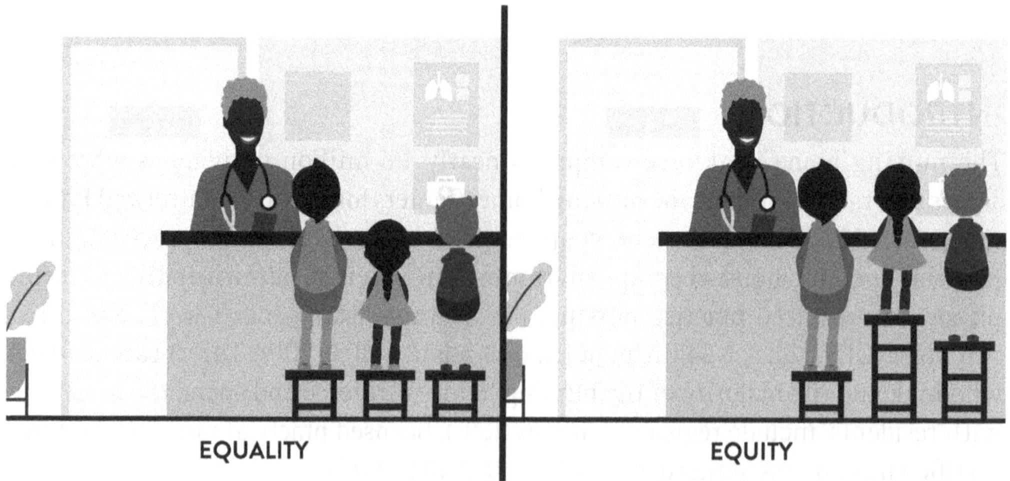

FIGURE 3.1 Equality versus equity. *From Thomas, 2021*

WHO AMONG THE NURSING HOME WORKFORCE EXPERIENCES INEQUITIES?

Inequities affecting the nursing home workforce have largely been described as disproportionately impacting the CNA workforce. Among the 600,000 CNAs employed in nursing homes, 90% are female; 50% identify as Black, Latino, or other; and 20% identify as an immigrant (CDC, 2004; PHI, n.d.).

A significant inequity that this workforce experiences is the pay gap. This group of workers is generally not able to make a living wage at a median pay of $15.99/hour (BLS, 2021b). In some states, CNAs are not entitled to a minimum wage because CNAs are not a recognized workforce for minimum wage in that state (US Department of Labor, 2013). Such low pay is insufficient in covering basic living expenses, such as rent/mortgage, transportation, utilities, and groceries. As a result, 18% of CNAs live in poverty, and 20% are uninsured or underinsured with regards to health coverage (PHI, n.d.). To fill the gaps in the low pay that CNAs receive, many must work second and third jobs (Baughman et al., 2022; Dill et al., 2022). During the pandemic, this practice was shown to increase the spread of COVID-19 infections and subsequent deaths (Baughman et al., 2022).

Another significant inequity experienced by CNAs is the way in which this workforce is treated. CNAs are often subjected to disrespect, racism, discrimination, and abuse from residents and families and are responsible for extremely high workloads (Travers, Teitelman, et al., 2020).

Experiences of racism have been cited as more prevalent in the nursing home setting than out in the community (Berdes & Eckert, 2001; Travers, Teitelman, et al., 2020). CNAs of racial and ethnic minoritized backgrounds are often victims of racial slurs and the recipients of differential negative treatment, such as fewer staff assigned when the majority of staff assigned that shift are people of color (Dodson & Zincavage, 2007; Travers, Teitelman, et al., 2020).

Regarding workload, CNAs often care for more than eight residents per shift, and during the COVID-19 pandemic, reports of residents not being seen for whole shifts because CNAs were responsible for an extremely high number of residents were common (Spanko, 2020). Lack of voice and power differentials that are at play in the nursing home setting deter CNAs from speaking up and being a part of important decision-making and resident care-planning activities (Travers, Teitelman, et al., 2020).

RNs are usually responsible for supervising CNAs; however, this relationship has been strained, likely because RNs are not educated on how best to foster a fruitful relationship with CNAs as well as how best to support CNAs, and they lack the competence to address issues of racial occurrences (Dodson & Zincavage, 2007; Foner, 1994; Holmberg et al., 2013). For example, CNAs have shared feelings of being unsupported, disrespected, and devalued, and they feel nursing home environments lack teamwork and supervisors fail to recognize them for their work. In recent years, CNAs have fought to create a voice for themselves through labor organizations and the National Association of Health Care Assistants.

Inequities are also prevalent in the promotion and support of nursing home jobs compared to other settings. For example, historically, education and the marketing of jobs for RNs have been directed primarily to acute care settings, with little focus on the nursing home setting. In 2010, the American Association of Colleges of Nursing (AACN) required nursing schools to include content on the older adult; however, content focused on the nursing home setting was not required (AACN, 2010). Some schools of nursing have taken the liberty to add this content and/or provide a real-world experience in the nursing home setting for students; however, this type of education remains very limited (John A. Hartford Foundation, n.d.).

Affinity toward acute care work versus nursing home work has also been driven by pay. For example, RNs can earn over $10,000 more working in a hospital versus a nursing home (BLS, 2021e). CNAs and primary care clinicians (physicians, nurse practitioners, and physician assistants) are also able to earn more working in a hospital versus a nursing home (BLS, 2021a, 2021b, 2021c, 2021d). This difference in pay across settings has created a shortage of RNs and CNAs who wish to work in nursing homes, which has increased the workload for these workers and resulted in subsequent poor care delivery for residents. A lack of investment in those who work in nursing home settings with regard to their pay, training, and education is likely also rooted in a disregard for the population being cared for in this setting.

OVERVIEW OF THE NURSING HOME RESIDENT POPULATION

Roughly 1.1 million residents reside in certified nursing homes (Kaiser Family Foundation, 2022; Michas, 2022). Over the years, there has been a racial and ethnic demographic shift in the use of nursing homes (Travers, Dick, et al., 2022). Along with this shift, disparities in care delivery and health outcomes have become more pervasive.

Black, Latino, and Native American older adults are particularly subject to inequitable access to high-quality healthcare services compared to non-Latino white and Asian-American older adults. To this end, the Institute of Medicine (IOM, now known as NASEM) has declared racial disparities in the quality of healthcare a high-priority problem (IOM, 2003).

Health Disparities Defined

Health disparities have been defined by the CDC (2017) as preventable differences in the burden of disease, injury, and violence or in opportunities to achieve optimal health experienced by socially disadvantaged racial, ethnic, and other minoritized population groups and communities.

Who Experiences Disparities and How?

Historically, non-Hispanic white older adults accounted for the majority of the nursing home population, nearing 90% in the year 2000 (Centers for Medicare & Medicaid Services [CMS], 2000). Native American older adults made up less than 1% of the nursing home population during this time and have been known to use the Indian Health Service system for necessary care (LaVeist, 2011). While this system provides health services to Native American older adults and is meant to decrease health disparities in care, it uses an acute model and lacks a sufficient structure to deliver services to older adults (Davis & Aguilar, 2008).

Black and Latino older adults made up 10.2% and 3.1% of the nursing home population, respectively, in the year 2000 (CMS, 2000). These two racial and ethnic groups have traditionally opted to reside in the community and utilize other long-term care services (primarily home health services and informal care) or have been found to face disproportionate access to nursing home services (Whitfield & Baker, 2013). The privatization of nursing home care has been partly responsible for the disproportionate access to nursing home services, as nursing homes prefer Medicare over Medicaid because of Medicare's higher reimbursement rate (American Council on Aging, 2022; Grabowski, 2022).

Private pay is subsequently associated with higher-quality nursing home care and more resources (e.g., staffing), as the majority of private payers are white residents

(Anderson et al., 1998; Grabowski, 2022; Mor et al., 2004; Spector & Takada, 1991). Alternatively, Medicaid payment for nursing home care has been associated with a lower quality of care and poorer health outcomes because resources from Medicaid do not translate into adequate funding. The majority of residents covered by Medicaid have been people belonging to racial and ethnic minoritized groups (Wodchis et al., 2007).

These differences in care seen as a result of differences in payment source have created a two-tiered system, with those who are disproportionately poor and of a racial or ethnic minoritized group predominantly residing in lower-tier facilities (Mor et al., 2004). However, in the most recent years of data collection by the Nursing Home Compendium, white older adults have been found to make up only 78% of the nursing home population, while the proportion of Black and Latino older adults has increased to 14% and 5%, respectively; Native American older adults have remained at less than 1% (CMS, 2015).

This racial and ethnic demographic shift has been said to be because of disparities in long-term care options, with an increased number of white older adults utilizing assisted living services that require private payments, while a large proportion of racial and ethnic minoritized groups are utilizing Medicaid for long-term care services. More white older adults are moving out of nursing homes, and as a result, occupancy rates in this setting are declining (Pruitt, 2013), creating an increased demand to fill beds with other racial and ethnic groups, further suggesting that nursing homes had increased selectivity in previous years.

Another disparity in access to care is related to decision-making. White older adults have been found to be more involved with the decision to be placed in a nursing home, while Black older adults have been found to have very little to no involvement in this decision (Dill et al., 2022; Travers, Hirschman, et al., 2020). Furthermore, Black older adults have shared reports of being tricked into a nursing home placement. It is important to consider the level of mistrust that might arise among older adults belonging to racial and ethnic minoritized groups.

These groups have been subjected to long-standing acts of manipulation in healthcare—such as being tricked in this case, or in other cases such as the Tuskegee syphilis study—that subsequently have placed stress on their ability to trust and comply with the healthcare system (Alsan & Wanamaker, 2018). Continued situations such as these will cause additional strain on the delivery of quality nursing home care, which is why the inclusion of both older adults of racial and ethnic minoritized groups and their families in all healthcare decisions when possible is critical (HealthinAging.org, 2015) to overcome recollections of the domination and coercion of older adults (Johnson et al., 2010; Travers, Hirschman, et al., 2020). This history has implications for how the healthcare system might look to address lack of acceptance to necessary and recommended care and treatment initiatives among Black older adults, for example, as a result of past wrongdoings.

In addition to decision-making processes, the way in which the preferences of residents are assessed and honored must also be revisited. Many residents in the nursing home setting speak different languages and have preferences for particular foods that are not honored as a result of lack of staff diversity, failure for staff to utilize interpretive resources, limited funds to provide diverse food options, or disinterest in directing funds toward diverse food options (Abbott et al., 2018; Bangerter et al., 2016; Debesay et al., 2022).

Residential and facility segregation also heavily impacts access to quality nursing home care (Falvey et al., 2021). The more segregated the nursing home is with Black residents, the greater the observed disparities across nursing homes when it comes to quality of care indicators such as pressure ulcers, pneumococcal and influenza vaccinations, and COVID-19 infections and deaths (Fennell et al., 2010; Mack et al., 2020; Travers et al., 2021; Travers, Dick, et al., 2018; Travers, Schroeder, et al., 2018). Researchers have found that all-white nursing homes have lower deficiency scores (Li & Mukamel, 2010). A greater percentage of all-white facilities have fewer or no instances of restraint use and have higher staffing levels dedicated to direct care and RNs when compared to nursing homes with less than 15% or equal or greater than 15% of Hispanic residents (Mor et al., 2004). Private pay was also found to be the most common form of compensation given by white older adults. The number of Medicaid-supported residents increased substantially as the number of Hispanic residents increased within the home.

Measuring performance indicators (deficiency citations, staffing levels, and financial viability of the nursing home), Hispanic older adults were found to be more likely to reside in poorly performing nursing homes compared to white older adults (Chisholm et al., 2013). Researchers reported that nursing homes with greater proportions of Black older adults had higher rates of pressure ulcers, activities of daily living decline, quality of care deficiencies, and harm citations compared with facilities that had no Black residents (Chang et al., 2012). Similarly, research has found that rates of pressure ulcers increased among nursing homes with higher numbers of Black residents, along with decreasing influenza and pneumococcal vaccination rates (Li & Mukamel, 2010; Li et al., 2011).

Other studies found that the relative risk of nursing home closure among freestanding facilities was greater in zip codes with the highest percentages of Black residents compared to zip codes with the lowest percentages of Black residents (Feng et al., 2011). Significant staffing disparities were also found within facilities located in severely deprived neighborhoods (Falvey et al., 2022).

Implications for Nursing Policy and Practice

Understanding current inequities and disparities occurring in the nursing home setting is important for nurses to explain, predict, advocate for, and address prevailing inequities and disparities that result in poor quality of care and health outcomes among disadvantaged groups. Moreover, nurses are in an important position to lead these efforts as RNs, preceptors, educators, managers, and directors of nursing. Many of these problems must be addressed by critically assessing the structures that continue to perpetuate them. Some of these solutions include requiring nursing programs to implement a curriculum that is inclusive of didactic and experiential learning focused on nursing homes.

Specific to nursing home policy, a possible solution could be to raise the reimbursement rate nursing homes receive so that differential care does not result from a lower financial credit line because nursing homes are taking on more Medicaid payments. In most cases, such payments are so low that the ability to invest in quality improvement, let alone adequate staffing, is heavily affected (Grabowski, 2001).

Furthermore, nursing homes could ensure that a certain proportion of funds go toward resident care and staff (e.g., increased pay and benefits), which some states have done (National Governors Association, 2022). The government can also make pay across work settings more equitable and/or incentivize and reframe nursing home work and aging.

Additionally, healthcare providers contribute significantly to the problem of inequities as a result of bias. It is important to increase awareness of these issues. *Implicit bias* refers to a lack of awareness of unconscious biases or attitudes that are difficult to acknowledge and control (Hall et al., 2015). Holding nursing homes accountable for the treatment of their staff and residents through alternative payment models that give added incentive payments to nursing homes that provide high-quality and cost-efficient care, for example, is an important consideration. Efforts to address equity issues should take into account resident and staff satisfaction surveys, the collection of baseline data, and the collection of demographic data—pre- and post- the implementation of these efforts so that their success can be tracked adequately.

Social workers and nurses are more involved in nursing home placement decisions for Black older adults compared to white older adults. While this support is essential, residents belonging to racial and ethnic minoritized groups are routinely sent to nursing homes of lower quality and poor performance (Grabowski & McGuire, 2009). When considering nursing home placement for such residents, it is important that these healthcare professionals are equipped with the tools, education, resources, and sensitivity to make the best placement decisions while concurrently considering the residents' preferences, finances, and health needs.

Promotores, Spanish-speaking community health workers, are essential in improving healthcare access and outcomes among the Latino community, as they understand the needs of Latino individuals and help them navigate the healthcare system (Bauer & Kantayya, 2010; Rosenthal et al., 2010).

Increased knowledge of DEI issues, bias training, and commitment to an environment that does not condone inequitable treatment are required at both the individual and system levels. The adoption of DEI content is especially important in nursing education curricular standards and certification requirements. The components of DEI are broken down in the sections that follow.

Diversity

Diversity is defined as a commitment to increasing the representation of individuals from diverse and/or underrepresented backgrounds (CDC, 2017). In other words, diversity means that everyone is invited to the party. Increasing the diversity of the nursing home workforce across positions and roles is important to foster diverse thinking and a welcoming environment. This means that workers of different races, ethnicities, genders, and sexual orientations should be found across roles to mirror the people who are being served. This will help with diversifying programming, food offerings, employee engagement, collaborations, and the development of materials and resources that are accessible to those who speak different languages and are from diverse backgrounds.

The NASEM 2022 report on nursing home quality noted the need to hire a workforce that is culturally congruent to the residents that are being served in nursing homes and are equipped to practice cultural humility and sensitivity (NASEM, 2022). To recruit this workforce, it is important to expose people from diverse cultures, races, ethnicities, and backgrounds to a variety of roles in nursing homes.

Equity

Equity is defined as a commitment to actively work to challenge and respond to the bias, harassment, and discrimination that occurs within an organization (University of Michigan, n.d.). Some approaches related to the promotion of equity include understanding the issues that are occurring among staff and residents of varied backgrounds so that one may know what efforts need to be developed and where they should be directed, such as increasing staffing, increasing wages, and incentivizing CNAs so that they do not have to work multiple jobs. Furthermore, different forms of support (e.g., mental, tangible, physical, and emotional) should be provided. It is also important to educate staff so that they know how to confront issues related to bias, harassment, and discrimination. Related to the delivery of equitable care, the NASEM report (2022) called for nursing homes to be accountable for the total cost of care and poor care delivery through alternative payment models.

Inclusion

Inclusion is defined as a commitment to pursuing deliberate efforts to ensure that an organization is a place where differences are welcomed, varying perspectives are respectfully heard, and every individual feels a sense of belonging and inclusion (University of Michigan, n.d.). Inclusion ensures that people do not feel "othered." Vital to efforts to enhance inclusivity is ensuring that all voices that need to be at the table are indeed at the table and feel empowered to speak up. This consists of inviting residents, all relevant staff, and families to resident care planning meetings, for example.

Another aspect of inclusion is ensuring that materials, resources, and offerings are accessible to people from diverse backgrounds. This might consist of providing education in languages that work best for CNAs and ensuring that CNAs understand the educational material (Andrulis & Brach, 2007). This can be accomplished by drawing on more visual resources and practical experiences, as well as by providing information that CNAs need in a way that they can understand. The diversity of the workforce influences the inclusivity of the environment, as a more diverse workforce is more in tune with the needs of the staff and residents, and they are able and willing to meet those needs. Recommendations from the NASEM report (2022) additionally included the following:

- Identifying care preferences (of residents) and implementing and monitoring corresponding care plans
- Understanding and honoring preferences among residents—language, food, religion, etc.

Other layers of inclusion include empowering CNAs through opportunities for advancement and ensuring that bidirectional communication with other healthcare staff is occurring. Furthermore, engagement with CNAs should be increased by including them in care teams and involving them in care plans.

A model in the nursing home space being used and is worth noting is inclusion, diversity, equality, and acceptance (Marselas, 2021). It involves bias training and cultural competency education for staff, leadership engagement to address challenging DEI issues, opportunities to spotlight staff with diverse backgrounds, and executives serving as thought leaders outside the senior living industry. The program sets goals and tracks metrics to ensure that the work done is more than lip service. Importantly, the program goes beyond making a statement; instead, it creates an operational plan that incorporates resources, tools, and activities to educate, engage, and equip its members to follow through on the stated values of DEI and belonging.

To guide the development of DEI policy, nursing homes might consider educational and/or informational events, such as town halls, webinars, and evidence-based articles, ensuring that DEI initiatives in the organization's policy agenda and data collection efforts are ongoing. A standing DEI committee with a chief diversity officer is also important in driving DEI initiatives (Jolley & Peck, 2022).

CASE STUDY Nursing Home DEI Initiative Aims to Increase Diversity, Promote Equity, and Enhance Inclusivity in the Workforce

ABC Nursing Home is a long-term care facility that serves a diverse population of residents. However, the workforce does not reflect the diversity of its residents, and the staff lacks the cultural competence necessary to provide equitable care to their entire resident population. As a result, ABC Nursing Home is struggling with issues related to staff turnover, low morale among staff, and poor quality of care delivery.

This lack of DEI not only affects the staff but also has a significant impact on the residents of ABC Nursing Home. Residents with diverse backgrounds and cultural experiences may feel isolated or misunderstood by staff who do not share their backgrounds or understand their cultural practices. This can lead to a lack of trust in the staff and a feeling of neglect or discrimination. Furthermore, residents who do not receive equitable care may experience adverse health outcomes or a decreased quality of life.

To address these issues, ABC Nursing Home's leadership team decided to implement a DEI initiative aimed at increasing diversity, promoting equity, and enhancing inclusivity in the workforce. The initiative involved the following steps:

1. **Assessing the current state:** ABC Nursing Home's leadership team conducted an assessment using the Cultural Competence Assessment instrument to determine the current state of cultural competence and DEI in the workforce. The assessment revealed that ABC Nursing Home's workforce lacked diversity, and the staff did not have the cultural competence or sensitivity necessary to provide equitable care to all residents. The residents also reported feeling isolated or misunderstood by the staff.
2. **Developing a DEI policy:** ABC Nursing Home's leadership team developed a DEI policy that outlined the organization's commitment to increasing diversity, promoting equity, and enhancing inclusivity in the workforce. The policy included a plan to recruit and retain a diverse workforce, provide cultural competence training to staff, and ensure that all residents receive equitable care specific to their needs and preferences. The policy also emphasized the importance of creating a welcoming and inclusive environment for residents.
3. **Implementing the DEI initiative:** ABC Nursing Home's leadership team implemented the DEI initiative by recruiting a diverse workforce, providing cultural competence training to staff from experts in this area, and involving residents,

families, and staff in care planning meetings. Recruitment efforts that ABC Nursing Home drew on included garnering referrals from staff already working at the nursing home, working with faith communities and people from diverse backgrounds who were connected to communities of diverse backgrounds, and providing benefits that appealed to people of diverse backgrounds such as child care and transportation. ABC Nursing Home also provided resources and materials in languages that CNAs and other staff could understand and created opportunities for advancement and bidirectional communication. The initiative also focused on creating a welcoming and inclusive environment for residents, including celebrating cultural events and providing culturally appropriate care, food, and activities.

4. **Measuring success:** The ABC Nursing Home's leadership team measured the success of the DEI initiative by tracking metrics related to DEI in the workforce. The metrics included the diversity of the workforce, the percentage of staff who completed cultural competence training, resident satisfaction with the care they received, and staff job satisfaction and retention rates.

The DEI initiative at ABC Nursing Home resulted in several positive outcomes, including an increase in staff morale and job satisfaction, a decrease in turnover, and an improvement in the quality of care provided to residents.

Increase in staff morale and job satisfaction:

1. With a more diverse workforce, staff members are likely to feel more valued and appreciated, which can lead to higher morale and job satisfaction.
2. Providing cultural competence training can also help staff feel more competent and confident in their ability to provide equitable care to all residents.
3. When staff members feel more satisfied with their jobs, they are more likely to stay with the organization and provide better care to residents.

Decrease in turnover:

1. With higher staff morale and job satisfaction, turnover rates are likely to decrease. This means that ABC Nursing Home can retain experienced staff members, reducing the need to constantly train new employees.
2. Lower turnover rates can also lead to more consistent care for residents, as staff members have more experience and knowledge of each resident's unique needs.

(continues)

(continued)

Improvement in the quality of care provided to residents:

1. A more diverse workforce with cultural competence training can provide more equitable care to all residents, regardless of their background or identity.
2. Involving residents, families, and staff in care planning meetings can help ensure that each resident's unique needs and preferences are taken into account when developing care plans.
3. Providing resources and materials in languages that CNAs can understand can also help ensure that all residents receive clear and accurate information about their care.
4. The ABC Nursing Home's leadership team attributed these positive outcomes to the organization's commitment to increasing diversity, promoting equity, and enhancing inclusivity in the workforce.

The case study of ABC Nursing Home illustrates the importance of DEI in the nursing home workforce for both staff and residents. By implementing a DEI initiative, ABC Nursing Home was able to recruit and retain a diverse workforce, provide culturally competent care, and enhance inclusivity in the workplace. The success of the initiative demonstrates that a commitment to DEI can lead to positive outcomes for both staff and residents in long-term care facilities.

SUMMARY

Leaders of nursing institutions must make DEI a goal with programs and initiatives that are a part of the culture of the organization to back it up. Furthermore, it is important to have DEI principles that are meant to enhance the care and work environment for residents and workers from diverse and underrepresented backgrounds. A focus on DEI, both in nursing schools and in nursing homes, will help to engage, educate, and equip nurses to deliver person-centered, culturally responsive care and to effectively recognize and respond to implicit bias in healthcare settings, which in turn will lead to a reduction in inequities and disparities experienced in the nursing home setting by workers and residents.

REFERENCES

Abbott, K. M., Heid, A. R., Kleban, M., Rovine, M. J., & Van Haitsma, K. (2018). The change in nursing home residents' preferences over time. *Journal of the American Medical Directors Association, 19*(12), 1092–1098. https://doi.org/10.1016/j.jamda.2018.08.004

Alsan, M., & Wanamaker, M. (2018). Tuskegee and the health of black men. *The Quarterly Journal of Economics, 133*(1), 407–455. https://doi.org/10.1093/qje/qjx029

American Association of Colleges of Nursing. (2010). *Recommended baccalaureate competencies and curricular guidelines for the nursing care of older adults.* https://www.aacnnursing.org/Portals/0/PDFs/CCNE/AACN-Gero-Competencies-2010.pdf

American Council on Aging. (2022, Dec. 26). *Medicaid coverage of nursing home care: When, where and how much they pay.* https://www.medicaidplanningassistance.org/medicaid-and-nursing-homes/

Anderson, R. A., Hsieh, P. C., & Su, H. F. (1998). Resource allocation and resident outcomes in nursing homes: Comparisons between the best and worst. *Research in Nursing & Health, 21*(4), 297–313. https://doi.org/10.1002/(sici)1098-240x(199808)21:4<297::aid-nur3>3.0.co;2-a

Andrulis, D. P., & Brach, C. (2007). Integrating literacy, culture, and language to improve health care quality for diverse populations. *American Journal of Health Behavior, 31*(Suppl. 1), S122–S133. https://www.ncbi.nlm.nih.gov/pmc/articles/PMC5091931/

Bangerter, L. R., Van Haitsma, K., Heid, A. R., & Abbott, K. (2016). "Make me feel at ease and at home": Differential care preferences of nursing home residents. *The Gerontologist, 56*(4), 702–713. https://doi.org/10.1093/geront/gnv026

Bauer, S., & Kantayya, V. S. (2010). Improving access to primary care and health outcomes in migrant farm worker populations: Challenges and opportunities. *Disease-a-Month, 56*(12), 706–718. https://doi.org/10.1016/j.disamonth.2010.10.004

Baughman, R. A., Stanley, B., & Smith, K. E. (2022). Second job holding among direct care workers and nurses: Implications for COVID-19 transmission in long-term care. *Medical Care Research and Review, 79*(1), 151–160. https://doi.org/10.1177/1077558720974129

Berdes, C., & Eckert, J. M. (2001). Race relations and caregiving relationships: A qualitative examination of perspectives from residents and nurse's aides in three nursing homes. *Research on Aging, 23*(1), 109–126. https://doi.org/10.1177/0164027501231006

Centers for Disease Control and Prevention. (2004). *National Nursing Assistant Survey.* https://www.cdc.gov/nchs/nnhs/nnas.htm

Centers for Disease Control and Prevention. (2017, Jan. 27). *Diversity and inclusion management.* http://medbox.iiab.me/modules/en-cdc/www.cdc.gov/minorityhealth/diversityandinclusion/index.html

Centers for Disease Control and Prevention. (2022, May). *Post-acute and long-term care providers and services users in the United States, 2017–2018.* https://www.cdc.gov/nchs/data/series/sr_03/sr03-047.pdf

Centers for Medicare & Medicaid Services. (2000). *Nursing home data compendium 2000.* https://www.cms.gov/Medicare/Provider-Enrollment-and-Certification/CertificationandComplianc/Downloads/NHDataComp2000_Part1.pdf

Centers for Medicare & Medicaid Services. (2015). *Nursing home data compendium.* https://www.cms.gov/Medicare/Provider-Enrollment-and-certification/CertificationandComplianc/Downloads/nursinghomedatacompendium_508-2015.pdf

Chang, Y. J., Siegel, B., & Wilkerson, G. (2012). Measuring healthcare disparities and racial segregation in Missouri nursing homes. *Journal for Healthcare Quality, 34*(1), 16–25. https://doi.org/10.1111/j.1945-1474.2011.00135.x

Chisholm, L., Weech-Maldonado, R., Laberge, A., Lin, F. C., & Hyer, K. (2013). Nursing home quality and financial performance: Does the racial composition of residents matter? *Health Services Research, 48*(6 Pt 1), 2060–2080. https://doi.org/10.1111/1475-6773.12079

Davis, M., & Aguilar, M. (2008). *Minority and multicultural health related sites.* Minnesota Department of Health.

Debesay, J., Arora, S., & Fougner, M. (2022). Organisational culture and ethnic diversity in nursing homes: A qualitative study of healthcare workers' and ward nurses' experiences. *BMC Health Services Research, 22*(1), 843. https://doi.org/10.1186/s12913-022-08184-y

Dill, J., Frogner, B., & Travers, J. (2022). Taking the long view: Understanding the rate of second job holding among long-term care workers. *Medical Care Research and Review, 79*(6), 844–850. https://doi.org/10.1177/10775587221089414

Dodson, L., & Zincavage, R. M. (2007). "It's like a family": Caring labor, exploitation, and race in nursing homes. *Gender & Society, 21*(6), 905–928. https://doi.org/10.1177/0891243207309899

Falvey, J., Hade, E., Friedman, S., Deng, R., & Travers, J. (2021). Impact of neighborhood socioeconomic disadvantage on staffing hours in US nursing homes. *Innovation in Aging, 5*(Suppl. 1), 979–980.

Falvey, J. R., Hade, E. M., Friedman, S., Deng, R., Jabbour, J., Stone, R. I., & Travers, J. L. (2022). Severe neighborhood deprivation and nursing home staffing in the United States. *Journal of the American Geriatrics Society, 71*(3), 1–9. https://doi.org/10.1111/jgs.17990

Feng, Z., Lepore, M., Clark, M. A., Tyler, D., Smith, D. B., Mor, V., & Fennell, M. L. (2011). Geographic concentration and correlates of nursing home closures: 1999–2008. *Archives of Internal Medicine, 171*(9), 806–813. https://doi.org/10.1001/archinternmed.2010.492

Fennell, M. L., Feng, Z., Clark, M. A., & Mor, V. (2010). Elderly Hispanics more likely to reside in poor-quality nursing homes. *HealthAffairs, 29*(1), 65–73. https://doi.org/10.1377/hlthaff.2009.0003

Foner, N. (1994). *The caregiving dilemma: Work in an American nursing home.* University of California Press. https://www.ucpress.edu/book/9780520203372/the-caregiving-dilemma

Grabowski, D. C. (2001, March). Does an increase in the Medicaid reimbursement rate improve nursing home quality? *The Journals of Gerontology: Series B, 56*(2), S84–S93. https://doi.org/10.1093/geronb/56.2.s84

Grabowski, D. C. (2022). Putting the nursing and home in nursing homes. *Innovation in Aging, 6*(4), igac029. https://doi.org/10.1093/geroni/igac029

Grabowski, D. C., & McGuire, T. G. (2009). Black-white disparities in care in nursing homes. *Atlantic Economic Journal, 37*(3), 299–314. https://doi.org/10.1007/s11293-009-9185-7

Hall, W. J., Chapman, M. V., Lee, K. M., Merino, Y. M., Thomas, T. W., Payne, B. K., Eng, E., Day, S. H., & Coyne-Beasley, T. (2015). Implicit racial/ethnic bias among health care professionals and its influence on health care outcomes: A systematic review. *American Journal of Public Health, 105*(12), e60–e76. https://doi.org/10.2105/AJPH.2015.302903

HealthinAging.org. (2015). *Eldercare at home: Choosing a nursing home: Caregiving how to's.* https://www.healthinaging.org/tools-and-tips/caregiver-guide-choosing-nursing-home

Holmberg, S. D., Spradling, P. R., Moorman, A. C., & Denniston, M. M. (2013). Hepatitis C in the United States. *The New England Journal of Medicine, 368*(20), 1859–1861. https://doi.org/10.1056/NEJMp1302973

Institute of Medicine (US) Committee on Understanding and Eliminating Racial and Ethnic Disparities in Health Care, Smedley, B. D., Stith, A. Y., & Nelson, A. R. (Eds.). (2003). *Unequal treatment: Confronting racial and ethnic disparities in health care.* National Academies Press.

Johnson, R., Popejoy, L. L., & Radina, M. E. (2010). Older adults' participation in nursing home placement decisions. *Clinical Nursing Research, 19*(4), 358–375. https://doi.org/10.1177/1054773810372990

Jolley, C. E., & Peck, L. P. (2022, May 31). Diversity, equity, & inclusion policies of national nursing organizations. *The Online Journal of Issues in Nursing, 27*(2), Manuscript 2.

The John A. Hartford Foundation. (n.d.). *Revisiting the teaching nursing home.* https://www.johnahartford.org/grants-strategy/revisiting-the-teaching-nursing-home

Kaiser Family Foundation (2022, July). *Total number of residents in certified nursing facilities.* https://www.kff.org/other/state-indicator/number-of-nursing-facility-residents/?currentTimeframe=1&sortModel=%7B%22colId%22:%22Location%22,%22sort%22:%22asc%22%7D

LaVeist, T. A. (2011). *Minority populations and health: An introduction to health disparities in the United States.* John Wiley & Sons.

Li, Y., & Mukamel, D. B. (2010). Racial disparities in receipt of influenza and pneumococcus vaccinations among US nursing-home residents. *American Journal of Public Health, 100* (Suppl. 1), S256–S262. https://doi.org/10.2105/AJPH.2009.173468

Li, Y., Yin, J., Cai, X., Temkin-Greener, J., & Mukamel, D. B. (2011). Association of race and sites of care with pressure ulcers in high-risk nursing home residents. *JAMA, 306*(2), 179–186. https://doi.org/10.1001/jama.2011.942

Mack, D. S., Jesdale, B. M., Ulbricht, C. M., Forrester, S. N., Michener, P. S., & Lapane, K. L. (2020). Racial segregation across U.S. nursing homes: A systematic review of measurement and outcomes. *The Gerontologist, 60*(3), e218–e231. https://doi.org/10.1093/geront/gnz056

Marselas, K. (2021, May 21). *'Put some meat on the bone' to create meaningful diversity programs.* McKnights Senior Living. https://www.mcknightsseniorliving.com/home/news/put-some-meat-on-the-bone-to-create-meaningful-diversity-programs/

Merriam-Webster Dictionary. (n.d.). *Inequity.* https://www.merriam-webster.com/dictionary/inequity

Michas, F. (2022, Oct. 10). *Number of residents in certified nursing facilities in the United States as of 2022, by state.* Statista. https://www.statista.com/statistics/1168843/number-residents-certified-nursing-facilities-state/

Mor, V., Zinn, J., Angelelli, J., Teno, J. M., & Miller, S. C. (2004). Driven to tiers: Socioeconomic and racial disparities in the quality of nursing home care. *The Milbank Quarterly, 82*(2), 227–256. https://doi.org/10.1111/j.0887-378X.2004.00309.x

National Academies of Sciences, Engineering, and Medicine. (2022). *The national imperative to improve nursing home quality: Honoring our commitment to residents, families, and staff.* National Academies Press. https://doi.org/10.17226/26526

National Academies of Sciences, Engineering, and Medicine, Health and Medicine Division; Board on Population Health and Public Health Practice; Committee on Community-Based Solutions to Promote Health Equity in the United States; Baciu, A., Negussie, Y., Geller, A., & Weinstein, J. N. (Eds.). (2017). *Communities in action: Pathways to health equity.* National Academies Press. PMID: 28418632

National Governors Association. (2022, Nov. 1). *Addressing wages of the direct care workforce through Medicaid policies.* https://www.nga.org/publications/addressing-wages-of-the-direct-care-workforce-through-medicaid-policies/

PHI. (n.d.). *U.S. nursing assistants employed in nursing homes: Key facts.* https://www.phinational.org/wp-content/uploads/legacy/phi-nursing-assistants-key-facts.pdf

Pruitt, N. (2013). *Quality of care in skilled nursing care centers.* American Health Care Association.

Rosenthal, E. L., Brownstein, J. N., Rush, C. H., Hirsch, G. R., Willaert, A. M., Scott, J. R., Holderby, L. R., & Fox, D. J. (2010). Community health workers: Part of the solution. *HealthAffairs, 29*(7), 1338–1342. https://doi.org/10.1377/hlthaff.2010.0081

Spanko., A. (2020, Oct. 26). *Lawmakers implement stricter nursing home staffing ratios in early COVID-19 hotspot.* Skilled Nursing News. https://skillednursingnews.com/2020/10/lawmakers-implement-higher-nursing-home-staffing-ratios-in-early-covid-19-hotspot/

Spector, W. D., & Takada, H. A. (1991). Characteristics of nursing homes that affect resident outcomes. *Journal of Aging and Health, 3*(4), 427–454. https://doi.org/10.1177/089826439100300401

Thomas, O. (2021, April 13). *What is health equity and why is it so important?* Nationwide Children's Hospital. https://www.nationwidechildrens.org/family-resources-education/700childrens/2021/04/health-equity-why-important

Travers, J. L., Agarwal, M., Estrada, L. V., Dick, A. W., Gracner, T., Wu, B., & Stone, P. W. (2021). Assessment of coronavirus disease 2019 infection and mortality rates among nursing homes with different proportions of Black residents. *Journal of the American Medical Directors Association, 22*(4), 893–898.e2. https://doi.org/10.1016/j.jamda.2021.02.014

Travers, J. L., Dick, A. W., & Stone, P. W. (2018). Racial/ethnic differences in receipt of influenza and pneumococcal vaccination among long-stay nursing home residents. *Health Services Research, 53*(4), 2203–2226. https://doi.org/10.1111/1475-6773.12759

Travers, J. L., Dick, A. W., Wu, B., Grabowski, D. C., Robison, J., Agarwal, M., Perera, G. U., & Stone, P. W. (2022). A profile of Black and Latino older adults receiving care in nursing homes: 2011–2017. *Journal of the American Medical Directors Association, 23*(11), 1833–1837.

Travers, J. L., Hirschman, K. B., & Naylor, M. D. (2020). Adapting Andersen's expanded behavioral model of health services use to include older adults receiving long-term services and supports. *BMC Geriatrics, 20*(1), 58. https://doi.org/10.1186/s12877-019-1405-7

Travers, J. L., Schroeder, K. L., Blaylock, T. E., & Stone, P. W. (2018). Racial/ethnic disparities in influenza and pneumococcal vaccinations among nursing home residents: A systematic review. *The Gerontologist, 58*(4), e205–e217. https://doi.org/10.1093/geront/gnw193

Travers, J. L., Teitelman, A. M., Jenkins, K. A., & Castle, N. G. (2020). Exploring social-based discrimination among nursing home certified nursing assistants. *Nursing Inquiry, 27*(1), e12315. https://doi.org/10.1111/nin.12315

University of Michigan. (n.d.). *Defining diversity, equity and inclusion.* https://diversity.umich.edu/about/defining-dei/

US Bureau of Labor Statistics. (2019, May). *Occupational employment and wage statistics: Nursing care facilities (skilled nursing facilities).* https://www.bls.gov/oes/2019/may/naics4_623100.htm

US Bureau of Labor Statistics. (2021a, May). *Occupational employment and wage statistics: Nurse practitioners.* https://www.bls.gov/oes/current/oes291171.htm

US Bureau of Labor Statistics. (2021b, May). *Occupational employment and wage statistics: Nursing assistants.* https://www.bls.gov/oes/current/oes311131.htm

US Bureau of Labor Statistics. (2021c, May). *Occupational employment and wage statistics: Physician assistants.* https://www.bls.gov/oes/current/oes291071.htm

US Bureau of Labor Statistics. (2021d, May). *Occupational employment and wage statistics: Physicians.* https://www.bls.gov/oes/current/oes291229.htm

US Bureau of Labor Statistics. (2021e, May). *Occupational employment and wage statistics: Registered nurses.* https://www.bls.gov/oes/current/oes291141.htm

US Department of Labor. (2013, September). *Home health care and the companionship services exemption under the Fair Labor Standards Act (FLSA).* https://www.dol.gov/agencies/whd/fact-sheets/25-flsa-home-healthcare

Whitfield, K. E., & Baker, T. A. (2013). *Handbook of minority aging.* Springer Publishing.

Wodchis, W. P., Hirth, R. A., & Fries, B. E. (2007). Effect of Medicaid payment on rehabilitation care for nursing home residents. *Health Care Financing Review, 28*(3), 117–129.

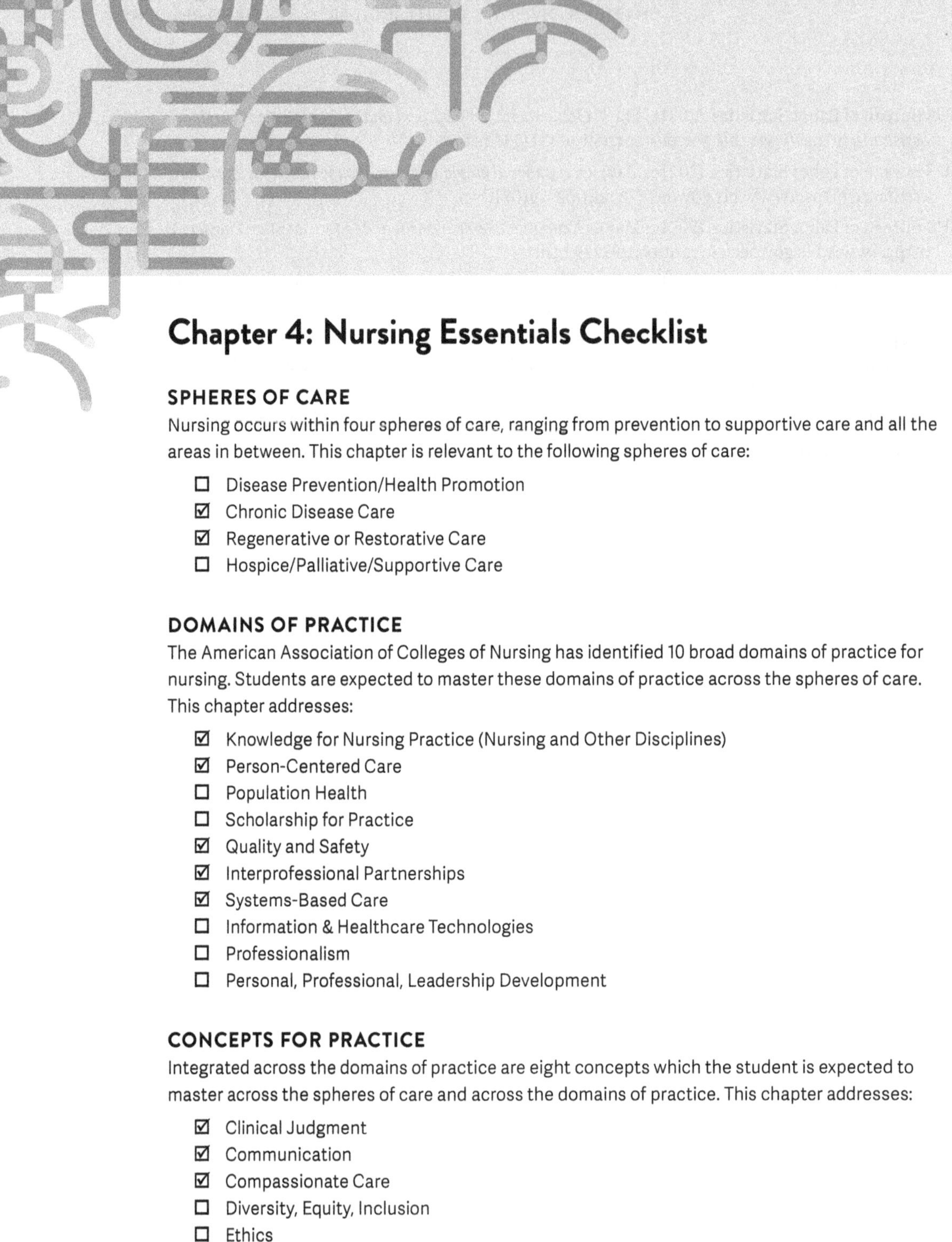

Chapter 4: Nursing Essentials Checklist

SPHERES OF CARE

Nursing occurs within four spheres of care, ranging from prevention to supportive care and all the areas in between. This chapter is relevant to the following spheres of care:

- ☐ Disease Prevention/Health Promotion
- ☑ Chronic Disease Care
- ☑ Regenerative or Restorative Care
- ☐ Hospice/Palliative/Supportive Care

DOMAINS OF PRACTICE

The American Association of Colleges of Nursing has identified 10 broad domains of practice for nursing. Students are expected to master these domains of practice across the spheres of care. This chapter addresses:

- ☑ Knowledge for Nursing Practice (Nursing and Other Disciplines)
- ☑ Person-Centered Care
- ☐ Population Health
- ☐ Scholarship for Practice
- ☑ Quality and Safety
- ☑ Interprofessional Partnerships
- ☑ Systems-Based Care
- ☐ Information & Healthcare Technologies
- ☐ Professionalism
- ☐ Personal, Professional, Leadership Development

CONCEPTS FOR PRACTICE

Integrated across the domains of practice are eight concepts which the student is expected to master across the spheres of care and across the domains of practice. This chapter addresses:

- ☑ Clinical Judgment
- ☑ Communication
- ☑ Compassionate Care
- ☐ Diversity, Equity, Inclusion
- ☐ Ethics
- ☑ Evidence-Based Practice
- ☐ Health Policy
- ☐ Social Determinants of Health

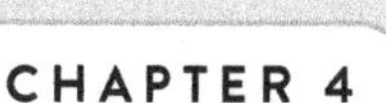

PERSON- AND FAMILY-CENTERED CARE: COMPREHENSIVE CARE PLANNING

Marie Boltz, PhD, GNP-BC, FGSA, FAAN
Katherine M. Abbott, PhD, MGS, FGSA
Amy Berman, RN, LDH(hon), FAAN
Sam Fazio, PhD
Sheila L. Molony, PhD, APRN, FAAN
Kim Ratliff, BSN, RN
Kimberly Van Haitsma, PhD , FGSA
Sheryl Zimmerman, PhD

OBJECTIVES

1. Define person- and family-centered care and the elements that comprise it.
2. Use tools to assess preferences for care and activities.
3. Adopt function-focused care as the foundation for nursing practice in nursing homes.

INTRODUCTION

Person- and family-centered care has been examined in the literature for many years, starting in the 1960s. The Institute for Healthcare Improvement (IHI) in partnership with the Institute for Patient- and Family-Centered Care, funded by the Robert Wood Johnson Foundation, created a program that incorporates reliable approaches that are evidence-based and can be measured. These two organizations have long been known as exceptional resources for how to define patient and family care and then build the momentum that's so necessary to achieve this work. A paper by Conway et al. (2006) provides a roadmap for how to achieve success in patient- and family-centered care.

Any of us who work in the clinical area know that this seemingly easy construct is challenging and at the same time incredibly rewarding.

Core concepts for this care include dignity and respect, information-sharing, participation, and collaboration (Johnson et al., 2009). We have come a long way since the 1960s toward achieving the integration of these concepts into practice. Back then, it was not unusual for a patient and family to have no access to their healthcare information or record. Sadly, very often the patient did not even know their diagnosis, especially if it was cancer. That information was kept from the patient for fear of scaring them. The Institute of Medicine report *Crossing the Quality Chasm* (2001) underscored the need for patient- and family-centered care and set forth principles to redesign and improve care, which included the following:

- Care based in continuous healing relationships
- Customization based on patient needs and values
- Patients as the source of control
- Shared knowledge in the free flow of information
- The need for transparency

Much of the literature has been written generally to address any care setting, but some have gone farther to document family-centered care in nursing homes and in particular for those with dementia (Lopez et al., 2013).

It is extremely important that we think about person- and family-centered care as a continuum no matter where the older person resides and no matter who is providing the care. Continuity is essential for the patient and the family for them to feel real trust and confidence in the healthcare team.

The purpose of this chapter is to review patient- and family-centered care with an emphasis on the long-term care setting and the way that setting serves as a hub for information translation and for fidelity to the patient's goals and preferences.

AACN ESSENTIALS

The American Association of Colleges of Nursing (AACN) "Essentials" (2021) outline several key competencies required for person-centered assessment and care. These include demonstrating empathy, compassionate care, and mutual respect with the individual and family. Establishing a relationship with the resident and family is essential to understand the values, beliefs, and personal histories that infuse artful nursing care. Empathy is cultivated by being fully present with other human beings and trying to understand their current experience or situation, through their eyes. Understanding what matters in a particular situation is essential to identify the possibilities for hope, healing, and well-being (Benner & Wrubel, 1989). The AACN Essentials (2021) highlight the role of skillful nursing assessment to gather the necessary data to provide excellent care. Person-centered care is informed by pre-assessment reflection where the nurse uses caring intention to focus on the experience of the other person. The nurse asks three self-reflective questions (Molony et al., 2018):

1. How will I demonstrate empathy and respect for this person's uniqueness and wholeness during the assessment process?
2. How will I demonstrate that I value therapeutic partnership with this person and family?
3. How will I demonstrate hope and therapeutic optimism for quality of living?

THE 4MS OF AGE-FRIENDLY CARE

The Age-Friendly Health System movement—led by IHI since 2016 in partnership with the American Hospital Association and the Catholic Health Association—is an exceptionally well-suited framework for addressing person- and family-centered care and comprehensive care planning. The essential elements of Age-Friendly care consist of a set of what is called the *4Ms: What Matters, Mentation, Medication, and Mobility.* The 4Ms have been published in the literature and have gotten exceptional traction in healthcare systems. The opportunity now is to ensure that the Age-Friendly Health System approach is reliable and consistent across any location of care, no matter who provides the care (Fulmer & Berman, 2016; Mate et al., 2018). Now in nearly 3,000 locations of care with over 400 nursing homes participating, the 4M set and concomitant measurement strategies create a perfect vehicle for ensuring a shared language across care settings for the benefit of patients and families.

Chapter 2 outlined the positive benefits of this approach, and the Revisiting the Teaching Nursing Home initiative in the state of Pennsylvania is advancing the evidence and knowledge needed to ensure that Age-Friendly care in nursing homes is patient- and family-centered and addresses what matters. The opportunity to get essential information from nursing assistants, the physical therapy team, the dietary team, the housekeeping team, and any other group of people interacting with the patient and family is imperative. A nursing home guide has been published by IHI (2020) that is readily accessible and provides clear steps to achieving evidenced-based 4M care in nursing homes. The 4Ms are being tested in the Revisiting the Teaching Nursing Home program, originally funded by the Robert Wood Johnson Foundation from 1982 to 1987.

The original program envisioned an embedded partnership between nursing homes and academic nursing schools (Shaughnessy et al., 1995). The program was discontinued in 1987 when funding was no longer available, but then the COVID-19 pandemic unveiled the dramatic need for new approaches to strengthening nursing home faculty and staff. This renewed approach is implementing a contemporary version of the Teaching Nursing Home model in three regions of Pennsylvania to demonstrate how enhanced partnerships between academic nursing schools and skilled nursing facilities can improve quality and cost outcomes. The project draws upon existing resources from the Age-Friendly Health Systems initiative (IHI, 2020) while integrating lessons learned and partnerships created through the COVID-19 pandemic and the original Teaching Nursing Home (Mezey et al., 2008) implementation from the 1980s.

The Pennsylvania State University College of Nursing, University of Pennsylvania School of Nursing (Penn Nursing), and University of Pittsburgh School of Nursing are each providing faculty and educational support to achieve the program goals. The Jewish Healthcare Foundation, Henry L. Hillman Foundation, and Independence Foundation co-fund this initiative, and partnerships are now taking place in this revised contemporary program. The advent of the internet and online learning as well as the capacity to hold meetings via interactive platforms have fundamentally changed the speed with which faculty and staff can communicate in real time.

Assessing Preferences for Care and Activities

For several years, there has been an ongoing effort to reframe Alzheimer's and dementia from a negative medicalized experience (i.e., one of inexorable loss) to one that is a social process (Gaugler et al., 2019). By reframing Alzheimer's and dementia as a social process, the emphasis shifts from the limitations of the person living with Alzheimer's and dementia to structural limitations of the physical and social environment that inhibit their ability to engage. Reframing Alzheimer's and dementia moves the narrative of Alzheimer's and dementia from solely a negative experience to one that also incorporates experiences where individuals continue to learn, make meaningful contributions, and age successfully.

At the same time, there has been an effort to move away from a deficit-based model of assessment, which is static and tends to predict and control, to a strength-based model, which is dynamic and encourages one to discover and adapt. A strength-based model focuses on what the individual can do rather than what they can't do and encourages us to explore possibilities for continued function, connection, and relationships. Using this information about who the person is and what they can do should inform our every interaction and experience.

Holism and holistic assessment are core values in nursing (Essential 2.3c; AACN, 2021). *Strengths-based nursing* is an approach inclusive of uniqueness, embodiment, subjective reality and created meaning, self-determination, collaborative partnership, health and healing, and learning, timing, and readiness (Gottlieb, 2014). Assessing individuals with or without a diagnosis of dementia warrants an understanding of the person's unique abilities, skills, and strengths, as well as their personal concerns, needs, and goals. These are often gathered in the context of the narrative life story (Mast, 2011). Tuning into the experiential world and subjective reality of the other person; spending time being with the person in a way that enables attunement to the signals from the body, mind, and spirit; and recognizing the importance of timing during care are all components of skillful, caring nursing processes.

Recognizing dementia as an experience of changing skill sets rather than as a disease helps optimize skills that remain strong (e.g., noticing beauty, reflecting others' emotions, experiencing joy) while supporting aspects of life that depend on ebbing skills (e.g., memory or problem-solving; Cornish, 2019). True collaboration and person-centered care means listening to the voices and expressions of individuals living with dementia and to the lived experience of living positively with dementia. Individuals and families living positively with dementia speak of love, humor, hope, giving thanks, seeking pleasure and enjoyment, as well as "still being me," growing, and transcending (Wolverson et al., 2016).

The Alzheimer's Association's dementia care practice recommendations (Fazio et al., 2018) for person-centered assessment and care planning include an emphasis on the dynamic, situational experience of the person with dementia and care partner (Molony et al., 2018). One of the most important domains of assessment is the inquiry into strengths and facilitators of well-being. What brings a sense of accomplishment? What is the person typically doing when having fun? What types of activities bring serenity, calmness, or a positive mood? What routines and rituals help the person to feel like themselves? What do they look forward to? The assessment guidelines also highlight many important issues inherent in the 4M model. Persons with cognitive impairment are at increased risk for excess disability due to the effects of polypharmacy, deliriogenic medicines, and medication adverse effects. The role of embodiment in dementia care requires comprehensive, skillful assessment for hidden conditions such as orthopnea with dyspnea at rest, undetected dental abscesses, or electrolyte imbalances that silently assail physical and cognitive function.

Timing and readiness are also relevant to strengths-based nursing. Living with dementia is dynamic and situational. What matters at a given point in time will change as the person's experience of the internal and external world changes. Fostering positive experiences within the physical, social, and existential environment requires humanistic approaches and artful nursing.

Another key element of strengths-based nursing is person-environment integration. People have the potential to thrive when there is harmony between the physical, social, and human environment (Gottlieb, 2014; Haight et al., 2002). Expanding the perspective of person-centered care to include person-environment-centered care provides another lens on "what matters."

Harmony between all levels of the environment is best encapsulated in the context of "person-environment fit"—the extent to which the characteristics of the individual and the environment match (Chaudhury & Oswald, 2019). If there is an optimal match, well-being will be maximized to the extent possible. For example, the availability of a walker and the absence of rugs on the floor promote mobility. Less evident is the consequence of poor fit in relation to mentation. Environmental characteristics may create "press" on an individual's psychological state (Lawton & Nahemow, 1973) and result in stress that exceeds the person's ability to cope (Smith et al., 2006) and unmet needs (Algase et al., 1996). Examples of poor fit in this context include an individual who resists care because bath water is too hot or the environment is too noisy (Scales et al., 2018). The utility of this framework is that it demonstrates that the environment is modifiable and should be considered in care assessment and planning.

Assessing and Cultivating At-Homeness

At-homeness is the human experience of person-environment integration and is an ongoing, dynamic process of reconnecting with self in the context of situational change (Molony, 2010). As health, function, residential dwelling, relationships, and/or sense of self change, reestablishing at-homeness requires acknowledging and honoring the most salient aspects of the situation from the point of view of the person experiencing it. At-homeness is strengthened by experiences that have personal significance to an individual in the context of their own self-concept, history, and physical and social world. At-homeness may be described using four experiential subdomains:

- **Personal power** includes autonomy, self-efficacy, and agency. It is amplified by perceived freedom and self-efficacy (Dawson et al., 2013; Molony et al., 2011).
- **Refuge** is an experience of comfort, safety, and wholeness in the context of perceived threats to self (physical, emotional, social, spatial, or spiritual). Refuge is strengthened by leaving and returning to a place of comfort and relaxation or by being protected from perceived threats to wholeness.
- **Relationship** encompasses the people, pets, possessions, places, values, cultural practices, symbols, and ideas that enable belonging, mutuality, and love. Relationship is strengthened by connection to loved others as well as to symbolic representations of cherished people, places, and ideas.
- **Self-reconciliation** means recognizing and reconnecting to oneself in the context of one's personal history, present situation, and anticipated future. This includes connecting with one's strengths as well as opening a space for new possibilities, new identities, hope, and growth. Self-reconciliation may be challenged by memory impairment that distances the person from their own history or impairs recognition of significant people or places (Zingmark et al., 1993).

Searching for home may be a process of finding existential belonging and comfort and restoring one's sense of emplacement in the world. Nursing assessment that includes personal knowing enlightens the situated possibilities for caring and restoring at-homeness and self-reconciliation, particularly after relocation to a new dwelling (Hertz et al., 2016; Hirschman & Hodgson, 2018).

Using tools such as the Preferences for Everyday Living Inventory (PELI, described later in the chapter) to identify meaningful preferences for living provides insight into the types of experiences that strengthen person-environment relationship and at-homeness. Using meaningful preferences to guide caring actions enables discrete experiences of at-homeness. Examples of additional assessment questions and actions that may enable at-homeness are shown in Table 4.1.

TABLE 4.1 Assessment Questions and Actions

	SAMPLE ASSESSMENT QUESTIONS	ENABLE/EMPOWER/OPTIMIZE
Empowerment—do what I want	How would you complete this sentence: "If I could do something that I really wanted to do I would . . ."	Providing meaningful choices; enabling hopes and dreams; supporting "speaking up."
Empowerment—mastery, feel useful	What helps you to feel a sense of accomplishment? What helps you to feel useful?	Supporting personally meaningful goals; enabling self-care; enabling the ability to feel useful and care for others and/or places or things; avoiding infantilizing speech.
Refuge	How would you complete this sentence: "I feel safe when . . ." or "I wish I had more privacy for . . ." Tell me about a time when you felt "at peace." (Questions in the PELI about favorite taste, smells, sounds, sights, and sensations are also relevant.)	Creating familiar, comfortable, relaxing spaces (indoor and out); providing "special places" that provide respite from "usual rules"; fostering ease of navigability and journeying; enabling privacy and a sense of security; treating pain; protecting possessions; preventing perception of imprisonment.
Relationship	Complete these sentences: "I feel attached to [ ]." "[ ] is just like family to me." Are there any objects or possessions that are important to you? (Ask about important people, animals, spaces/places, values/beliefs, views/vistas/landscapes.)	Welcoming spaces, events, and opportunities for loved ones to gather meaningful possessions and meaningful symbols; removing acoustic and geographic barriers to forming new friendships.
Self-reconciliation	What are some of the important things to know about your life story? Complete these sentences: "I feel most like myself when . . ." or "I like to reminisce about . . ." or "I look forward to . . ."	Supporting routines or rituals of personal importance; aesthetic experiences; familiar objects, photos, music; telling one's story; restoring health after illness exacerbation.

	SAMPLE ASSESSMENT QUESTIONS	ENABLE/EMPOWER/OPTIMIZE
Person-environment integration	Tell me about an experience where you felt truly "at home in the world" or about an experience where you lost track of time. Do you have any favorite rituals? Are there any small everyday experiences that make you feel comforted?	Tracking positive experiences and signs of positive emotions, serenity, joy, and relaxation; sharing situational details with the team and using small trials to enhance these experiences; using evidence-based relocation guidelines to provide transitional care before, during, and after relocations to establish equilibrium and at homeness.

Persons with dementia or primary progressive aphasia may not be able to provide answers to these questions, as communicative skills are affected. Family members and carers may be able to provide insight, but it is also crucial for nurses to use presencing and collaborative partnership to sense and appreciate emotional and behavioral cues that convey pleasure, displeasure, frustration, interest, vitality, and boredom.

At-homeness is cultivated by attending to both the physical environment and the experiential environment (Molony & Rabig, 2023). Nurses' advocacy (Essential 9.3a; AACN, 2021) may be used to support architectural and design insights that provide humanistic dwellings and alternatives to hospital-inspired structures (Ferdous & Roberts, 2023). Intentional presence, empathy, and caring (Essentials 9.2a, b, and c; AACN, 2021) may be used to inform ongoing experiential assessment and person-centered care planning. The role of therapeutic design in supporting positive outcomes for people with dementia has been studied for many years (Calkins, 2018; Day et al., 2000). The physical design of a nursing home can empower or constrain independence, socialization, mobility, and sensory or experiential comfort, and efforts to redesign the long-term care environment to improve these structures are in process. Innovative models such as Green House (introduced in Chapter 1) or small house nursing homes are built from the ground up to prioritize these experiences.

The experience of at-homeness is not restricted to particular types of dwellings, however. These experiences may be enabled by places where people experience a sense of belonging, comfort, love, agency, and self-coherence. In a small, mixed-methods longitudinal study that explored trajectories of at-homeness during transitions to a small house model nursing home, some residents chose not to move to the new environment because they already experienced high levels of person-environment harmony in their current residence. For others, experiences of at-homeness were simply not perceived as possible in the physical, social, and experiential environment of the traditional long-term care setting (Molony et al., 2011).

Approaches to Care

Think for a moment about your daily routine. Are you an early riser or do you prefer to sleep in? Do you like to read, listen to particular music, or spend time with one person or in a larger group? These preferences, often lifelong, provide a source of pleasure, meaning, and autonomy. While these preferences do not disappear once someone moves into a nursing home, it can be difficult to convey important preferences to care team members. Federal regulations mandate a focus on person-centered care based on knowing and honoring resident preferences. Yet despite good intentions, preferences are often overlooked in the day-to-day press of nursing home life. When preferences are honored, residents report greater satisfaction with care. Staff may report higher job satisfaction when they know and honor resident preferences. However, experience shows providers need streamlined tools to capture and act upon these preferences to improve quality of care.

Fundamentally, good nursing care (Essential 2.1; AACN, 2021) considers what matters most to that person as a unique individual. This can be complex in caring for any individual, but it is especially so when a nurse is providing care to someone living with dementia. Crafting an approach to care involves four basic tasks (AACN, 2021):

1. Gathering information about how the person prefers to live their daily life (Essential 2.3)
2. Communicating those preferences to all who interact with that person (Essentials 2.2 and 2.9)
3. Using evidence and strength-based approaches to honor that individual's preferences for how they wish to live their daily life (Essential 2.5)
4. Continuously evaluating the quality of the individualized care approaches (Essential 2.7)

We will briefly review examples of each step in the process using older adults living in nursing homes as an example.

Gathering Information About How a Person Prefers to Live Their Life

We don't often stop to consider the specifics of what daily routines and activities are important to us and make us feel a sense of comfort and meaning in our daily life. Perhaps one of the main reasons we don't think much about it is that we may be physically, cognitively, and functionally able to act autonomously. Older adults who live in nursing homes face challenges to engaging autonomously in their daily life preferences, in part because of physical, cognitive, and functional limitations in their ability to act independently. But they also face challenges in living in a shared living environment where systems and routines may be aligned to act in accordance with organizational efficiencies rather than flex with individual preferences for each older adult residing there.

As a starting point, nurses need to have tools to more easily assess what matters to the older adults they care for. In the nursing home, the Minimum Data Set (MDS) 3.0, Section F is a good starting point (Saliba & Buchanan, 2008). This tool asks residents a total of 16 questions designed to assess aspects of both personal care and recreational activities that the resident may prefer.

In work that expands upon the MDS assessments, the PELI (Van Haitsma et al., 2013) is a questionnaire written in conversational language that helps nursing home staff understand what type of care would be responsive to individual preferences to people living in nursing homes (see Table 4.2). The inventory is constructed in such a way to allow a staff member to ask about anywhere from one to 72 types of daily preferences for living across five domains (Carpenter et al., 2000). Substantial work has been done to ensure that these preferences are asked in the voice of the resident and that the content covers major domains of everyday life (Abbott, Heid, et al., 2018; Abbott, Klumpp, et al., 2018; Van Haitsma et al., 2014).

There are many training materials (tip sheets, webinars, and videos) designed to help facilitate competencies in assessing preferences (see www.preferencebasedliving.com). Training materials cover complex areas such as engaging family and staff when the resident can't self-report their own preferences (Heid et al., 2017) and better understanding the circumstances around which a resident may change their minds about what is important to them (Heid et al., 2016).

TABLE 4.2 Domains and Example PELI

DOMAIN	EXAMPLE: HOW IMPORTANT IS IT TO YOU TO . . .
Social contact	Spend time one on one with someone?
Growth activities	Learn about topics that interest you?
Leisure activities	Be involved in cooking?
Self-dominion	Choose how you care for your hair?
Caregivers and care	Choose whether your daily caregiver is male or female?

Communicating Knowledge About Individual Resident Preferences to All Who Provide Care

Once a staff member completes the preference assessment and has gained important information about how that individual wants to live their daily life, the next step is to make sure every staff member that comes into regular contact with residents (e.g., housekeeping and maintenance) is knowledgeable about each resident's preferences. Preference information can be discussed in care planning meetings, shared in team huddles, or communicated during shift changes.

One technique that has been found to be useful and feasible is the creation of Preferences for Activities and Leisure (PAL) cards (Abbott, Heppner, et al., 2022). An example of a PAL card is shown in Figure 4.1, and Figure 4.2 shows how one might be used. PAL cards provide an easy tool to exchange information at a glance about a resident's background and important daily recreational and leisure preferences. Nursing homes that have used PAL cards have found that they promote more individualized care and spark conversations between staff, volunteers, and community members, contributing to a greater sense of connectedness. Training materials on how to create and use a PAL card can be found at https://www.preferencebasedliving.com/webinars/the-pal-card-quality-improvement-project/.

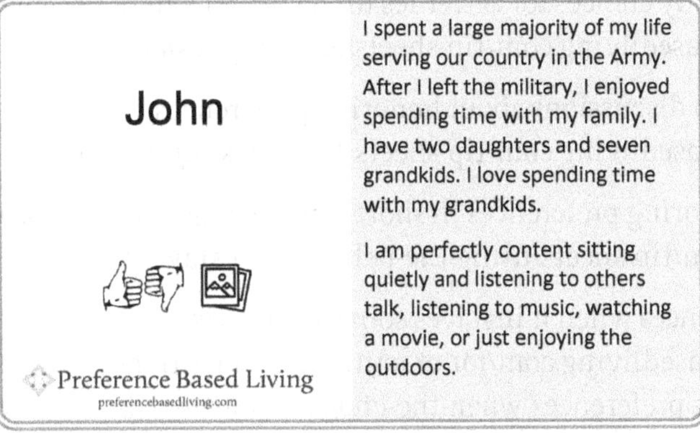

John

Preference Based Living
preferencebasedliving.com

I spent a large majority of my life serving our country in the Army. After I left the military, I enjoyed spending time with my family. I have two daughters and seven grandkids. I love spending time with my grandkids.

I am perfectly content sitting quietly and listening to others talk, listening to music, watching a movie, or just enjoying the outdoors.

Religion	Outdoor Activities
I am a devout Presbyterian. I love to spend my time listening to sermons or Christian music.	I enjoy spending time outside whenever possible, regardless of the weather. I would prefer just to sit outside and enjoy the fresh air and listen to nature.
Activities	**Socializing**
I enjoy spending time around children, either watching them play or listening to their stories.	I enjoy being around my family because they make me feel at home. I don't mind being around other people, but I probably won't engage in conversation.
TV & Music	**Communication Preferences**
I love to watch old Western movies, especially John Wayne movies. I also love to listen to big band music or Christian music.	When communicating with me, please use simple gestures or simple pictures to help me understand you and make choices.

FIGURE 4.1 Sample PAL card.

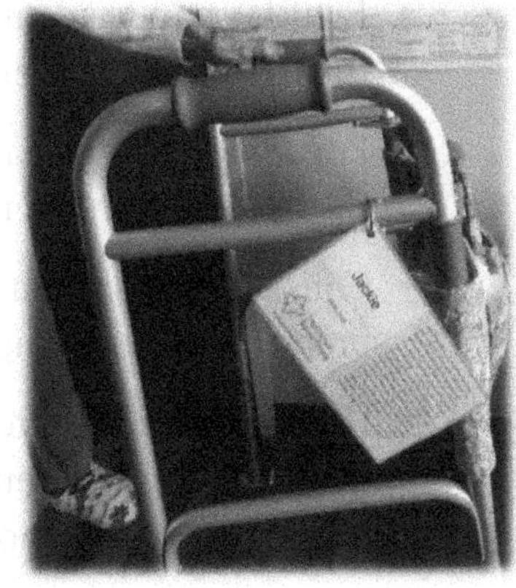

FIGURE 4.2 Sample PAL card in action.

Evidence-Based Innovative Approaches to Empowering Staff to Honor Residents' Wishes

Once community members are all aware of the important daily preferences for residents, the next step is to integrate and honor those preferences in day-to-day care delivery. Integrating preferences into care is no easy task, but again, many evidence-based approaches have been developed to make this easier to accomplish in the busy clinical environments of nursing homes. Approaches are available that help in the following areas:

- Integrating a resident's daily preferences into care plans (https://www.preferencebasedliving.com/tip-sheets/integrating-preferences-into-care-plans/)

- Facilitating a resident's daily choices for activities to the fullest extent possible (https://www.preferencebasedliving.com/tip-sheets/ensuring-resident-choice/)
- Engaging the care team in discussions about honoring preferences (https://www.preferencebasedliving.com/tip-sheets/helping-staff-engage/)
- Considerations when honoring preferences in short-stay settings (https://www.preferencebasedliving.com/tip-sheets/using-the-peli-in-short-stay-settings/)
- Honoring resident preferences when it involves some level of risk (https://www.preferencebasedliving.com/for-practitioners/practitioner/care-integration/honoring-preferences-when-the-choice-involves-risk/)
- Special considerations when honoring preferences during a pandemic quarantine (https://www.preferencebasedliving.com/tip-sheets/honoring-preferences-during-quarantine/)

One program that provides an excellent example of how to assess, honor, and evaluate the integration of preferences into care is called the brief Individualized Positive Psychosocial Interaction (IPPI) program (Van Haitsma et al., 2015). The IPPI program provides a step-by-step guide for care partners as they engage people living with dementia in positive ways that enhance the well-being of both the resident and the care partner. Numerous IPPI protocols and training materials show effective techniques to lead brief (about 10 minutes in length) personal care and leisure activities specially designed to build on the remaining strengths of persons living with dementia in the nursing home (Van Haitsma et al., 2015). Program materials are built around a simple framework of planning the interaction, doing the activity, gathering feedback from both residents and staff about the usefulness of the IPPIs, and ongoing quality improvement efforts to continuously adapt and improve the quality of the program over time.

Another example of how to honor resident's preferences for daily life is to examine how modifications of the physical environment may help to improve a resident's quality of life (Harrison et al., 2017). For example, to encourage food intake, make sure the person's favorite snack is available, that there is not too much distracting noise around the person, etc. (Herke et al., 2018).

Evaluating the Quality of Individualized Care via Quality Improvement Processes

After what matters most has been assessed, communicated, and integrated into care, the final step is to ensure that system-level processes are all working together to produce high quality of life and quality of care in the nursing home environment.

Developing competencies in performance improvement activities has been the focus of many efforts designed to create sustainable, high-quality care in nursing homes. For example, Abbott, Hulshult, et al. (2022) provided a detailed case example for how to integrate "agile" methods into nursing home care delivery. There have also been efforts to create pragmatic approaches to better understanding how to evaluate whether care is in alignment with resident preferences—e.g., making sure the daily care activities align with resident preferences (Van Haitsma et al., 2016). Finally, efforts are underway to develop a mobile responsive application to address paperwork burden in managing preference assessment (https://www.preferencebasedliving.com/compass/); see Table 4.3.

TABLE 4.3 Managing Preference Assessment

	ASSESSMENT	EVALUATION	OUTCOMES
Measure	Measures important resident preferences on how the resident would like to live daily life. Probing questions assist with learning specifics of ways to meaningfully integrate preferences into care.	Measures how often a person attends a preferred recreational activity in a given month. Individual reporting provides feedback on resident's level of participation in the life of the community. Audit tools assist with ensuring that plans of care reflect important preferences.	Resident satisfaction: Measures how satisfied a person may be with the fulfillment of an important preference. Resident engagement: Measures how engaged a resident is at preferred activities.
Benefit	Provides organization with a structured approach to honoring resident choice. Provides real-time tools to assist staff with creative ways to enhance resident engagement and streamlines planning to assist with prioritizing resident top interests.	Provides organizations with a tangible metric for demonstrating the provision of person-centered care. Provides reporting tools that pinpoint program strengths and opportunities for improving person-centered care programming.	Ensures high-quality person-centered recreational programming that reflects the needs and preferences of resident population.

CASE STUDY Putting Resident Preferences Into Action

Scenario 1

This event occurred when we started to focus on what matters. Our enhanced living coordinator started asking what brings our residents joy both when interviewing residents and also during resident council meetings. One resident said it was important to her to have her mother's sweet potato pie. The enhanced living staff arranged to have an activity where they made the sweet potato pie. The resident was thrilled to have the pie and share it with all her friends. This journey has enhanced the quality of life of residents through defining what is important to them.

Scenario 2

An independent living resident came to skilled nursing for rehabilitation after being hospitalized. Unfortunately, she was unable to return to her prior level of functioning and required 24-hour care and assistance with transfers. Her mobility was so impaired that she was also ineligible to go to personal care. As we discussed her living in skilled nursing, more discussions about what mattered to her came to light, which pushed us all out of our comfort zone. Her desire was to remain as active in the independent living community as she possibly could, which included having dinner in the main dining room, being involved in independent activities and committees, and going on trips with the independent residents.

These activities would not only take her outside of the supervision of the skilled nursing staff but also caused all departments to come together to figure out how to manage her requests. After re-adjusting our procedures, this resident is able to eat dinner with her friends at night, gather with her friends in the common area most of the day, and go on trips to various restaurants in the community. She returns to skilled nursing various times during the day for care and a little rest, and then she goes back out with her friends. She is living the life she desires while living in a skilled nursing facility where she receives the care she needs.

FUNCTION-FOCUSED CARE APPROACH

Physical function is considered to be a critical marker of health and influence upon quality of life. Older people have described the preservation of functional capability as even more important than longevity (National Institute for Health and Care Excellence, 2015). Physical function refers to activities of daily living (ADLs: bathing, dressing, transferring, continence, feeding) and instrumental activities of daily living (IADLs: cooking, cleaning, using transportation, laundry, managing finances).

Decline in physical function and physical activity is common in older adults and varies in its degree considerably from person to person. Over 80% of nursing home residents need help with three or more ADLs (Harris-Kojetin et al., 2019). Experts believe that a great deal of the functional loss results from inactivity and lack of engagement in self-care (Meneguci et al., 2021). Residents who have functional loss are at risk for persistent deconditioning, which then causes depression and negatively impacts cognition, further increasing functional decline (Colon-Emeric et al., 2013).

A significant challenge to promoting engagement in physical activity and self-care is the common perception that nursing home residents can't participate due to physical or cognitive limitations. Formal and informal caregivers tend to provide "total care" to the resident by focusing on task completion, thus taking away the person's ability to be as independent as possible (Resnick, Galik, et al., 2013). This focus on task completion does not acknowledge underlying capability and robs the resident of their remaining capabilities, resulting in further deconditioning and functional decline.

In contrast, a re-ablement philosophy focuses on the abilities and resources of older people to overcome losses, adapt, and maintain independence (Metzelthin et al., 2022). Similarly, *function-focused care* (FFC) is a philosophy of care that offers practical approaches to help the person restore lost function or optimize current function. FFC emphasizes assessing the person's capability and helping the person achieve or maintain their highest functional level by integrating physical activity into routine care interactions. Table 4.4 provides examples of FFC activities.

TABLE 4.4 Examples of Function-Focused Care Activities

Communication	Knowing the residents—their background, preferences, what matters—and using that information to encourage and motivate them Making sure hearing and vision devices, if needed, are accessible Focusing on emotions: Show empathy and affection with eye contact, smiling, listening, and validating For the person with dementia, use prompting, verbal cues, physical cues, modeling, and hand over hand as indicated Encouraging and supporting social connection with family and friends, including other residents Motivating the resident includes: • Social conversation and humor • Reminding: "You can do it" • Review the benefits of activity and remind them of how they are getting stronger • Celebrating success
Activities of daily living	Encouraging the resident to help move themselves in bed rather than automatically moving them Encouraging the use of the toilet rather than bedpans, urinals, and commodes; avoiding catheters whenever possible; prompted voiding Motivating and encouraging residents to participate in bathing, dressing, and grooming; consulting with rehab for assistive devices Motivating residents to walk more by having them walk to the dining room or activities (stopping to rest as needed rather than using a wheelchair) Encouraging residents to wheel themselves if a wheelchair is required Support self-feeding: Evaluate seating at meal, consult with occupational therapy if needed for seating and assistive devices; use prompts, hand over hand, finger foods for the person living with dementia if indicated
Physical activity	Encourage sit to stand exercises three times a day Assist/encourage exercise groups Provide/encourage lifting light weights while watching TV or waiting for an appointment Encourage participation in active games, dancing/movement, gardening, etc., based on preferences

The benefits of physical activity and FFC include improved mood, increased sense of well-being, less pain, and enhanced quality of life (Lee et al., 2019). Residents who have experienced a decline in their function during an illness and/or due to hospitalization can be helped to get back to baseline function by providing FFC activities (Boltz et al., 2014).

FFC is a systemic approach that addresses the barriers to FFC, which include:

1. Intrapersonal factors such as fear of falling, anxiety, depression, pain and other uncontrolled symptoms, cognitive impairment, underlying medical conditions such as anemia, and lack of motivation
2. Interpersonal factors including communication and interaction with staff and family, which discourages physical activity and self-care, staff knowledge about function, and how to promote it
3. Environmental factors such as unsafe walking areas, poor lighting, lack of assistive devices (e.g., walkers, glasses, hearing devices), beds that are too high or too low, etc.
4. Policy factors including the use of restraints and tethering devices (e.g., chair alarms and indwelling urinary catheters)

The FFC philosophy is incorporated into the direct care of residents including assessment and care planning as well as organizational approaches (environmental and policy modifications and staff, resident, and family education).

Assessment of Function

Medical diagnoses alone do not provide a reliable measure of physical function. In fact, a lengthy list of medical problems may not correlate at all with the degree of functional loss, as the older adult may have adapted to manage daily life with the diagnosed illnesses. Sources of adaptation include social support and engagement, optimal medical care, preserved cognition, a positive environment, and resilience (Colon-Emeric et al., 2013). The physical, cognitive, emotional, and social functioning of the older adult are all closely related and thus need to be assessed in tandem. The 4Ms provide a framework (Fulmer & Li, 2018) to assess the resident in order to develop a person-centered, FFC plan (see Table 4.5).

TABLE 4.5 Function-Focused Care Assessment Within the 4Ms Framework

M	DESCRIPTION
What matters	Information on the person's background, important relationships, and preferences for daily care, activities, and everyday routine are important to establish individualized goals and communicate in a positive manner. This data also guides a respectful approach, optimizes resident/staff relationships, conveys encouragement, and motivates the person to engage in function-promoting activity.
Mind/Mentation	The person's cognitive status and mood impact the person's ability to establish goals, follow directions, act with safety awareness, and follow through on a plan. Thus, periodic screenings for depression, delirium, and cognitive loss are essential components of a function-focused assessment. Also, fear of falling is a leading cause of immobility, which in turn increases the risk for falls. (See Chapter 6 for more information.) To develop a plan of care that promotes safe mobility, relevant questions include: Have you fallen before? Are you afraid of falling again?
Medications	Drugs that cause sedation or mobility problems or contribute to fall risk should be evaluated on an ongoing basis. These include benzodiazepines, antipsychotics, antidepressants, opioids, anticholinergics, and any medication that affects blood pressure (deVries et al., 2018; Seppala, van de Glind, et al., 2018; Seppala, Wermelinket et al., 2018). Medications to manage pain and other symptoms require diligent monitoring of their effectiveness and side effects.
Mobility and ADL	In the nursing home setting, the MDS reports on ADL functional performance (eating, oral hygiene, toileting hygiene, showering/bathing self, upper and lower body dressing, putting/taking off footwear, and personal hygiene) and need for help or assistance. Mobility (bed mobility, transfers, and walking) is also reported. It is important for the nurse to assess performance rather than rely on the reports of others and to evaluate ability, since performance does not always reflect ability. The Timed Up and Go test assesses the time that a person takes to rise from a chair, walk 3 meters, turn around 180 degrees, walk back to the chair, and sit down while turning 180 degrees (Podsiadlo & Richardson, 1991). The Basic Physical Capability Scale evaluates overall range of motion in all major upper and lower extremity joints; cognition (ability to follow a multiple step command); and muscle performance and balance (ability to get up from a chair; Resnick, Boltz, et al., 2013).

Function-Focused Care Planning and Interventions

Person-centered FFC plans are grounded in the assessment of the resident and are based on goals developed by the resident, the resident's preferred family, and the interdisciplinary team, including the nursing assistant. Function-focused goals address

ADLs (including self-personal care, mobility, meals, and toileting) and engagement in preferred activities. The SMART goal framework helps make goals more concrete and achievable. Using the acronym SMART, these goals are specific, measurable, attainable, relevant, and time-based (Gregory, 2018). Relevant goals reflect what matters to the resident. *What matters* guides the plan to meet goals and provides motivation to meet the goals. What matters goals may include, for example, regaining continence or being able to get in and out of a car to visit a family member's home. Care plan interventions should include what staff will do and what the resident will do and include family as indicated. Following is an example of a SMART goal with care plan interventions.

SMART goal that reflects *what matters*:

> "Within 90 days, I (the resident) will walk 300 feet to the dining room and back so that I will be able to walk down the aisle at my great-granddaughter's wedding."

Interventions:

1. The nursing assistant will provide contact-guard assistance for the resident to do sit to stands (10 repetitions) three times a day in the hallway using the grab-bar.
2. The resident will walk to the dining room three times a day with the nursing assistant following with a wheelchair, allowing stops to rest as needed, and the resident's daughter will provide encouragement and reminders about the upcoming wedding as a motivator.
3. The nurse will monitor blood pressure twice a week for orthostasis (a side effect of furosemide and carvedilol) and the need for acetaminophen for arthritic hip pain.
4. Physical therapy will monitor progress and increase prescribed walking distance when indicated.
5. Activities staff will encourage and assist to attend preferred physical activities (exercise bingo, daily dancing, balloon volleyball) and social /cognitive activities (daily current events, resident volunteer program).

The resident living with dementia requires adapted communication to accommodate impairments in memory, recall, executive function, and other challenges. These include communication that is brief and task-segmented (one step at a time), tactile (such as hand over hand technique), and includes the use of verbal or physical cues, chaining (getting the resident started with the activity), and modeling. These approaches should be utilized during all care interactions, including ADLs and meals. A consistent, structured daily routine that includes self-care, physical activity, and meaningful activities is important to promote optimal physical, social, and emotional function and a sense of security and well-being in the resident living with dementia. Continence can be promoted with a consistent toileting plan based on the resident's pattern of elimination. Physical activity, including walking, has been shown to decrease behavioral symptoms of distress while optimizing physical function. "Helping" activities such as vacuuming, dusting, and folding towels promote physical activity while increasing self-esteem in some residents (Boltz, 2020).

Environmental Approaches

In addition to the environmental considerations that accommodate age-related changes (e.g., adequate lighting and even non-glare flooring), there are specific approaches that align with FFC. They include walking areas that include pleasant destinations and rest spots, environmental cues, and equipment that supports activity and engagement in function such as appropriate chair, bed, and toilet height (80%–120% of lower leg length). Also, a relaxing environment that is consistent and free of distractions (e.g., a dining room that limits noise and foot traffic) supports emotional well-being so that the resident can focus on the task at hand and optimize their function.

Policies That Support FFC

Policies that support physical activity include those focused on safe mobility rather than merely fall prevention. The policy should emphasize identifying risk factors for falls (e.g., problems with gait and balance, medication use, medical problems, decreased safety awareness) and the interventions to mitigate risk. Other important policies that support FFC are those that guide and monitor pressure injury prevention and avoidance of restraints, indwelling urinary catheters, and other "tethers" such as chair alarms (Resnick et al., 2012).

Meals are especially important to both residents' health and quality of life. They provide not only nutritional sustenance but also a pleasant sensory experience and connection with staff and other residents (Liu et al., 2020). Function-focused policies maximize independence in eating and offer alternatives to hand feeding such as the use of assistive devices and food modification (e.g., finger foods that can be easily managed). In many nursing homes, residents are involved in setting up and clearing tables and baking and snack preparation (with assistance to implement infection control practices; Liu et al., 2015).

Over-reliance on wheelchairs is a concern in the nursing home, as residents may be encouraged to use wheelchairs out of expediency. Encouraging and assisting residents to walk whenever possible (e.g., "walk to dine" policy with groups of residents) helps maintain ambulation skills. For those residents who require wheelchairs, encouraging them to self-propel and transfer to a regular chair in the dining room promotes range of motion and strengthening. A policy that supports periodic assessment by physical and occupational therapy promotes their critical involvement in care planning, provision of modalities such as electrical stimulation for pain management, and the offering of function-promoting equipment such as adapted seating, grab-bars, mobility devices, and assistive devices for meals, bathing, and dressing.

FFC Education

Finally, staff, resident, and family training on FFC provided at their respective orientations and annual updates helps support a function-focused culture. The FFC training emphasizes a commitment to optimize the residents' function and promote their self-direction and describes the roles of the resident, family, and team members. FFC is promoted as a more effective and dignity-promoting alternative to restrictive policies for fall prevention such as restraint use and limiting mobility.

Organizational approaches are implemented so that FFC should be provided for every resident, every day, and with every encounter between the staff and the resident and between the family and the resident. A function-focused philosophy requires the involvement of the entire nursing home community—residents, families, and staff in all departments and roles.

Negotiated Risk

A barrier to honoring an individual's preferences is that staff may perceive the choice as risky. If you think about it, we all take risks every day. Why are we unwilling to allow for risk in the nursing home setting? Many will argue that nursing home providers have been tasked with keeping individuals in their care "safe." There is an inherent fear of being cited by surveyors if a resident is allowed to engage in something that may hurt them. For example, what if someone wants to eat a food that could present a choking hazard or go outside without a caregiver? How do you balance the tension between something that brings a resident joy but may also carry risk?

Fortunately, there are several tools that can be used to help mitigate potential risks associated with choices and preferences that may involve risk. The Preference Based Living website has a toolkit (see https://www.preferencebasedliving.com/for-practitioners/practitioner/care-integration/honoring preferences-when-the-choice-involves-risk/) that includes a guidebook, training video, infographics, and an interview with Liza Behrens, PhD, RN, who is leading efforts to advance our scientific understanding of pervasive risk avoidance (Behrens et al., 2020). The four-step guide includes:

1. Identify and understand the person's choice.
2. Discuss the choice and options with the person.
3. Develop a plan to honor the choice.
4. Carry out the plan and follow up.

PARTNERING WITH FAMILY AS TEAM MEMBERS

When a resident is admitted to the nursing home, family involvement changes but does not end. Families can play a critical role in assessment and the planning and delivery of care. They also provide visits/companionship, advocate for the resident, and in some instances help with personal care, meals, and activities. When needed, families provide vital information on the residents' preferences, health history, and functional status. Family involvement can promote positive relationships between staff and residents. Studies describe how families can ensure care quality and provide a touchstone to the resident's life, giving the resident a sense of self and identity and a sense of order and control (Gaugler & Mitchell, 2022). Residents have also reported relief from boredom when families visit and a sense of competence and achievement when maintaining family relationships (Graffigna et al., 2020; Puurveen et al., 2019). Family involvement in care also has been found to increase staff job satisfaction (Nguyen et al., 2015).

An understanding of the family response to the nursing home admission can help nurses support both the family and the resident. Family members are often dealing with a range of emotions at this time. They may be experiencing grief, guilt, and stress that can be significant enough to cause physical and psychological co-morbidity (Boltz & Galvin, 2013; Gaugler & Mitchell, 2022; Høgsnes et al., 2014). Priorities expressed by family members include sharing information and being involved in decision-making (Reid & Chappell, 2017). They have described barriers to communication with nursing home staff, including fears of being labeled as a "whiner" if they express worry or fears of retaliation if they complain. Lack of information is also described as a barrier to a positive relationship with both staff and the resident (Baumbusch & Phinney, 2014).

Upon admission of the resident, an important discussion about preferred family involvement should include both the resident and the family members. Opportunities for ongoing involvement include engagement in assessment, care planning, and decision-making; participation in activities and outings, laundry, and appointments; and helping with ADLs (eating, drinking, moving, bathing, toileting, or dressing) and behavioral manifestations of distress (Baumbusch & Phinney, 2014; Boogaard et al., 2017). Positive communication supports positive relationships with family members and includes:

- Positive informal communication, including greeting the family member and inquiring about their well-being and any concerns or worries. These conversations help make the family member feel welcome when visiting and make it easier for them to talk to staff (Hoek et al., 2021).
- Active listening and validation of family emotions without judgment (Aschieri et al., 2021).
- Avoiding descriptions of the resident using negative terms such as "difficult" or "combative."
- Avoiding the use of technical jargon (Puurveen et al., 2019).
- Communicating the successes and positive experiences of residents in addition to the problems (Hoek et al., 2021).

Additional strategies to support family members' effectiveness as members of the care team include:

- With the resident's agreement, consistently updating the family of changes in the resident's healthcare condition (Aschieri et al., 2021).
- Including the nursing assistant in care planning and updates to promote the relationship with family and resident (Nguyen et al., 2015).
- Avoiding the use of rigid, predetermined agendas at care conferences that prevent family from expressing their views (Puurveen et al., 2019).

Family members are integral to person-centered care. When nurses show concern and respect for them and include them in resident care, the resident and the entire nursing community benefit.

SUMMARY

There are several tenets guiding person- and family-centered care in the nursing home. The first is the concept of at-homeness which includes four dimensions: 1) personal power (resident autonomy, self-efficacy, and agency); 2) refuge (comfort, safety, and an environment that supports wholeness in health-physical, emotional, social, spatial, and spiritual); 3) relationship (the people, pets, possessions, places, values, cultural practices, symbols, and ideas that enable belonging, mutuality, and love); and 4) self-reconciliation (acknowledging strengths as well as potential for new possibilities, new identities, hope, and growth). At-homeness provides a philosophical base for person-centered care, and attention to its dimensions promotes the physical, psychological, and social well-being of the resident.

Another tenet is the commitment to honoring the preferences of the resident. In order to provide effective, individualized care, the nurse needs to understand the background, values, and preferences of the resident. "What Matters" to the resident should drive both the goals and associated care plan interventions including those that support optimized Mobility, Medication use, and Mentation/mind (the "4Ms"). The tenet of function-focused care (FFC) is based on the principle of strength-based care, wherein the nurse collaborates with other disciplines to integrate physical and cognitive activity and opportunities for meaningful socialization into the resident's daily routine. FFC recognizes the capabilities of the resident and emphasizes "doing with" rather than "doing for" the resident. The positive outcomes include lowered risk for functional decline, falls, depression, and other avoidable complications.

Finally, the residents' families are essential members of the nursing home team and are integral to person-centered care. They provide emotional security and connectivity to family and help the resident maintain a sense of identity. When nurses show concern and respect for families, provide information and education, and include them as desired by the resident in care, the resident, family, and entire nursing home community benefits.

REFERENCES

Abbott, K. M., Heid, A. R., Kleban, M., Rovine, M. J., & Van Haitsma, K. (2018, December). The change in nursing home residents' preferences over time. *The Journal of Post-Acute and Long-Term Care Medicine, 19*(12), 1092–1098. https://doi.org/10.1016/j.jamda.2018.08.004

Abbott, K. M., Heppner, A., Hicks, N., Hermesch, A., & Van Haitsma, K. (2022). Evaluating the implementation of a pragmatic person-centered communication tool for the nursing home setting: PAL cards. *Clinical Gerontologist, 45*(3), 634–646. https://doi.org/10.1080/07317115.2021.1929632

Abbott, K. M., Hulshult, A., Eshraghi, K., Heppner, A., Crumbie, V., Heid, A. R., Madrigal, C., Spector, A., & Van Haitsma, K. (2022, September). Applying agile methodology to reengineer the delivery of person-centered care in a nursing home: A case study. *The Journal of Post-Acute and Long-Term Care Medicine, 23*(9), 1442–1447. https://doi.org/10.1016/j.jamda.2022.05.012

Abbott, K. M., Klumpp, R., Leser, K. A., Straker, J. K., Gannod, G. C., & Van Haitsma, K. (2018, February). Delivering person-centered care: Important preferences for recipients of long-term services and supports. *The Journal of Post-Acute and Long-Term Care Medicine, 19*(2), 169–173. https://doi.org/10.1016/j.jamda.2017.10.005

Algase, D. L., Beck, C., Kolanowski, A., Whall, A., Berent, S., Richards, K., & Beattie, A. (1996). Need-driven dementia-compromised behavior: An alternative view of disruptive behavior. *American Journal of Alzheimer's Disease & Other Dementias, 11*(6). https://doi.org/10.1177/153331759601100603

American Association of Colleges of Nursing. (2021). *The essentials: Core competencies for professional nursing education.* https://www.aacnnursing.org/Portals/42/AcademicNursing/pdf/Essentials-2021.pdf

Aschieri, F., Barello, S., & Durosini, I. (2021, January). "Invisible voices": A critical incident study of family caregivers' experience of nursing homes after their elder relative's death. *Journal of Nursing Scholarship, 53*(1), 65–74. https://doi.org/10.1111/jnu.12610

Baumbusch, J., & Phinney, A. (2014, February). Invisible hands: The role of highly involved families in long-term residential care. *Journal of Family Nursing, 20*(1), 73–97. https://doi.org/10.1177/1074840713507777

Behrens, L. L., Boltz, M., Kolanowski, A., Sciegaj, M., Madrigal, C., Abbott, K., & Van Haitsma, K. (2020, Nov. 23). Pervasive risk avoidance: Nursing staff perceptions of risk in person-centered care delivery. *Gerontologist, 60*(8), 1424–1435. https://doi.org/10.1093/geront/gnaa099

Benner, P. E., & Wrubel, J. (1989). *The primacy of caring: Stress and coping in health and illness.* Addison-Wesley Pub. Co.

Boltz, M. (2020). Dementia assessment and care strategies. In M. Boltz, E. Capezuti, D. Zwicker, & T. Fulmer (Eds.), *Evidence-based geriatric nursing protocols for best practice* (6th ed., pp. 331–352). Springer.

Boltz, M., & Galvin, J. (2013). Post-acute needs of the person with dementia and their family caregivers [Abstract]. *The Gerontologist, 53.*

Boltz, M., Resnick, B., Chippendale, T., & Galvin, J. (2014). Testing a family-centered intervention to promote functional and cognitive recovery in hospitalized older adults. *Journal of the American Geriatrics Society, 62*(12), 2398–2407.

Boogaard, J. A., Werner, P., Zisberg, A., & van der Steen, J. T. (2017, December). Examining trust in health professionals among family caregivers of nursing home residents with advanced dementia. *Geriatrics & Gerontology International, 17*(12), 2466–2471. https://doi.org/10.1111/ggi.13107

Calkins, M. P. (2018). From research to application: Supportive and therapeutic environments for people living with dementia. *The Gerontologist, 58*(Suppl. 1), S114–S128. https://doi-org.libraryproxy.quinnipiac.edu/10.1093/geront/gnx146

Carpenter, B. D., Van Haitsma, K., Ruckdeschel, K., & Lawton, M. P. (2000). The psychosocial preferences of older adults: A pilot examination of content and structure. *The Gerontologist, 40,* 335–348. https://doi.org/10.1093/geront/40.3.335

Chaudhury, H., & Oswald, F. (2019). Advancing understanding of person-environment interaction in later life: One step further. *Journal of Aging Studies, 51,* 100821. https://doi-org.libraryproxy.quinnipiac.edu/10.1016/j.jaging.2019.1008

Colon-Emeric, C. S., Whitson, H. E., Pavon, J., & Hoenig, H. (2013). Functional decline in older adults. *American Family Physician, 88*(6), 388–394.

Conway, J., Johnson, B., Edgman-Levitan, S., Schlucter, J., Ford, D., Sodomka, P., & Simmons, L. (2006). *Partnering with patients and families to design a patient- and family-centered health care system: A roadmap for the future: A work in progress.* Institute for Family-Centered Care.

Cornish, J. (2019). *Dementia with dignity: Living well with Alzheimer's or dementia using the DAWN Method.* CreateSpace Publishing.

Dawson, N. T., Powers, S. M., Krestar, M., Yarry, S. J., & Judge, K. S. (2013, October). Predictors of self-reported psychosocial outcomes in individuals with dementia. *The Gerontologist, 53*(5), 748–759. https://doi.org/10.1093/geront/gns137

Day, K., Carreon, D., & Stump, C. (2000). The therapeutic design of environments for people with dementia: A review of the empirical research. *The Gerontologist, 40*(4), 397–416. https://doi-org.libraryproxy.quinnipiac.edu/10.1093/geront/40.4.397

de Vries, M., Seppala L. J., Daams J. G., van de Glind, E. M. M., Masud, T., van der Velde, N., & EUGMS Task and Finish Group on Fall-Risk-Increasing Drugs. (2018). Fall-risk-increasing drugs: A systematic review and meta-analysis: I. Cardiovascular Drugs. *Journal of the American Medical Directors Association, 19*(4), 371.e1–371.e9.

Fazio, S., Pace, D., Maslow, K., Zimmerman, S., & Kallmyer, B. (2018, Jan. 18). Alzheimer's Association dementia care practice recommendations. *The Gerontologist, 58*(Suppl. 1), S1–S9. https://doi.org/10.1093/geront/gnx182

Ferdous, F., & Roberts, E. (2023). *(Re)designing the continuum of care for older adults: The future of long-term care settings.* Springer.

Fulmer, T., & Berman, A. (2016, Nov. 13). *Age-Friendly Health Systems: How do we get there?* HealthAffairs. http://healthaffairs.org/blog/2016/11/03/age-friendly-health-systems-how-do-we-get-there/

Fulmer, T., & Li, N. (2018). Age-Friendly Health Systems for older adults with dementia. *The Journal for Nurse Practitioners, 14*(3), 160–165.

Gaugler, J. E., Bain, L. J., Mitchell, L., Finlay, J., Fazio, S., Jutkowitz, E., & Alzheimer's Association Psychosocial Measurement Workgroup. (2019). Reconsidering frameworks of Alzheimer's dementia when assessing psychosocial outcomes. *Alzheimer's Dementia Translational Research and Clinical Interventions, 5*(1), 388–389. https://doi.org/10.1016/j.trci.2019.02.008

Gaugler, J. E., & Mitchell, L. L. (2022, February). Reimagining family involvement in residential long-term care. *Journal of the American Medical Directors Association, 23*(2), 235–240. https://doi.org/10.1016/j.jamda.2021.12.022

Gottlieb, L. N. (2014, August). Strengths-based nursing. *American Journal of Nursing, 114*(8), 24–32. https://doi.org/10.1097/01.NAJ.0000453039.70629.e2

Graffigna, G., Barello, S., Morelli, N., Gheduzzi, E., Corbo, M., Ginex, V., Ferrari, R., Lascioli, A., Feriti, C., & Masella, C. (2020, Aug. 11). Place4Carers: A mixed-method study protocol for engaging family caregivers in meaningful actions for successful ageing in place. *BMJ Open, 10*(8), e037570. https://doi.org/10.1136/bmjopen-2020-037570

Gregory, A. (2018). *SMART goal setting 101*. The Balance. https://www.thebalancesmb.com/smart-goal-setting-101-2951829

Haight, B. K., Barba, B. E., Tesh, A. S., & Courts, N. F. (2002, March). Thriving: A life span theory. *Journal of Gerontological Nursing, 28*(3), 14–22. https://doi.org/10.3928/0098-9134-20020301-05

Harris-Kojetin, L., Sengupta, M., Lendon, J. P., Rome, V., Valverde, R., & Caffrey, C. (2019). Long-term care providers and services users in the United States, 2015–2016. National Center for Health Statistics. *Vital Health Statistics, 3*(43).

Harrison, S. L., Dyer, S. M., Laver, K. E., Milte, R. K., Fleming, R., & Crotty, M. (2017, December). Physical environmental designs in residential care to improve quality of life of older people. *Cochrane Database of Systematic Reviews*, CD012892. https://doi.org/10.1002/14651858.CD012892.pub2

Heid, A. R, Bangerter, M. A., Abbott, K. M., & Van Haitsma, K. (2017). Do family proxies get it right? Concordance in reports of nursing home residents' everyday preferences. *Journal of Applied Gerontology, 36*(6), 667–691. https://doi.org/10.1177/0733464815581485

Heid, A. R., Eshraghi, K., Duntzee, C., Abbott, K. M., Curyto, K., & Van Haitmsa, K. (2016). 'It depends': Reasons why nursing home residents change their minds about care preferences. *The Gerontologist, 56*(2), 243–255. https://doi.org/10.1093/geront/gnu040

Herke, M., Fink, A., Langer, G., Wustmann, T., Watzke, S., Hanff, A. M., & Burckhardt, M. (2018, July 18). Environmental and behavioural modifications for improving food and fluid intake in people with dementia. *Cochrane Database of Systematic Reviews, 7*(7), CD011542. https://doi.org/10.1002/14651858.CD011542.pub2

Hertz, J. E., Koren, M. E., Rossetti, J., & Tibbits, K. (2016, Nov. 1). Management of relocation in cognitively intact older adults. *Journal of Gerontological Nursing, 42*(11), 14–23. https://doi.org/10.3928/00989134-20160901-05

Hirschman, K. B., & Hodgson, N. A. (2018, Jan. 18). Evidence-based interventions for transitions in care for individuals living with dementia. *The Gerontologist, 58*(Suppl._1), S129–S140. https://doi.org/10.1093/geront/gnx152

Hoek, L. J., van Haastregt, J. C., de Vries, E., Backhaus, R., Hamers, J. P., & Verbeek, H. (2021, July). Partnerships in nursing homes: How do family caregivers of residents with dementia perceive collaboration with staff? *Dementia (London), 20*(5), 1631–1648. https://doi.org/10.1177/1471301220962235

Høgsnes, L., Melin-Johansson, C., Norbergh, K. G., & Danielson, E. (2014). The existential life situations of spouses of persons with dementia before and after relocating to a nursing home. *Aging & Mental Health, 18*(2), 152–160. https://doi.org/10.1080/13607863.2013.818100

Institute for Healthcare Improvement. (2020). *Age-Friendly Health Systems: Guide to using the 4Ms in the care of older adults.* https://www.ihi.org/Engage/Initiatives/Age-Friendly-Health-Systems/Documents/IHIAgeFriendlyHealthSystems_GuidetoUsing4MsCare.pdf

Institute of Medicine. (2001). *Crossing the quality chasm: A new health system for the 21st century.* National Academies Press. https://www.ncbi.nlm.nih.gov/books/NBK222274/

Johnson, B. H., Abraham, M. R., & Shelton, T. L. (2009). Patient- and family-centered care: Partnerships for quality and safety. *North Carolina Medical Journal, 70*(2), 125–130.

Lawton, M. P., & Nahemow, L. (1973). Ecology and the aging process. In *The psychology of adult development and aging* (pp. 619–674). American Psychological Association. https://doi-org.libraryproxy.quinnipiac.edu/10.1037/10044-020

Lee, S. J., Kim, M. S., Jung, Y. J., & Chang, S. O. (2019). The effectiveness of function-focused care interventions in nursing homes: A systematic review. *Journal of Nursing Research, 27*(1), e9.

Liu, W., Galik, E., Boltz, M., Nahm, E. S., & Resnick, B. (2015). Optimizing eating performance for older adults with dementia living in long-term care: A systematic review. *Worldviews on Evidence-Based Nursing, 12*(4), 228–235.

Liu, W., Perkhounkova, E., Williams, K., Batchelor, M., & Hein, M. (2020). Food intake is associated with verbal interactions between nursing home staff and residents with dementia: A secondary analysis of videotaped observations. *International Journal of Nursing Studies, 109*, 103654.

Lopez, R. P., Mazor, K. M., Mitchell, S. L., & Givens, J. L. (2013). What is family-centered care for nursing home residents with advanced dementia? *American Journal of Alzheimer's Disease & Other Dementias, 28*(8), 763–768.

Mast, B. (2011). *Whole person dementia assessment.* Health Professions Press.

Mate, K. S., Berman, A., Laderman, M., Kabcenell, A., & Fulmer, T. (2018). Creating Age-Friendly Health Systems: A vision for better care of older adults. *Healthcare, 6*(1), 4–6.

Meneguci, C. A. G., Meneguci, J., Sasaki, J. E., Tribess, S., & Júnior, J. S. V. (2021) Physical activity, sedentary behavior and functionality in older adults: A cross-sectional path analysis. *PLoS One, 16*(1), e0246275.

Metzelthin, S. F., Rostgaard, T., Parsons, M., & Burton, E. (2022). Development of an internationally accepted definition of reablement: A Delphi study. *Ageing & Society, 42*, 703–718.

Mezey, M. D., Mitty, E. L., & Burger, S. G. (2008). Rethinking Teaching Nursing Homes: Potential for improving long-term care. *The Gerontologist, 48*(1), 8–15.

Molony, S. L. (2010, October). The meaning of home: A qualitative meta-synthesis. *Research in Gerontological Nursing, 3*(4), 291–307. https://doi.org/10.3928/19404921-20100302-02

Molony, S. L., Evans, L. K., Jeon, S., Rabig, J., & Straka, L. A. (2011, August). Trajectories of at-homeness and health in usual care and small house nursing homes. *The Gerontologist, 51*(4), 504–515. https://doi.org/10.1093/geront/gnr022

Molony, S. L., Kolanowski, A., Van Haitsma, K., & Rooney, K. E. (2018, Jan. 18). Person-centered assessment and care planning. *The Gerontologist, 58*(Suppl. 1), S32–S47. https://doi.org/10.1093/geront/gnx173

Molony, S. L., & Rabig, J. (2023). A theory of creating *at-homeness* across the long-term care continuum. In F. Ferdous & E. Roberts (Eds.), *(Re)designing the continuum of care for older adults*. Springer. https://doi.org/10.1007/978-3-031-20970-3_5

National Institute for Health and Care Excellence. (2015). *Older people: Independence and mental wellbeing*. https://www.nice.org.uk/guidance/NG32/chapter/recommendations

Nguyen, M., Pachana, N. A., Beattie, E., Fielding, E., & Ramis, M. A. (2015, November). Effectiveness of interventions to improve family-staff relationships in the care of people with dementia in residential aged care: A systematic review protocol. *Joanna Briggs Institute Database of Systematic Reviews and Implementation Reports, 13*(11), 52–63. https://doi.org/10.11124/jbisrir-2015-2415

Podsiadlo, D., & Richardson, S. (1991). The timed "up & go": A test of basic functional mobility for frail elderly persons. *Journal of the American Geriatrics Society, 39*(2),142–148. doi: 10.1111/j.1532- 5415.1991.tb01616.x

Puurveen, G., Cooke, H., Gill, R., & Baumbusch, J. (2019, Sep. 17). A seat at the table: The positioning of families during care conferences in nursing homes. *The Gerontologist, 59*(5), 835–844. https://doi.org/10.1093/geront/gny098

Reid, R. C., & Chappell, N. L. (2017, August). Family involvement in nursing homes: Are family caregivers getting what they want? *Journal of Applied Gerontology, 36*(8), 993–1015. https://doi.org/10.1177/0733464815602109

Resnick, B., Boltz, M., & Wells, C. (2013). Physical capability scale: Psychometric testing. *Clinical Nursing Research, 22*(1), 7–29.

Resnick, B., Galik, E., & Boltz, M. (2013). Function focused care approaches: Literature review of progress and future possibilities. *Journal of the American Medical Directors Association, 14*(5), 313–318.

Resnick, B., Galik, E., Boltz, M., & Pretzer-Aboff, I. (2012). *Restorative care nursing for older adults: A guide for all care settings* (2nd ed.). Springer.

Saliba, D., & Buchanan, J. (2008). *Development and validation of a revised nursing home assessment tool: MDS 3.0.* Report for Centers for Medicare & Medicaid Services. https://www.cms.gov/Medicare/Quality-Initiatives-Patient-Assessment-Instruments/NursingHomeQualityInits/downloads/MDS30FinalReport.pdf

Scales, K., Zimmerman, S., & Miller, S. J. (2018). Evidence-based nonpharmacological practices to address behavioral and psychological symptoms of dementia. *The Gerontologist, 58*(Suppl. 1), S88–S102. https://doi-org.libraryproxy.quinnipiac.edu/10.1093/geront/gnx167

Seppala, L. J., van de Glind, E. M. M., Daams, J. G., Ploegmakers, K. J., de Vries, M., Wermelinket, A. M. A. T., van der Velde, N., & EUGMS task and finish group on fall-risk-increasing drugs. (2018). Fall-risk-increasing drugs: A systematic review and meta-analysis: Others. *Journal of the American Medical Directors Association, 19*(4), 372.e1–372.e8. doi: 10.1016/j.jamda.2017.12.099

Seppala L. J., Wermelinket, A. M. A. T., de Vries, M., Ploegmakers, K. J., van de Glind, E. M. M., Daams, J. G., van der Velde, N., & EUGMS task and finish group on fall-risk-increasing drugs. (2018). Fall-risk-increasing drugs: A systematic review and meta-analysis: Psychotropics. *Journal of the American Medical Directors Association, 19*(4), 371.e11–371.e17. doi: 10.1016/j.jamda.2017.12.098

Shaughnessy, P. W., Kramer, A. M., Hittle, D. F., & Steiner, J. F. (1995). Quality of care in teaching nursing homes: Findings and implications. *Health Care Financing Review, 16*(4), 55.

Smith, M., Hall, G. R., Gerdner, L., & Buckwalter, K. C. (2006). Application of the progressively lowered stress threshold model across the continuum of care. *Nursing Clinics of North America, 41*(1), 57–58.

Van Haitsma, K. S., Abbott, K. M., Heid, A. R., Carpenter, B., Curyto, K., Kleban, M., & Spector, A. (2014). The consistency of self reported preferences for everyday living: Implications for person-centered care delivery. *Journal of Gerontological Nursing, 40*, 34–46. https://doi.org/10.3928/00989134-20140820-01

Van Haitsma, K. S., Abbott, K. M., Heid, A. R., Spector, A., Eshraghi, K., Duntzee, C., Humes, S., Crumbie, V., Crespy, S., & Valkenburgh-Schultz, M. V. (2016). Honoring nursing home resident preferences for recreational activities to advance person-centered care. *Annals of Long-Term Care and Aging, 24*(2), 25–33.

Van Haitsma, K. S., Curyto, K., Abbott, K. M., Towsley, G. L., Spector, A., & Kleban, M. (2015, January). A randomized controlled trial for an individualized positive psychosocial intervention for the affective and behavioral symptoms of dementia in nursing home residents. *The Journals of Gerontology Series B: Psychological Sciences and Social Sciences, 70*(1), 35–45. https://doi.org/10.1093/geronb/gbt102

Van Haitsma, K. S., Curyto, K., Spector, A., Towsley, G., Kleban, M., Carpenter, B., Koren, M. J. (2013). The preferences for everyday living inventory: Scale development and description of psychosocial preferences responses in community-dwelling elders. *The Gerontologist, 53*, 582–595. doi:10.1093/geront/gns102

Wolverson, E. L., Clarke, C., & Moniz-Cook, E. D. (2016). Living positively with dementia: A systematic review and synthesis of the qualitative literature. *Aging & Mental Health, 20*(7), 676–699. https://doi-org.libraryproxy.quinnipiac.edu/10.1080/13607863.2015.1052777

Zingmark, K., Norberg, A., & Sandman, P. O. (1993). Experience of at-homeness in patients with Alzheimer's disease. *American Journal of Alzheimer's Care and Related Disorders and Research, 8*, 10–16. https://doi.org/https://doi.org/10.1177/153331759300800302

RESOURCES

Dementia Care Central: dementiacarecentral.com

Function Focused Care website: https://functionfocusedcare.wordpress.com/

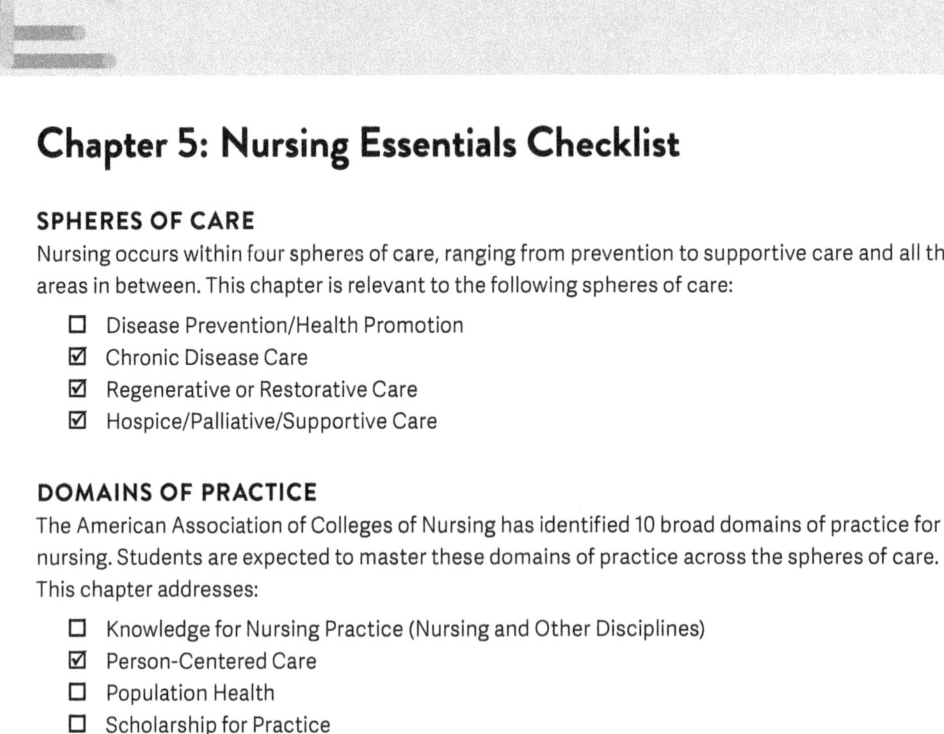

Chapter 5: Nursing Essentials Checklist

SPHERES OF CARE

Nursing occurs within four spheres of care, ranging from prevention to supportive care and all the areas in between. This chapter is relevant to the following spheres of care:

- ☐ Disease Prevention/Health Promotion
- ☑ Chronic Disease Care
- ☑ Regenerative or Restorative Care
- ☑ Hospice/Palliative/Supportive Care

DOMAINS OF PRACTICE

The American Association of Colleges of Nursing has identified 10 broad domains of practice for nursing. Students are expected to master these domains of practice across the spheres of care. This chapter addresses:

- ☐ Knowledge for Nursing Practice (Nursing and Other Disciplines)
- ☑ Person-Centered Care
- ☐ Population Health
- ☐ Scholarship for Practice
- ☐ Quality and Safety
- ☑ Interprofessional Partnerships
- ☑ Systems-Based Care
- ☐ Information & Healthcare Technologies
- ☐ Professionalism
- ☑ Personal, Professional, Leadership Development

CONCEPTS FOR PRACTICE

Integrated across the domains of practice are eight concepts which the student is expected to master across the spheres of care and across the domains of practice. This chapter addresses:

- ☐ Clinical Judgment
- ☑ Communication
- ☑ Compassionate Care
- ☐ Diversity, Equity, Inclusion
- ☐ Ethics
- ☐ Evidence-Based Practice
- ☐ Health Policy
- ☐ Social Determinants of Health

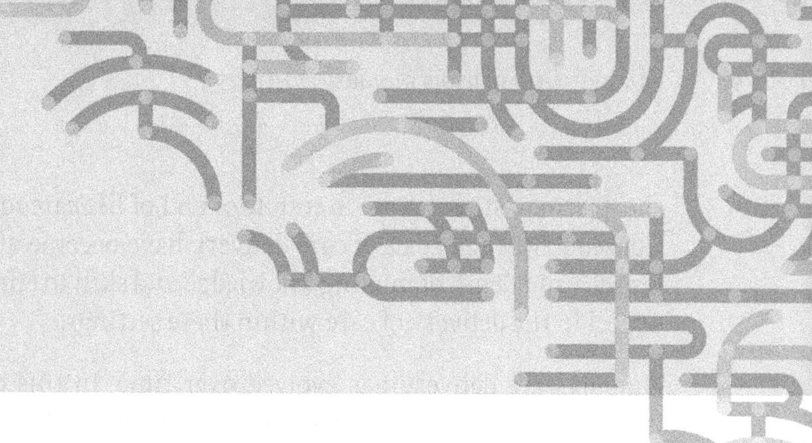

CHAPTER 5

MODELS OF NURSING CARE DELIVERY

Ann Kolanowski, PhD, RN, FAAN
Barbara J. Bowers, PhD, RN, FAAN
Joan G. Carpenter, PhD, CRNP, ACHPN, FPCN
Andrea Gilmore-Bykovskyi, PhD, RN
Laura Block, BS, BSN, RN

OBJECTIVES

1. List care-delivery models (CDMs) common in nursing practice.
2. Describe the nursing role in palliative and end-of-life CDMs.
3. Outline the nursing role in transitional CDMs.
4. Summarize the nursing role in dementia CDMs.

INTRODUCTION

Care-delivery models (CDMs) are infrastructures for organizing and providing care to people in a healthcare setting, the skill sets required of people who deliver that care, the context of care, and the expected outcomes of care (Duffield et al., 2010). CDMs are embedded in broader models of care, such as the medical, biopsychosocial, or quality-of-life models described in Chapter 1. In that chapter you learned that nursing homes have changed dramatically over the past century since their inception as almshouses for the poor. There are now national and international initiatives that call for more holistic, person-centered approaches to care in these settings. Additionally, nursing homes now serve a heterogeneous population, from people needing short-term post-acute care to respite or end-of-life care to long-term care and support. Consequently, the goals of care delivery have become quite varied and require great breadth and depth of nursing knowledge and skill to effectively support what people expect in the delivery of care within these settings.

Nursing care delivery has evolved over time. In this chapter we begin by briefly describing the traditional hierarchical CDM that has been prominent in nursing homes during the past century. We then focus on elements of CDMs that are relevant for today's nursing home and the leadership best practices that promote staff agency for providing quality care and supporting resident quality of life. Additionally, there is an in-depth discussion of CDMs that are relevant for groups of individuals in nursing homes with special needs: end-of-life care, transitional care, and dementia care. Chapter 5 provides a solid foundation for understanding the critical characteristics of CDMs in nursing homes that require transformative nursing leadership for the implementation of high-quality, person-centered care. More specifically, the content in this chapter will help you develop greater competency in chronic disease and hospice/palliative/supportive care; the domains of person-centered care; interprofessional partnerships; personal, professional, and leadership development; and the practice concepts of communication and compassionate care (American Association of Colleges of Nursing, 2021).

NURSING CARE-DELIVERY MODELS

Nursing care is essential to the services provided by a nursing home because of its direct impact on the quality of care residents receive, their quality of life, and the goals of care they identify as important to them. This contrasts somewhat with the acute-care setting, where, understandably, the emphasis is more narrowly focused on biomedical health outcomes.

Unlike other providers, nursing staff have a 24-hour presence in nursing homes. An adequate staff mix, defined as an adequate ratio of licensed to unlicensed personnel with appropriate and sufficient knowledge and skills, is essential to quality care delivery (Harrington et al., 2000). Given the existing payment models for nursing home care, most of the direct care in nursing homes is currently delivered by nursing assistants (PHI, 2019). This necessitates an approach to care delivery where the role of the professional nurse is to function as a team leader who supervises, coaches, and mentors the staff who deliver direct care and personal assistance to residents. To a large extent, nurses are working through the direct-care staff.

What constitutes an adequate staff mix in nursing homes has occupied national attention for many years. We know that staffing ratios and mix have been linked to quality of care and quality of life outcomes; that is, the higher the ratio of licensed to unlicensed nursing staff and the more highly educated the nurses are, the better the resident outcomes (Kim et al., 2009). And while the number, type, and preparation of staff available for resident care is in turn linked to the financial resources made available for that care, there is much that professional nurses can do to improve care delivery within the context of existing resources (Siegel et al., 2023). Instituting a nursing CDM that supports person-centered care is one such example.

Nursing CDMs define how staff are assigned and care is organized to meet the needs of residents. These models include total patient care, primary nursing, functional care, and team nursing (Fawcett, 2021). The demands and character of the work environment have largely determined which CDM is most appropriate and efficient for the setting in which it is applied. Table 5.1 gives a brief description of each type of CDM.

TABLE 5.1 Nursing Care-Delivery Models

CDM	DESCRIPTION
Total patient care	The oldest method of organizing care such that one care provider carries out all care requirements.
Primary nursing	A method of organizing care in which one nurse is responsible for the total nursing care of one or more patients 24 hours a day, seven days a week from the time of admission to discharge. This CDM is most often used in hospitals.
Functional nursing	A method of organizing care such that care providers deliver care based on the complexity of the task and their ability to carry out the task.
Team nursing	A method of organizing care that uses a team leader and team members to provide various aspects of care to a group of patients.

Care-Delivery Models Used in Today's Nursing Homes

Two of these models are used in nursing homes today: the functional and team CDMs. The functional CDM came into prominence in the 1930s to deal with nursing staff shortages and was based on the premise that nurses engaged with care recipients on a task-by-task basis and were evaluated based on task completion (Fairbrother et al., 2015). This nursing CDM is consistent with a biomedical model and its emphasis on biological health. In this approach to care delivery, staff are assigned to residents based on the complexity of their *care tasks* (dressings, tube feedings, intravenous antibiotic administration) and not their *care needs* (facilitating social interaction, promoting function, implementing preferences for care). In this model, there is little differentiation between the roles of RNs and LPNs, while it fosters a hierarchical relationship between licensed staff and nursing assistants who often work independently with inadequate supervision or mentoring. Research has shown that minimal mentoring of and communication with the direct-care team members leads to high staff turnover and lack of consistency in resident assignments, which, in turn, threatens the ability to deliver person-centered care (Bowers et al., 2003).

Team nursing emerged following World War II because of the desire for a more humanistic approach to care than functional nursing offered (Lambertsen, 1958). Team nursing assumes that the efforts of a diverse group of people result in better outcomes than the efforts of one individual. The success of the model depends on an educationally and experientially well-prepared professional nurse who assumes the team leader role (Sherman, 1990). The team leader is expected to use a participative style of leadership and to have effective communication skills to ensure continuity of care. In this model, input from all team members is expected and valued. Team nursing has many advantages and efficiencies as a CDM for the nursing home setting (the unit nurse working through certified nursing assistants to meet the needs of many residents), but a study of nursing home care models found that few staff report working in a team model (Temkin-Greener et al., 2009). The most common CDM in nursing homes today continues to be the functional CDM.

The functional CDM, with its emphasis on procedures and tasks rather than resident goals, preferences, and priorities, is not consistent with the current culture change movement focusing on person-centered care. It persists, in part, because professional nurses have not been educationally prepared to deliver person-centered care within a team context using leadership skills to delegate appropriately as well as develop and mentor the staff who are assigned to the residents under their care. So, how can the professional nurse align nursing care delivery in the nursing home with the goal of achieving high-quality, person-centered care?

Person-Centered Care Requires a Transformational Leader

At its core, person-centered care is about building positive relationships not only with residents and their family members but also with the staff. Evidence indicates that high-quality, person-centered care is more likely to be achieved when the culture of care delivery is characterized by healthy communication patterns, an empowered staff, a coaching/mentoring style of supervision, opportunities for professional growth, and family involvement as members of the healthcare team. These characteristics are indicators of positive relationships that help reduce staff turnover and develop direct-care staff for delivery of optimal resident care (Siegel et al., 2023).

Building and implementing this CDM (understood as relationship-based team nursing) requires a transformational leader, one who inspires and catalyzes staff to achieve quality person-centered care (McBride, 2019). The following evidence-based leadership practices help transform the CDM so that staff become empowered and person-centered care becomes a reality. The transformational leader will (Dellefield & Madrigal, 2022):

- Hire staff who are committed to a shared goal of quality care for resident quality of life
- Set clear expectations for the team
- Get to know the unique differences and capabilities of each staff member
- Institute the practice of consistent assignment of residents
- Be visible and accessible
- Build trust
- Develop feasible methods for exchanging communication between and among the staff, family, and residents
- Seek input on resident issues from all staff
- Engage in shared governance
- Move from conflict to collaboration
- Act as a mentor/coach to staff

Table 5.2 lists resources that will enhance your skills as a transformational leader who can implement a nursing CDM that inspires and catalyzes staff to deliver person-centered care.

TABLE 5.2 Resources for Leaders Promoting Person-Centered Care

CHARACTERISTICS OF NURSING CDM THAT PROMOTE PERSON-CENTERED CARE	RESOURCE
Leadership	Kouzes, J., & Posner, B. (2016). *Learning Leadership: The Five Fundamentals of Becoming an Exemplary Leader.* Wiley. Harris, M., Kolanowski, A., & Greenberg, S. (Eds.). (2022). Nursing Leadership in Long-Term Care. *Nursing Clinics of North America, 57*(2), 171–314. McBride, A. (2020). *The Growth and Development of Nurse Leaders* (2nd ed.). Springer Publishing Co. Wealth in Diversity Consulting: Transforming Leaders and Teams: http://www.wealthindiversity.com/index.html
Healthy communication patterns	AHRQ Module 4: Teamwork and Communication: https://www.ahrq.gov/hai/quality/tools/cauti-ltc/modules/implementation/long-term-modules/module4/mod4-facguide.html AHRQ Improving Patient Safety and Team Communication Through Daily Huddles: https://psnet.ahrq.gov/primer/improving-patient-safety-and-team-communication-through-daily-huddles
Empowered staff and shared governance	ANCC Pathways to Excellence in Long-Term Care: https://www.nursingworld.org/organizational-programs/pathway/overview/pathway-to-excellence-in-long-term-care/
Coaching/mentoring style of supervision	Bergstedt, K., & Wei, H. (2020). Leadership Strategies to Promote Frontline Nursing Staff Engagement. *Nursing Management, 51*(2), 48–53. https://doi.org/10.1097/01.NUMA.0000651204.39553.79
Opportunities for professional growth	Healthcare Academy: https://healthcareacademy.com/ National Association of Health Care Assistants: https://www.nahcacna.org/resources/
Family involvement	The National Consumer Voice for Quality Long-Term Care: https://theconsumervoice.org/uploads/files/issues/family-involvement-in-nursing-home-care-factsheet-final.pdf Centers for Medicare & Medicaid Services Resident and Family Engagement in Nursing Home Quality: https://www.cms.gov/Medicare/Provider-Enrollment-and-Certification/QAPI/Downloads/QAPI-Consumer-Factsheet.pdf Ohio Department of Aging Resident and Family Council Toolkit: https://aging.ohio.gov/care-and-living/get-help/get-an-advocate/resident-family-council-toolkit

We will now turn our attention to three specific CDMs that are relevant for groups of individuals in nursing homes with special needs: palliative and end-of-life care, transitional care, and dementia care. Each of these CDMs is based on a team approach with the goal of delivering person-centered care.

MODELS OF PALLIATIVE AND END-OF-LIFE CARE

Many nursing home residents live with serious illness and functional debility coupled with multiple chronic conditions including cognitive impairment. Together, these conditions place residents at risk for health-related decline. Approximately 25% of residents receiving Medicare-paid care in nursing homes spend their final days there, and one-third of older adults will receive care in a nursing home in the last three months of life (Teno et al., 2018). It is important that nurses attend to the myriad physical, psychosocial, and spiritual symptoms that residents experience and provide care consistent with what is most important to them throughout serious illness and as they approach end of life. However, this can be challenging in nursing homes, where residents experience an uncertain illness trajectory (Carpenter et al., 2018). Nurses often must use their intuitive experiences to identify residents' signs of approaching end of life (Johnson et al., 2014). For example, a resident with congestive heart failure may experience frequent hospitalizations and frailty that places them at risk for further decline and death (Carpenter et al., 2017). In addition, residents are particularly disadvantaged and vulnerable because of the relative isolation and lack of palliative care resources for staff and palliative trained practitioners in this environment (Lester et al., 2016).

Palliative Care

Some have argued that nursing home care is fundamentally palliative (Ersek & Carpenter, 2013; Ersek et al., 2022). *Palliative care* is resident- and family-centered care that provides an essential layer of support for people living with serious illness. It can be applied at any point in the illness trajectory and is not limited to those who are approaching the end of life, as is hospice care. Palliative care incorporates open communication about goals of care and treatment preferences, heightened attention to symptom assessment and management, and psychosocial and spiritual support.

Hospice Care

The most commonly used end-of-life care model in nursing homes is hospice. *Hospice* is a Medicare-paid benefit that has eligibility requirements that include a six-month prognosis, decisions to forgo "curative" treatments, and resident/family agreement to hospice instead of other Medicare-covered treatments for their illness. The hospice agency oversees a resident's plan of care in the nursing home and provides all medications and supplies related to their illness while the nursing home continues to provide day-to-day nursing and residential care. The Medicare hospice benefit does not pay for a resident's room and board during their long-term stay. Only in rare circumstances does it pay for hospice care during the Medicare post-acute care benefit (e.g., skilled nursing care and rehabilitation), such as when the hospice diagnosis and the post-acute care illness are not related.

There are many benefits of hospice in nursing homes. Hospice care improves symptom assessment and management, especially for pain and shortness of breath (Parast et al., 2021). Hospice helps to reduce potentially burdensome treatments and is associated with a lower risk of end-of-life hospitalization (Cai et al., 2018). Hospice also offers support and benefits to family care partners including the ability to adjust positively after the resident's death (Currow et al., 2020; Gage et al., 2016). Despite these benefits, past research has found that family members report confusion over their role in collaborating with the hospice providers and nursing home staff (Gage et al., 2016). Therefore, it is important that nurses prioritize communication among all team members and the resident's family.

CASE STUDY Facilitating Communication Regarding a Hospice Patient in a Nursing Home

Mr. G is an 85-year-old nursing home resident who is receiving hospice care from a community-based hospice program. He has a hospice diagnosis of congestive heart failure, with hypertensive heart disease and dependence on supplemental oxygen. He also is diagnosed with chronic renal failure, peripheral vascular disease, and osteoarthritis. The nursing home nurse noted an increase in lower extremity edema, cough, and lung sounds with wheezes, and that Mr. G was less responsive than usual. Upon noticing these signs, the nurse called the hospice agency and talked with Mr. G's primary nurse to report the change in status. The hospice nurse consulted the hospice nurse practitioner, who ordered a diuretic for suspected worsening congestive heart failure. The nursing home nurse then called

Mr. G's daughter and informed her of the changes, documented the events in a progress note, called and informed the nursing home primary care provider, and increased monitoring of Mr. G for comfort. The nursing home nurse also informed the supervisor and made a note for shift change. All these steps helped to facilitate communication using written documentation and verbal updates to communicate changes to Mr. G's plan of care.

External Palliative Care Consultations

For residents who do not qualify for or choose not to receive hospice care, another model for palliative care in nursing homes is *external palliative care consultations* (Lima & Miller, 2018). These services may be provided by an individual clinician with a specialty practice in palliative care or an extension of an interdisciplinary hospice team. External palliative care consultants make recommendations for a resident's care, most often focused on advance care planning or symptom management.

Studies have shown that there are many benefits to external palliative care consultation, including reduction in residents' hospitalizations and emergency department visits, enhanced symptom management, and increases in advance care planning, documentation of treatment preferences, and referrals to hospice care (Miller et al., 2016, 2017; Morris & Galicia-Castillo, 2017).

Some challenges exist to external palliative care consultations:

- Less than one-third of community palliative care programs serve nursing homes, leading to a lack of specialist providers to meet residents' needs (Lupu et al., 2018).
- Nursing home staff are unclear about how to decide a resident is "eligible" for palliative care and what guidelines should be used in the nursing home setting (ElMokhallalati et al., 2020).
- Consultations may be complex, and recommendations may not be implemented by primary care providers or followed through by staff in the nursing home environment (Carpenter et al., 2017).

Nurses play a key role in overcoming these challenges by using evidence based palliative care resources, including the *Clinical Practice Guidelines for Quality Palliative Care*, 4th Edition (National Coalition for Hospice and Palliative Care, 2018).

Primary Palliative Care

Another model of care for people living with serious illness in nursing homes is *primary palliative care,* also known as *internal* or *integrated palliative care.* There are aspects of the nursing home environment that support palliative care practices, including ongoing strong relationships between direct-care workers and residents, the interdisciplinary team, and quarterly care planning meetings (Park et al., 2021). Nursing home staff are often "like family" to residents. In particular, nursing assistants spend more time with residents and providing hands-on care (24 hours/day) than any other staff in nursing homes (PHI, 2019). Nursing assistants have a critical role observing residents for changes and alerting nurses to signs that may indicate palliative care needs (e.g., uncontrolled symptoms, distress, changes in status).

The interdisciplinary team in nursing homes is similar to that of the hospice and palliative care team; the interdisciplinary team meets during regularly scheduled care plan meetings to share information with residents and families. During these meetings, staff review current conditions and any changes residents have experienced. Care plan meetings can support advance care planning conversations. Some researchers have used written and video decision aids to enhance goals of care discussions and support decisions around life-sustaining treatments with varied success (Hanson et al., 2017; Hickman et al., 2016; Moyo et al., 2022).

There are challenges to primary palliative care, including facility and staff investment in initiatives to enhance palliative services and staff turnover (Currow et al., 2020). Nursing homes often have multiple quality improvement processes, required training, and mandatory inservices being implemented at any given time that may detract from one another. Staff turnover requires that educational programs be offered continually and the new skills practiced consistently to maintain knowledge and skill set. As a result, optional initiatives such as palliative care programs may not gain traction. However, research has shown that educating nursing home staff in palliative care helps to enrich their skill set (Lamppu et al., 2019).

Resources for Palliative and Hospice Care

There are three commonly recognized models for serious illness care in nursing homes: hospice care for residents whose life expectancy is six months or less, and external consultation teams and primary palliative care for residents at any stage of illness. Each nursing home setting offers a unique environment where one palliative or end-of-life care model may be implemented successfully and another may not. Nurses need to recognize both the facility resources and staff capacity to support implementation of hospice and palliative care services in nursing homes. Many professional and advocacy groups have developed curricula, websites, and other resources to support nurses delivering palliative care services in nursing homes (see Table 5.3).

TABLE 5.3 Nursing Homes Palliative and Hospice Care Resources for Nurses

RESOURCE	TITLE	TYPE	URL
Center to Advance Palliative Care (CAPC)	Online Clinical Training Courses for All Clinicians	Website with education programs	https://www.capc.org/training/
CAPC	Designing a Long-Term Care Palliative Care Program	Website with resources	https://www.capc.org/toolkits/designing-a-long-term-care-palliative-care-program/
Get Palliative Care	A Quality Life podcasts	Podcast	https://soundcloud.com/get-palliative-care
National Hospice and Palliative Care Organization (NHPCO)	NHPCO Resources	Website	https://www.nhpco.org/resources/
NHPCO	NHPCO podcasts	Podcast	https://www.nhpco.org/resources/nhpco-podcasts/
Hospice and Palliative Nurses Association	Advance Care Planning Resources	Website with resources, education programs, professional development	https://www.advancingexpertcare.org/practice-research/resource-pages/advance-care-planning/
American Association of Colleges of Nursing	End-of-Life Nursing Education Consortium	Website with resources, education programs, professional development	https://www.aacnnursing.org/ELNEC

MODELS OF TRANSITIONAL CARE

Nursing home residents experience a high number of transitions within and between care settings, including moving frequently between community settings, post-acute rehabilitative and/or skilled nursing, emergency departments, and hospital settings. Regardless of whether a resident is in a nursing home environment for rehabilitative, post-acute, or long-term care, most residents enter into the nursing home environment through a hospital discharge or transfer (Goodwin et al., 2011). Unfortunately, research suggests that nearly one in four individuals will return to the hospital within 30 days of their discharge to a nursing home (Burke et al., 2016; Mor et al., 2010), with hospitalizations often preceded by emergency department visits.

From a resident and family perspective, hospitalizations and emergency visits can be extremely disruptive to daily lives and routines. It is important to recognize that hospitalization as a common precipitating factor to nursing home admission is a clinically significant event for older adults, exposing them to heightened risk for iatrogenic events and accelerated functional decline.

From a nursing home staff perspective, hospitalizations and emergency visits can create a feeling of a "revolving door" or "churn" of nursing home residents, which can challenge establishment of a therapeutic relationship or progress toward goals of care. Nursing home residents also experience transitions to assisted living facilities or areas discharged to the community. These transitions are often considered "favorable" as they mark movement toward more independent settings of care.

The experience of transitions for residents is often complex and often involves multiple transfers between settings or levels of care (see Figure 5.1). Many nursing home residents will experience more than two transitions in care in a 30-day time frame.

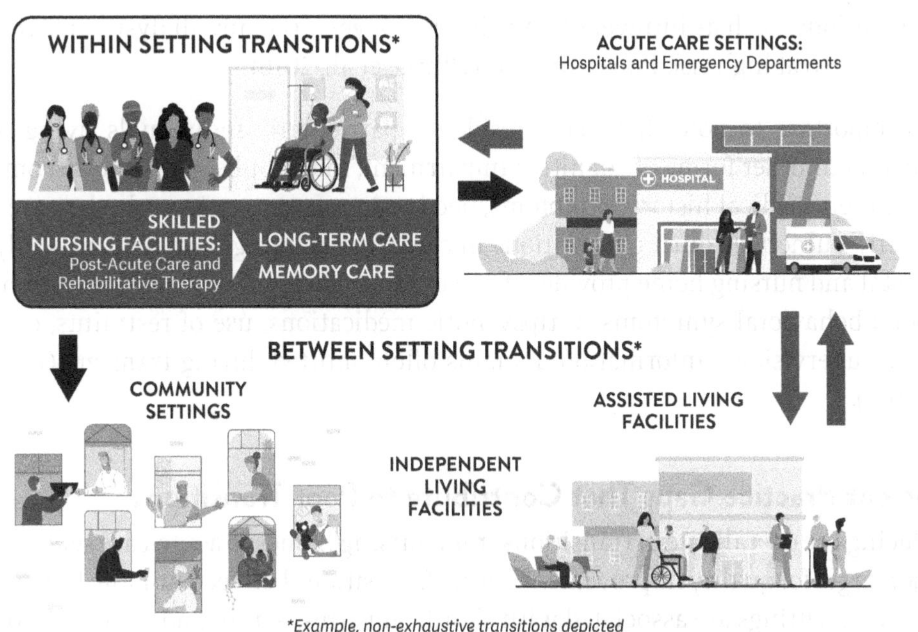

FIGURE 5.1 Experience of transitions.

A Closer Look at Hospital Readmissions: Are They Avoidable?

Individuals are at highest risk for a transition in care immediately after a hospitalization event—half of nursing home-to-hospital readmissions occur during the first 14 days (about two weeks) of a nursing home stay, and most happen in just the first few days (Burke et al., 2016). A return to the hospital or a readmission within 30 days is largely considered a marker of missed or poor care during the transitional period from hospital to nursing home. However, hospital readmissions may also signal critical thinking and decision-making on behalf of nurses who are using the information and resources they have at hand. While most hospital readmissions are needed based on the resident's condition at the moment, a significant number of readmissions are considered avoidable or preventable had the early signs of changing condition been detected and treated.

Individuals most at risk for hospital readmission are those with multiple comorbidities, recent and longer hospitalizations, cognitive impairment, and diagnoses of congestive heart failure, infections and sepsis, or electrolyte imbalances (Burke et al., 2016). In general, individuals experiencing greater levels of acuity and corresponding interventions, such as intravenous antibiotics, oxygen therapy, dialysis, and wound care, are also at high risk for readmission (Burke et al., 2016).

It is important to note that many residents, particularly individuals living with dementia or other forms of cognitive impairment, may not be able to fully communicate their medical history, symptoms, needs, or preferences. As such, they are particularly vulnerable during transitions in care. People living with dementia rely on hospital and nursing home providers for accurate transfer of information, especially around behavioral symptoms, antipsychotic medications, use of restraints, or one-to-one supervision—information domains often omitted during transfers (King et al., 2013).

Current Practice Gaps That Contribute to Poor Transitions

Reducing the overall rate of transitions from nursing homes to acute-care settings is a major target for quality improvement efforts. Transitions between nursing homes and acute-care settings are associated with significant stress/strain and expose residents to heightened risk for iatrogenic events such as medication errors, unwanted or invasive interventions, and hospital-related complications such as delirium (Dwyer et al., 2014; Tjia et al., 2009). Many of these transitions are potentially avoidable through improved inter-setting communication, continuity in care, and detection and management of acute changes in condition.

While the following list is not exhaustive, it highlights key system pressures and practice gaps that researchers have identified contribute to poor transitions in care. Subsequently, we will describe efforts to address these gaps:

- Researchers have found gaps in inter-setting communication between hospital and nursing home providers (e.g., the written discharge summary, warm handoffs, shared clinicians). Hospital discharge papers are often delayed and found to be incomplete or inaccurate, particularly in medication and behavioral status domains (Adler-Milstein et al., 2021). When attempting to provide a warm handoff to nursing home providers, it can be challenging to reach them by phone (Britton et al., 2017). Altogether, this can hinder creation of a care plan by nursing home providers.
- Research has consistently documented that hospital providers do not fully understand the nursing home care environment (Britton et al., 2017).

Therefore, decisions on placement appropriateness may not be fully informed, and correspondingly, hospital providers may not sufficiently communicate their rationale for placement and the patient's needs to nursing home providers. Greater investment in relationships and communication between nursing homes and local hospitals to build situational awareness of each environment is needed.

- There is an overall trend toward shorter lengths of stay in acute-care settings such as hospitals that shifts greater acuity to post-acute care settings such as nursing homes. Yet, nursing homes have very different staffing structures compared to hospitals, often functioning with higher patient-to-staff ratios and lacking onsite clinicians, pharmacists, and laboratory testing. These system pressures combine with a lack of training and tools for nursing home staff, leading to inadequate prevention, detection, and management of acute changes in condition, which contribute to risk for hospital readmission. Inadequate symptom monitoring, medication errors, and breaches in infection control are direct contributors (Ouslander et al., 2010, 2016). Nursing home staff and attending clinicians, particularly those who may have less familiarity with the resident, may opt to utilize acute-care resources for management of changes in condition to mitigate lack of resources and associated risk (Marincowitz et al., 2022).
- Residents and their families also play an important role in decisions around transitions in care, with their perspectives prioritized by nursing home staff (Marincowitz et al., 2022). Residents and family members often request a hospital readmission or, in the absence of advance care planning, hospital readmission may be indicated (Jacobsen et al., 2017; Ouslander et al., 2016).

Transitional Care Interventions

In the past two decades, there has been a concerted effort to understand what makes a transition between care settings successful, and eight core essentials have been identified (Naylor et al., 2017):

- Patient engagement
- Caregiver engagement
- Complexity and medication management

- Patient education
- Caregiver education
- Patients' and caregivers' well-being
- Care continuity
- Accountability

Several interventions have been developed to target transitions in care among nursing home residents, particularly targeting hospital to nursing home transitions and reducing rehospitalization.

A major initiative in this area is the Interventions to Reduce Acute Care Transfers (INTERACT) program. INTERACT is a comprehensive quality improvement program that provides a suite of tools to support identification and management of acute changes in condition among nursing home residents to reduce hospitalization. Tools focus on four areas:

1. Quality improvement
2. Communication
3. Decision support
4. Advance care planning

INTERACT has been integrated successfully within other initiatives, such as the Missouri Quality Initiative for nursing homes, or MOQI. MOQI supports integration of advanced practice registered nurses and structured tools that together support early identification of changes in condition and transitions between settings. MOQI provides INTERACT resources and coaches, along with resources around health information technology, care coordination, and advance care planning. MOQI resulted in a reduction in hospitalizations (Rantz et al., 2017).

Common features of transitional care interventions include:

- Integration of providers across acute, post-acute, and primary care settings, both structurally and with improved tools for communication
- Improved discharge planning in the hospital setting, including structured tools, interoperable health information technology, and warm handoffs

- Integration of advanced care practitioners in the nursing home environment
- Medication reconciliation
- Advance care planning

CASE STUDY Caring for a Patient Transitioning From Hospitalization to Rehabilitative Care

SG is a 78-year-old who is being admitted to your facility for rehabilitative care following hospitalization for acute calculous cholecystitis (inflammation of the gallbladder). SG was considered too unstable for cholecystectomy (surgical removal of the gallbladder), and instead, percutaneous drainage of the gallbladder was performed. The plan is to perform a cholecystectomy once inflammation and infection have resolved and SG has regained some strength. SG is being treated with intravenous antibiotics.

The Director of Nursing at your facility coordinated with the hospital on SG's admission and gave you a brief report on SG's condition toward the beginning of your evening shift. The Director of Nursing also started a paper chart for SG that includes her hospital discharge summary and paperwork on code status and advanced directives, and entered the orders from the hospital discharge papers into the electronic medical records your facility uses.

You learn that SG has a history of diabetes mellitus II, hypercholesterolemia, hypertension, atrial fibrillation, myocardial infarction, and heart failure. Her medications include metformin, insulin glargine, insulin lispro, atorvastatin, metoprolol, aspirin, famotidine, and losartan. You learn that prior to hospitalization, SG was living at home with daily support from her daughter. SG is alert and oriented to person, place, time, and situation (AOx4), and because of functional decline during her hospital stay, she currently requires two-person assist with a wheeled walker (2A with WW). She is on room air.

SG has a peripherally inserted central catheter line in her left upper arm. You are to administer piperacillin-tazobactam (Zosyn) 3.375 grams intravenously q6h. The Director of Nursing confirms the medication will be delivered by the off-site pharmacy during their 2200 dropoff.

SG arrives by medical transport at 1800. You introduce yourself, help her settle into her room, orient her to the unit and call light, and take a set of admission vitals.

(continues)

(continued)

SG's vitals are as follows: BP 122/83, HR 93, RR 19, T 99.1, SpO2 97% on room air. SG rates 4/10 pain in her right upper quadrant. She states, "I just feel crummy." You conduct a head-to-toe assessment and do not find any other notable concerns.

STOP & REFLECT

- What factors heighten SG's risk for a nursing home-to-hospital readmission?
- Do you see any practice gaps affecting the quality of SG's transition to the nursing home? Consider practice gaps on both the sending (hospital) and receiving (nursing home) side. What system-level factors might also be at play in this case study?
- What actions would you take next to address SG's situation?
    - You check and see SG does not have orders for pain medication. You are concerned about her slightly elevated temperature and general malaise. The Director of Nursing is no longer at the facility, nor is the nurse practitioner who visits throughout the week. You look through the hospital discharge paperwork and do not find any information on her condition at discharge or vital signs for comparison. The intravenous antibiotics are overdue for administration but have not yet arrived from the off-site pharmacy.
    - You decide to call an on-call physician to discuss SG's situation. It has been an hour since you last checked SG's vitals, as you have also been assisting the other residents under your care, and you find her temperature is now 99.7 and her pain is rated at 5/10. You have confirmed with SG that she would like to have you discuss her situation with the on-call physician rather than visiting the emergency department. You have also called SG's daughter per SG's request to keep her informed.
    - You use SBAR (Situation, Background, Assessment, Recommendation) to report your findings to the on-call physician. SBAR is a framework for communication between members of the healthcare team about a patient's condition and involves the following:
        1. **S = Situation:** SG has elevated temperature, malaise, and reports pain.
        2. **B = Background:** SG is a 78-year-old admitted following hospital stay for acute calculous cholecystitis. There is no order for pain medication

or elevated temperature, and the antibiotic that was ordered has not arrived yet.

3. **A = Assessment:** SG needs pain relief and an antibiotic administered.
4. **R = Recommendation:** Ask for pain medication that will also reduce temperature and request that antibiotic be administered immediately upon arrival.

SG's physician feels the presenting symptoms may be expected given the gallstone was not removed and antibiotic therapy has been delayed because of the hospital-to-nursing home transition. The physician orders vital checks q4h, acetaminophen 650 mg q6h prn, and that the antibiotics be administered immediately upon receipt. The physician also requests that you call back with any worsening symptoms, including nausea and vomiting, yellowing of the skin or eyes, or sweating.

You administer acetaminophen prn immediately, and upon reassessment, SG's temperature is 98.9 and pain 4/10. You later administer the intravenous Zosyn, and SG's vital signs further stabilize.

STOP & REFLECT

The nurse in this case study made several key decisions:

- What would you have done similarly and what would you have done differently?
- Can you imagine a situation in which you may have needed to transfer SG back to the emergency department for further assessment and care? What may have influenced this decision? Would such an emergency department visit be avoidable?
- How do you think the use of standardized tools and templates might have facilitated improved transfer of care for SG? What should have been communicated on such tools or templates?

DEMENTIA CARE MODEL

More than half of nursing home residents are living with dementia, and therefore understanding and meeting their medical, psychosocial, and functional care needs is integral to the role of all nursing home staff.

Care Needs of People Living With Dementia in Nursing Homes

Nursing homes are a particularly important care environment for people living with dementia, not only providing post-acute and long-term care services but also specialized memory care and end-of-life care supports (Callahan et al., 2012).

Dementia is a syndrome characterized by changes in memory, thinking, language, communication, and executive functioning that impact daily living. Many different underlying etiologies contribute to the development of dementia, the most common of which is Alzheimer's disease (present in 60%–80% of dementia cases).

As dementia progresses, it increasingly impacts an individual's capacity to identify, communicate, and meet their medical, psychosocial, and functional needs. As a result, persons living with dementia often need support performing activities of daily living (e.g., bathing, dressing, and eating) and fostering positive engagement in meaningful activities, supportive relationships, security, autonomy, and respect—all of which are central to the increasing focus on living well with dementia as identified by individuals living with cognitive symptoms and their care partners (Jennings et al., 2017; Kolanowski et al., 2018).

Adopting a strength-based approach to care for people living with dementia is critical to supporting well-being. Strength-based approaches emphasize identifying, maintaining, and utilizing an individual's unique abilities and strengths rather than focusing solely on their losses or deficits. Each individual's specific strengths, cognitive resilience, and underlying pathological brain changes vary considerably; therefore, specific care needs and retained abilities are unique to each individual person.

In advanced stages of dementia, individuals often experience a significant decline in communication and functional abilities and may experience changes such as incontinence and difficulty swallowing. Additionally, virtually all people living with dementia will experience behavioral and psychological symptoms of dementia, such as the following:

- Aggression
- Agitation
- Anxiety
- Apathy
- Care resistance
- Changes to appetite
- Changes in sleep
- Delusions
- Depression
- Hallucinations
- Irritability
- Repetitive questions
- Wandering

Behavioral and psychological symptoms of dementia, also referred to as *expressions of unmet need*, behavioral expressions, and responsive behaviors are a heterogenous group of symptoms associated with dementia (Kovach et al., 2005). Effectively preventing and responding to behavioral and psychological symptoms of dementia requires understanding them as attempts to communicate unmet needs, such as pain, loneliness, or overstimulation, particularly as dementia progression impairs language and communication abilities.

In other words, people living with dementia are not intentionally aggressive or agitated because of underlying hostility, but rather because of an underlying need to communicate discomfort, fear, or another unmet need. Management of these symptoms, through attention to identifying and addressing unmet needs they serve to communicate, is often a major focus of care for people living with dementia in nursing home environments and a target for dementia-specific care interventions.

Dementia-Specific Care Models and Interventions

Structurally, nursing homes can provide care for individuals living with dementia either in an integrated fashion (residents with and without dementia receiving care in the same area of the nursing home) or in special units or households that are dedicated to residents with dementia. Dedicated dementia-specific units are often known as dementia special care units (SCUs) or memory care units. Approximately one in five long-term care communities have an SCU (Park et al., 2013). Within SCUs, nursing homes may require a locked entry to the unit and doors with alarms, offer dementia-specific programming, and have staff with additional training.

Beyond structure, there are many different models of care and interventions for people living with dementia. Across models of care and interventions, there is a shared recognition that nursing home residents living with dementia have distinct cognitive, functional, behavioral, and social care needs that require specialized staff training, modified environments, and involvement of caregivers. These care models also attempt to address the range of adverse outcomes nursing home residents with dementia are often at heightened risk for, including falls, delirium, pressure ulcers, underrecognized and undertreated pain, neglect, and physical and chemical restraints.

In Table 5.4, we highlight a few major initiatives specific to nursing home residents living with dementia that have been well-studied. Nurses' roles across these interventions include but are not limited to:

- Identifying residents who may benefit from tailored interventions
- Recommending specific interventions or care approaches based on knowledge of the resident's needs or preferences (e.g., tailored music program for resident who often taps fingers when background music is played, or scheduled acetaminophen for resident who has arthritis diagnosis documented in their chart)
- Collaborating with an interdisciplinary team to update care plan and orders as necessary and with therapists, nursing aides, and other staff on delivery of intervention
- Directly trialing different care approaches and monitoring their effectiveness

TABLE 5.4 Nonpharmacological Interventions for Symptoms

MODEL	BRIEF DESCRIPTION	CORE COMPONENTS
Music Therapy (e.g., music & memory)	Music therapy recognizes that certain symptoms (e.g., behavioral symptoms, pain) are a result of a lack of sensory stimulation. Music therapy has demonstrated a positive effect among people with dementia, for example, reducing agitation during mealtime and baths.	Listening to music Singing Playing instruments Dancing
Tailored Activity Program (TAP)	TAP is a model that focuses on assessment of behavioral symptoms and the strengths and capabilities of the person living with dementia to deliver individualized activities. Example activities can include reminiscence and photo activities, instrumental or household activities (folding towels, sorting envelopes), games and recreation, arts and crafts, and exercise/physical activity.	Assessment of behavioral symptoms and preserved capabilities, with recognition that these may vary across disease type and stage Customization of activities instead of using a one-size-fits-all approach Incorporation of family and environment

MODEL	BRIEF DESCRIPTION	CORE COMPONENTS
Serial Trial Intervention (STI)	STI is a model that focuses on identification and treatment of pain, behavioral symptoms, and unmet needs among nursing home residents with dementia through repeat or serial assessment and treatment with incorporation of pharmacological and nonpharmacological interventions. This model recognizes behavioral symptoms as communication of unmet need.	Routine identification of behavioral symptoms as form of communication, wherein onset of changes in behavior triggers a protocol of assessment and treatment Physical needs assessment Affective needs assessment with focus on environment, sensory stimulation, meaningful engagement Nonpharmacological interventions and environmental modifications Analgesic trials if indicated Consultation with specialist providers and trial of psychotropics as needed
Staff Training in Assisted Living Residencies (STAR)	STAR is a model that focuses on providing assisted living workforce with dementia-specific education and that strengthens staff-resident interactions through a focus on the person-environment fit and the social learning theory.	Training on the ABCs (activators, behaviors, consequences) of dementia-related behaviors to help staff respond to dementia-specific needs Knowledge and skill enhancement around the basics of dementia, resident communication, collaboration with staff and families, and meaningful activities A focus on dignity
Describe, Investigate, Create, and Evaluate (DICE)	DICE is a model that incorporates a stepwise approach to nonpharmacological responses to behavioral symptoms. There is attention to understanding context and expectations around behavioral symptoms as well as potential biopsychosocial contributors.	Caregiver describes behavioral symptoms including the context, environment, and degree of distress Causes of behavioral symptoms are investigated, including physiological causes such as pain or medication side effects, caregiver expectations or needs, social engagement, physical environment, and culture Co-creation of a care plan with incorporation of treatment for physical causes and nonpharmacological interventions surrounding caregiver support, meaningful engagement, simplification of tasks, safe environment, and appropriate degrees of stimulation Evaluate effectiveness of treatment; depending on safety and acuteness of behavioral symptoms, psychotropics may be considered

Additionally, models focused on environment and organizational culture have demonstrated benefit for residents living with dementia. For example, the neighborhood or household model can provide residents living with dementia with opportunities for physical activity and social connection, while the Eden Alternative and Green House models alike focus on identifying individuals' abilities rather than losses. Wellspring communities have focused on creating a village environment and memory care neighborhoods with integrated social programs and dementia-trained staff (Fazio, Pace, Flinner, et al., 2018).

Across these models, there is an emphasis on creating a home-like environment—with private and shared spaces; opportunity for preferred activities, music, and food; appropriate stimuli; safe access to the outdoors; and controlled entry and exit points to ensure residents' security.

The Key Essentials of Dementia Care

We would like to wrap up this section by distilling the key essentials of dementia care (Fazio, Pace, Maslow, et al., 2018; see Figure 5.2), which are relevant for all nurses regardless of the model of care, interventions, or staffing structures that may be in place in their setting.

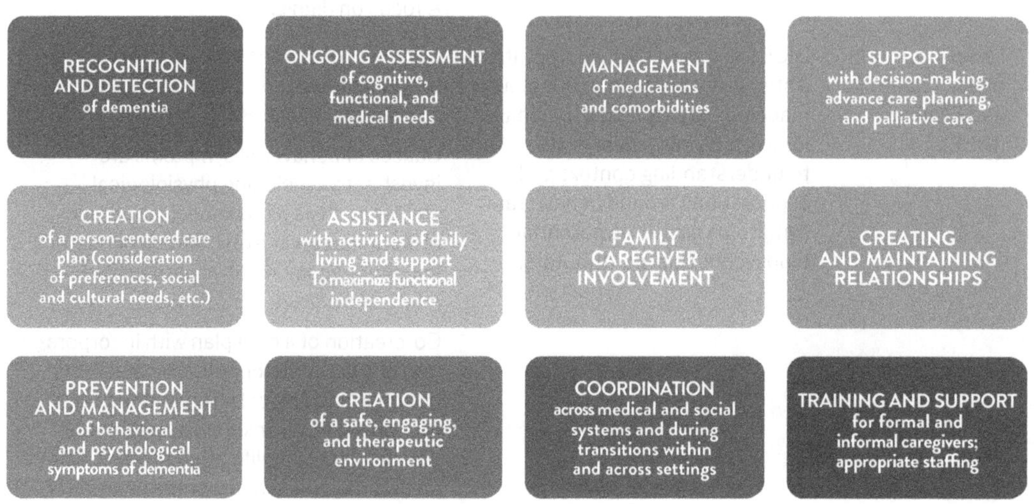

FIGURE 5.2 Essentials of dementia care in nursing homes.

A few essentials of dementia care deserve further attention, particularly for the role in shaping nursing home care.

Helping Residents With Dementia Maintain a Sense of Self

Person-centered care is a broadly endorsed priority across models of dementia care and generally describes attention to the individual beyond the task of care through valuation of their unique identity and worthiness and engaging meaningfully in relationship with others. It is posited that person-centered care approaches influence individuals living with dementia both through neurobiological impacts and impact on identity.

One's sense of self is intricately related to the esteem and value conferred on the self through relationships and by society. This sense of self is threatened by depersonalizing actions others take when interacting with individuals with dementia, such as infantilizing talk (e.g., "sweetie," "Did you behave yourself?", describing adults as "cute" or "adorable," exaggerated tone, use of words such as "diaper" rather than "underwear") and the stigma society places upon dementia. Infantilizing talk is also sometimes referred to as "elderspeak" and has been shown in research to lead to care resistance and agitation (Herman & Williams, 2009).

Therefore, person-centered care promotes maintaining a sense of self through active inclusion in life and relationships, meaningful engagement in activities, and experiencing the world alongside people with dementia from their point of view. To do this, it is important to actively initiate and observe your interactions with residents with dementia across care tasks and in focused one-to-one engagement:

- Do they turn away their head and body when you approach from a certain side? Perhaps they do not recognize you or your intent for approaching them.
- Is there a certain resident who becomes particularly anxious in the afternoon? Perhaps they are in pain from sitting in their chair for an extended period of time or fearful of the separation that occurs each night when they leave the common room and go to their own room.

Understanding a person's background and preferences is also essential to your efforts to truly getting to know a resident. For example, maybe the resident who is anxious at night spent over 80 years of their life in the company of family and thus fears the separation and loneliness that comes with the nursing home's routine of moving them from the common room back into their own room each evening.

Seeing Behavioral and Psychological Symptoms of Dementia as Forms of Communication

Within a person-centered care framework, behavioral and psychological symptoms of dementia are considered a form of meaningful communication, as they are often a response to unmet physical, social, emotional, or environmental needs. Assuming that behaviors are a form of hostile or ill-intended communication or action by the person living with dementia is more likely to result in the following:

- Caregiver burnout: For example, a resident's delusion that you are going to harm them may feel emotionally hurtful to the nurse if interpreted as a personal and intentional action.
- Responses that are ineffective: For example, reprimanding the person with dementia for thinking that a nurse would cause harm.

Nonpharmacological interventions—such as the use of individualized music, reminiscence therapy, or physical activity—have demonstrated effectiveness in preventing and managing behavioral and psychological symptoms of dementia and pose minimal to no risks.

Being Responsive to the Perspectives of People Living With Dementia

Finally, and importantly, dementia-specific care must also be responsive to the perspectives of people living with dementia themselves, who have historically had very little opportunity to share their thoughts on nursing home care. When people living with dementia have been engaged in research on this topic, they have shared the importance of having a personal space, sharing their story and reflecting on memories, and engaging in meaningful activities (Mjørud et al., 2017). They also talk about the sense of loss that they often experience and the continued adjustment to the nursing home (Mjørud et al., 2017). This research underscores the importance of relationships, with family members and staff alike.

CASE STUDY Caring for a Resident in a Memory Care Unit

MT is an 88-year-old resident who has been residing within a specialized memory care unit for the past three years. Prior to that, MT had been living with his wife at home with support from their children and home healthcare. MT experienced several falls and hospitalizations, and together with their care team, MT's family decided to pursue long-term nursing home care.

MT worked in construction for over 40 years, is known for his barbecues and love of jazz, and has two children and five grandchildren who visit him regularly alongside his wife. However, MT's wife recently experienced a decline in her health and has not visited in several weeks.

MT's diagnoses include Alzheimer's type dementia, hypertension, osteoarthritis, and depression. His medications include donepezil, memantine, losartan, aspirin, sertraline, calcium with vitamin D, acetaminophen (scheduled and prn), polyethylene glycol (prn), and bisacodyl (prn). MT is oriented to himself and recognizes family as well as nurses and nursing aides who work with him frequently. He is generally aware he is not at home but is not able to remember where he is or why he is there. MT uses a wheelchair and a sit-to-stand aid with one assist and gait belt during transfers. His knees often bother him. MT fell three days ago and has a small skin tear to his left forearm that is covered with a transparent film dressing to be changed every three days and as needed.

Your facility protocol requires 72 hours of neurological assessment, vitals monitoring, and skin checks, and these have been completed with no additional abnormal findings beyond the skin tear and some slight bruising around it.

During shift change report, you learn that MT did not sleep well during the night, was attempting to get out of bed without assistance, and was calling out for his wife. The nurse reports that MT was able to get some sleep from 0400–0700. As you begin your shift, the nursing aide reports to you that MT does not wish to get out of bed to have breakfast in the dining room, nor does he wish for his breakfast to be brought to him. You discuss with the nursing aide that MT did not sleep well and that you and the nursing aide can check back in with him in an hour. An hour later, MT wishes to get up and eat. However, he does not wish to take his morning medications and raises his voice when you attempt to assess his left forearm skin tear.

(continues)

(continued)

STOP & REFLECT

- Which behavioral and psychological symptoms of dementia is MT experiencing? Are any of them potentially problematic? Try using the DICE (Describe, Investigate, Create, and Evaluate—refer to Table 5.4) approach to try to better understand each behavior.
- What feelings do you think MT may be experiencing? Does he have any physical needs that are unaddressed? Think about pain and physical needs around toileting, hunger, thirst, physical comfort, and vital signs.
- As a nurse, what is within your scope of practice to address regarding MT's situation, and how can you leverage your interdisciplinary team members to meet his needs?

You ask MT if he is experiencing any pain, and in response, he turns his body away. You decide to use the Pain Assessment in Advanced Dementia Scale to assess his pain and find the following: normal breathing, repeated calling out, frowning facial expression, tense body language, and unable to console, distract, or reassure. This equals a score of 5, which indicates moderate pain.

MT may be experiencing pain in his left forearm and could also be experiencing pain due to his arthritis, particularly with decreased mobility post-fall. He is also experiencing some agitation and calling out, and resistance to care. He may also be experiencing the desire to leave his bed and seek a personal or comfort item or avoid disturbances.

You feel that resistance to care is currently posing a problem to being able to assess and address MT's pain, which could be contributing to his agitation and calling out. You know that resistance to care can be caused by pain but also by your approach. You decide that you will first take a small break and try again by reducing the noise in his room, sitting down next to him, validating his feelings, and facilitating independence. MT agrees to acetaminophen only.

When lunch nears, he agrees to join fellow residents in the dining room and take the rest of his medications. Upon assessment, he now rates his pain verbally by saying, "No, I feel good." You feel it is important to continue to address MT's needs to continue promoting his well-being and to prevent further behavioral and psychological symptoms into the evening and night.

You hypothesize that MT's agitation and calling out may be due to not only pain but also feelings of loneliness and boredom given his increased isolation post-fall and with fewer family visitors. After lunch, you ask the recreational aide to offer him some individualized music therapy, remembering his love of jazz. You hope that addressing his pain and offering meaningful engagement might also promote more alertness during the day and better sleep at night. Though your shift is nearing its end, you provide the next nurse with details on your assessment, interventions, and MT's response. You also brainstorm other potential strategies. The oncoming nurse agrees that she will facilitate a phone call between MT and his wife and reach out to other family to inquire if they may be able to bring photos for reminiscence therapy. You leave a voicemail for the nurse practitioner to report some medication resistance (a comprehensive medication review given polypharmacy/medication burden) and inquire about additional pain management strategies alongside protective arm sleeves and fall mats.

STOP & REFLECT

- How do you see the essentials of dementia care at play in this case study?
- What resources do you feel are needed to facilitate comprehensive dementia care for MT?

SUMMARY

Models of care delivery provide the infrastructure for organizing and providing care to residents in nursing homes. They contribute to the quality of care that staff deliver and residents receive. There are now national and international calls for transforming care delivery so that it supports the delivery of person-centered care. We have seen that high-quality, person-centered care is more likely to be achieved when there is strong professional leadership and when the culture of care delivery is characterized by healthy communication patterns, an empowered staff, a coaching/mentoring style of supervision, opportunities for professional growth, and family involvement as members of the healthcare team. These characteristics are indicators of positive relationships that help reduce staff turnover and develop direct-care staff for delivery of optimal resident care. The CDMs we reviewed in this chapter (relationship-based team nursing, palliative and end-of-life care, transitional care, and dementia-care) have these characteristics and are more likely to result in positive resident outcomes (e.g., greater care preference congruence, fewer avoidable hospitalizations, and better management of medical conditions) than more traditional CDMs. As a professional nurse leader, you will want to ensure that the CDM you adopt is consistent with best organizational practices for quality care delivery.

REFERENCES

Adler-Milstein, J., Raphael, K., O'Malley, T. A., & Cross, D. A. (2021, Jan. 4). Information sharing practices between US hospitals and skilled nursing facilities to support care transitions. *JAMA Network Open, 4*(1), e2033980. https://doi.org/10.1001/jamanetworkopen.2020.33980

American Association of Colleges of Nursing. (2021). *The essentials: Core competencies for professional nursing education.* https://www.aacnnursing.org/Portals/42/AcademicNursing/pdf/Essentials-2021.pdf

Bowers, B. J., Esmond, S., & Jacobson, N. (2003, March). Turnover reinterpreted: CNAs talk a bout why they leave. *Journal of Gerontological Nursing, 29*(3), 36–43. https://doi.org/10.3928/0098-9134-20030301-09

Britton, M. C., Ouellet, G. M., Minges, K. E., Gawel, M., Hodshon, B., & Chaudhry, S. I. (2017, November). Care transitions between hospitals and skilled nursing facilities: Perspectives of sending and receiving providers. *The Joint Commission Journal on Quality and Patient Safety, 43*(11), 565–572. https://doi.org/10.1016/j.jcjq.2017.06.004

Burke, R. E., Whitfield, E. A., Hittle, D., Min, S. J., Levy, C., Prochazka, A. V., Coleman, E. A., Schwartz, R., & Ginde, A. A. (2016, March 1). Hospital readmission from post-acute care facilities: Risk factors, timing, and outcomes. *Journal of the American Medical Directors Association, 17*(3), 249–255. https://doi.org/10.1016/j.jamda.2015.11.005

Cai, S., Miller, S. C., & Gozalo, P. L. (2018). Nursing home–hospice collaboration and end-of-life hospitalizations among dying nursing home residents. *Journal of the American Medical Directors Association, 19*(5), 439–443. https://doi.org/https://doi.org/10.1016/j.jamda.2017.10.020

Callahan, C. M., Arling, G., Tu, W., Rosenman, M. B., Counsell, S. R., Stump, T. E., & Hendrie, H. C. (2012, May). Transitions in care for older adults with and without dementia. *Journal of the American Geriatrics Society, 60*(5), 813–820. https://doi.org/10.1111/j.1532-5415.2012.03905.x

Carpenter, J. G., Berry, P. H., & Ersek, M. (2017). Nursing home care trajectories for older adults following in-hospital palliative care consultation. *Geriatric Nursing, 38*(6), 531–536. https://doi.org/10.1016/j.gerinurse.2017.03.016

Carpenter, J. G., Berry, P. H., & Ersek, M. (2018, April). Care in nursing facilities after palliative consult. *Journal of Hospice & Palliative Care Nursing, 20*(2), 153–159. https://doi.org/10.1097/njh.0000000000000420

Currow, D. C., Agar, M. R., & Phillips, J. L. (2020, March 20). Role of hospice care at the end of life for people with cancer. *Journal of Clinical Oncology, 38*(9), 937–943. https://doi.org/10.1200/jco.18.02235

Dellefield, M. E., & Madrigal, C. (2022, June). Nursing leadership – Transforming the work environment in nursing homes. *Nursing Clinics of North America, 57*(2), 299–314. https://doi.org/10.1016/j.cnur.2022.02.008

Duffield, C., Roche, M., Diers, D., Catling-Paull, C., & Blay, N. (2010, August). Staffing, skill mix and the model of care. *Journal of Clinical Nursing, 19*(15–16), 2242–2251. https://doi.org/10.1111/j.1365-2702.2010.03225.x

Dwyer, R., Gabbe, B., Stoelwinder, J. U., & Lowthian, J. (2014, November). A systematic review of outcomes following emergency transfer to hospital for residents of aged care facilities. *Age and Ageing, 43*(6), 759–766. https://doi.org/10.1093/ageing/afu117

ElMokhallalati, Y., Bradley, S. H., Chapman, E., Ziegler, L., Murtagh, F. E., Johnson, M. J., & Bennett, M. I. (2020, September). Identification of patients with potential palliative care needs: A systematic review of screening tools in primary care. *Palliative Medicine, 34*(8), 989–1005. https://doi.org/10.1177/0269216320929552

Ersek, M., & Carpenter, J. G. (2013, October). Geriatric palliative care in long-term care settings with a focus on nursing homes. *Journal of Palliative Medicine, 16*(10), 1180–1187. https://doi.org/10.1089/jpm.2013.9474

Ersek, M., Unroe, K. T., Carpenter, J. G., Cagle, J. G., Stephens, C. E., & Stevenson, D. G. (2022, February). High-quality nursing home and palliative care—One and the same. *Journal of the American Medical Directors Association, 23*(2), 247–252. https://doi.org/10.1016/j.jamda.2021.11.027

Fairbrother, G., Chiarella, M., & Braithwaite, J. (2015, November). Models of care choices in today's nursing workplace: Where does team nursing sit? *Australian Health Review, 39*(5), 489–493. https://doi.org/10.1071/AH14091

Fawcett, J. (2021, July). Thoughts about models of nursing practice delivery. *Nursing Science Quarterly, 34*(3), 328–330. https://doi.org/10.1177/08943184211010460

Fazio, S., Pace, D., Flinner, J., & Kallmyer, B. (2018, Jan. 18). The fundamentals of person-centered care for individuals with dementia. *The Gerontologist, 58*(Suppl._1), S10–S19. https://doi.org/10.1093/geront/gnx122

Fazio, S., Pace, D., Maslow, K., Zimmerman, S., & Kallmyer, B. (2018, Jan. 18). Alzheimer's Association dementia care practice recommendations. *The Gerontologist, 58*(Suppl._1), S1–S9. https://doi.org/10.1093/geront/gnx182

Gage, L. A., Washington, K., Oliver, D. P., Kruse, R., Lewis, A., & Demiris, G. (2016, May). Family members' experience with hospice in nursing homes. *American Journal of Hospice and Palliative Medicine, 33*(4), 354–362. https://doi.org/10.1177/1049909114560213

Goodwin, J. S., Howrey, B., Zhang, D. D., & Kuo, Y. F. (2011, December). Risk of continued institutionalization after hospitalization in older adults. *The Journals of Gerontology Series A: Biological Sciences & Medical Sciences, 66*(12), 1321–1327. https://doi.org/10.1093/gerona/glr171

Hanson, L. C., Zimmerman, S., Song, M.-K., Lin, F.-C., Rosemond, C., Carey, T. S., & Mitchell, S. L. (2017). Effect of the goals of care intervention for advanced dementia: A randomized clinical trial. *JAMA Internal Medicine, 177*(1), 24–31. https://doi.org/10.1001/jamainternmed.2016.7031

Harrington, C., Kovner, C., Mezey, M., Kayser-Jones, J., Burger, S., Mohler, M., Burke, R., & Zimmerman, D. (2000, February). Experts recommend minimum nurse staffing standards for nursing facilities in the United States. *The Gerontologist, 40*(1), 5–16. https://doi.org/10.1093/geront/40.1.5

Herman, R. E., & Williams, K. N. (2009). Elderspeak's influence on resistiveness to care: Focus on behavioral events. *American Journal of Alzheimer's Disease & Other Dementias, 24*(5), 417–423. https://doi.org/10.1177/1533317509341949

Hickman, S. E., Unroe, K. T., Ersek, M. T., Buente, B., Nazir, A., & Sachs, G. A. (2016, November). An interim analysis of an advance care planning intervention in the nursing home setting. *Journal of the American Geriatrics Society, 64*(11), 2385–2392. https://doi.org/10.1111/jgs.14463

Jacobsen, J. M. L., Schnelle, J. F., Saraf, A. A., Long, E. A., Vasilevskis, E. E., Kripalani, S., & Simmons, S. F. (2017, Nov. 10). Preventability of hospital readmissions from skilled nursing facilities: A consumer perspective. *The Gerontologist, 57*(6), 1123–1132. https://doi.org/10.1093/geront/gnw132

Jennings, L. A., Palimaru, A., Corona, M. G., Cagigas, X. E., Ramirez, K. D., Zhao, T., Hays, R. D., Wenger, N. S., & Reuben, D. B. (2017, March). Patient and caregiver goals for dementia care. *Quality of Life Research, 26*(3), 685–693. https://doi.org/10.1007/s11136-016-1471-7

Johnson, M., Attree, M., Jones, I., Al Gamal, E., & Garbutt, D. (2014, June). Diagnosis, prognosis and awareness of dying in nursing homes: Towards the gold standard? *International Journal of Older People Nursing, 9*(2), 95–105. https://doi.org/10.1111/opn.12024

Kim, H., Harrington, C., & Greene, W. H. (2009, February). Registered nurse staffing mix and quality of care in nursing homes: A longitudinal analysis. *The Gerontologist, 49*(1), 81–90. https://doi.org/10.1093/geront/gnp014

King, B. J., Gilmore-Bykovskyi, A. L., Roiland, R. A., Polnaszek, B. E., Bowers, B. J., & Kind, A. J. (2013, July). The consequences of poor communication during transitions from hospital to skilled nursing facility: A qualitative study. *Journal of the American Geriatrics Society, 61*(7), 1095–1102. https://doi.org/10.1111/jgs.12328

Kolanowski, A., Fortinsky, R. H., Calkins, M., Devanand, D. P., Gould, E., Heller, T., Hodgson, N. A., Kales, H. C., Kaye, J., Lyketsos, C., Resnick, B., Schicker, M., & Zimmerman, S. (2018, December). Advancing research on care needs and supportive approaches for persons with dementia: Recommendations and rationale. *Journal of the American Medical Directors Association, 19*(12), 1047–1053. https://doi.org/10.1016/j.jamda.2018.07.005

Kovach, C. R., Noonan, P. E., Schlidt, A. M., & Wells, T. (2005). A model of consequences of need-driven, dementia-compromised behavior. *Journal of Nursing Scholarship, 37*(2), 134–140. https://doi.org/10.1111/j.1547-5069.2005.00025_1.x

Lambertsen, E. C. (1958). *Education for nursing leadership*. Lippincott.

Lamppu, P. J., Laurila, J., Finne-Soveri, H., Laakkonen, M. L., Kautiainen, H., & Pitkälä, K. H. (2019, August). Training nursing home staff to improve residents' end-of-life care: Design and baseline findings from a randomized controlled trial. *European Geriatric Medicine, 10*(4), 649–657. https://doi.org/10.1007/s41999-019-00200-5

Lester, P. E., Stefanacci, R. G., & Feuerman, M. (2016, March). Prevalence and description of palliative care in US nursing homes: A descriptive study. *American Journal of Hospice and Palliative Medicine, 33*(2), 171–177. https://doi.org/10.1177/1049909114558585

Lima, J. C., & Miller, S. C. (2018, February). Palliative care consults in U.S. nursing homes: Not just for the dying. *Journal of Palliative Medicine, 21*(2), 188–193. https://doi.org/10.1089/jpm.2017.0099

Lupu, D., Quigley, L., Mehfoud, N., & Salsberg, E. S. (2018, April). The growing demand for hospice and palliative medicine physicians: Will the supply keep up? *Journal of Pain and Symptom Management, 55*(4), 1216–1223. https://doi.org/10.1016/j.jpainsymman.2018.01.011

Marincowitz, C., Preston, L., Cantrell, A., Tonkins, M., Sabir, L., & Mason, S. (2022). What influences decisions to transfer older care-home residents to the emergency department? A synthesis of qualitative reviews. *Age and Ageing, 51*(11), afac257. https://doi.org/10.1093/ageing/afac257

McBride, A. B. (2019). *The growth and development of nurse leaders* (2nd ed.). Springer Publishing.

Miller, S. C., Lima, J. C., Intrator, O., Martin, E., Bull, J., & Hanson, L. C. (2016, November). Palliative care consultations in nursing homes and reductions in acute care use and potentially burdensome end-of-life transitions. *Journal of the American Geriatrics Society, 64*(11), 2280–2287. https://doi.org/10.1111/jgs.14469

Miller, S. C., Lima, J. C., Intrator, O., Martin, E., Bull, J., & Hanson, L. C. (2017, July). Specialty palliative care consultations for nursing home residents with dementia. *Journal of Pain and Symptom Management, 54*(1), 9–16.e15. https://doi.org/10.1016/j.jpainsymman.2017.03.005

Mjørud, M., Engedal, K., Røsvik, J., & Kirkevold, M. (2017). Living with dementia in a nursing home, as described by persons with dementia: A phenomenological hermeneutic study. *BMC Health Services Research, 17*(1), 93. https://doi.org/10.1186/s12913-017-2053-2

Mor, V., Intrator, O., Feng, Z., & Grabowski, D. C. (2010). The revolving door of rehospitalization from skilled nursing facilities. *HealthAffairs, 29*(1), 57–64. https://doi.org/10.1377/hlthaff.2009.0629

Morris, D. A., & Galicia-Castillo, M. (2017, June). Caring about residents' experiences and symptoms (CARES) program: A model of palliative care consultation in the nursing home. *American Journal of Hospice and Palliative Medicine, 34*(5), 466–469. https://doi.org/10.1177/1049909116641606

Moyo, P., Loomer, L., Teno, J. M., Gutman, R., McCreedy, E. M., Bélanger, E., Volandes, A. E., Mitchell, S. L., & Mor, V. (2022, March). Effect of a video-assisted advance care planning intervention on end-of-life health care transitions among long-stay nursing home residents. *Journal of the American Medical Directors Association, 23*(3), 394–398. https://doi.org/10.1016/j.jamda.2021.09.014

National Coalition for Hospice and Palliative Care. (2018). *Clinical practice guidelines for quality palliative care* (4th ed.). https://www.nationalcoalitionhpc.org/wp-content/uploads/2020/07/NCHPC-NCPGuidelines_4thED_web_FINAL.pdf

Naylor, M. D., Shaid, E. C., Carpenter, D., Gass, B., Levine, C., Li, J., Malley, A., McCauley, K., Nguyen, H. Q., Watson, H., Brock, J., Mittman, B., Jack, B., Mitchell, S., Callicoatte, B., Schall, J., & Williams, M. V. (2017, June). Components of comprehensive and effective transitional care. *Journal of the American Geriatrics Society, 65*(6), 1119–1125. https://doi.org/10.1111/jgs.14782

Ouslander, J. G., Lamb, G., Perloe, M., Givens, J. H., Kluge, L., Rutland, T., Atherly, A., & Saliba, D. (2010, April). Potentially avoidable hospitalizations of nursing home residents: Frequency, causes, and costs [see editorial comments by Drs. Jean F. Wyman and William R. Hazzard, pp. 760–761]. *Journal of the American Geriatrics Society, 58*(4), 627–635. https://doi.org/10.1111/j.1532-5415.2010.02768.x

Ouslander, J. G., Naharci, I., Engstrom, G., Shutes, J., Wolf, D. G., Alpert, G., Rojido, C., Tappen, R., & Newman, D. (2016, March 1). Root cause analyses of transfers of skilled nursing facility patients to acute hospitals: Lessons learned for reducing unnecessary hospitalizations. *Journal of the American Medical Directors Association, 17*(3), 256–262. https://doi.org/10.1016/j.jamda.2015.11.018

PHI. (2019). *U.S. nursing assistants employed in nursing homes: Key facts.* https://www.phinational.org/resource/u-s-nursing-assistants-employed-in-nursing-homes-key-facts-2019/

Parast, L., Tolpadi, A. A., Teno, J. M., Elliott, M. N., & Price, R. A. (2021, April). Hospice care experiences among cancer patients and their caregivers. *Journal of General Internal Medicine, 36*(4), 961–969. https://doi.org/10.1007/s11606-020-06490-x

Park, M. S., Lee, S. J., Choi, Y. R., & Chang, S. O. (2021, April 9). Exploring a nursing home-specific, interdisciplinary, function-focused, communicative framework based on Situation, Background, Assessment, and Recommendation. *Journal of Nursing Research, 29*(3), e151. https://doi.org/10.1097/jnr.0000000000000428

Rantz, M. J., Popejoy, L., Vogelsmeier, A., Galambos, C., Alexander, G., Flesner, M., Crecelius, C., Ge, B., & Petroski, G. (2017, Nov. 1). Successfully reducing hospitalizations of nursing home residents: Results of the Missouri Quality Initiative. *Journal of the American Medical Directors Association, 18*(11), 960–966. https://doi.org/10.1016/j.jamda.2017.05.027

Sherman, R. O. (1990, November). Team nursing revisited. *Journal of Nursing Administration, 20*(11), 4346. https://www.ncbi.nlm.nih.gov/pubmed/2231014

Siegel, E. O., Kolanowski, A. M., & Bowers, B. J. (2023). A fresh look at the nursing home workforce crisis: Transforming nursing care delivery models. *Research in Gerontological Nursing, 16*(1), 5–13. https://doi.org/10.3928/19404921-20230104-01

Temkin-Greener, H., Cai, S., Katz, P., Zhao, H., & Mukamel, D. B. (2009, February). Daily practice teams in nursing homes: Evidence from New York state. *The Gerontologist, 49*(1), 68–80. https://doi.org/10.1093/geront/gnp011

Teno, J. M., Gozalo, P., Trivedi, A. N., Bunker, J., Lima, J., Ogarek, J., & Mor, V. (2018, July 17). Site of death, place of care, and health care transitions among US Medicare beneficiaries, 2000–2015. *Journal of the American Medical Association, 320*(3), 264–271. https://doi.org/10.1001/jama.2018.8981

Tjia, J., Bonner, A., Briesacher, B. A., McGee, S., Terrill, E., & Miller, K. (2009). Medication discrepancies upon hospital to skilled nursing facility transitions. *Journal of General Internal Medicine, 24*(5), 630–635. https://doi.org/10.1007/s11606-009-0948-2

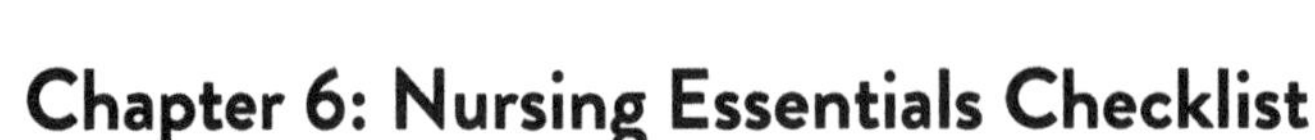

Chapter 6: Nursing Essentials Checklist

SPHERES OF CARE

Nursing occurs within four spheres of care, ranging from prevention to supportive care and all the areas in between. This chapter is relevant to the following spheres of care:

- ☑ Disease Prevention/Health Promotion
- ☑ Chronic Disease Care
- ☑ Regenerative or Restorative Care
- ☐ Hospice/Palliative/Supportive Care

DOMAINS OF PRACTICE

The American Association of Colleges of Nursing has identified 10 broad domains of practice for nursing. Students are expected to master these domains of practice across the spheres of care. This chapter addresses:

- ☑ Knowledge for Nursing Practice (Nursing and Other Disciplines)
- ☑ Person-Centered Care
- ☐ Population Health
- ☐ Scholarship for Practice
- ☑ Quality and Safety
- ☐ Interprofessional Partnerships
- ☐ Systems-Based Care
- ☐ Information & Healthcare Technologies
- ☐ Professionalism
- ☐ Personal, Professional, Leadership Development

CONCEPTS FOR PRACTICE

Integrated across the domains of practice are eight concepts which the student is expected to master across the spheres of care and across the domains of practice. This chapter addresses:

- ☑ Clinical Judgment
- ☑ Communication
- ☐ Compassionate Care
- ☐ Diversity, Equity, Inclusion
- ☐ Ethics
- ☑ Evidence-Based Practice
- ☐ Health Policy
- ☐ Social Determinants of Health

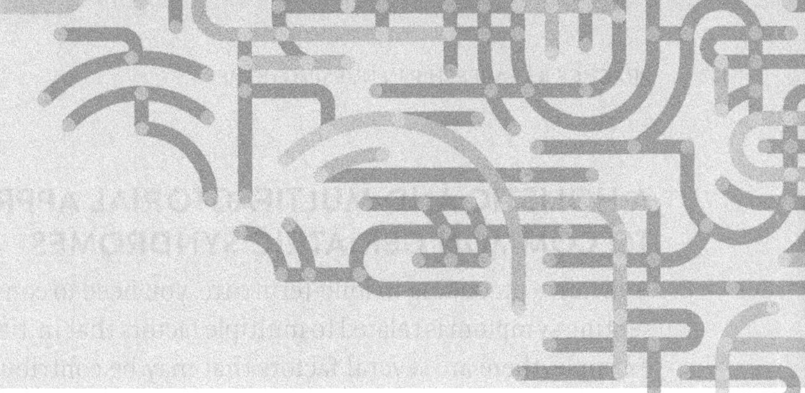

CHAPTER 6

COMMON GERIATRIC SYNDROMES

Elizabeth Galik, PhD, CRNP, FAAN, FAANP

OBJECTIVES

1. Describe geriatric syndromes common among older adults in nursing homes.
2. Distinguish acute and chronic presentations of cognitive impairment.
3. Appreciate that, although common, geriatric syndromes are not inevitable consequences of aging.
4. Develop nursing care plans to prevent geriatric syndromes and restore optimal function and quality of life.

INTRODUCTION

Geriatric syndromes are common health problems experienced by older adults that often have multiple causes and are not specific to one organ system. Geriatric syndromes in the nursing home setting that will be discussed in this chapter include cognitive impairment, nutritional deficits, frailty, falls, and urinary incontinence. Geriatric syndromes can be challenging to assess and treat because the presenting symptom may not be directly related to the underlying physical problem. For example, a nursing home resident experiences urinary incontinence as a new symptom that may or may not be related to an underlying disease of the genitourinary system, such as urinary stress incontinence or a urinary tract infection. Assessment and treatment of geriatric syndromes requires you to take a more holistic and multifactorial approach to adequately assess and intervene on the resident's behalf.

A HOLISTIC AND MULTIFACTORIAL APPROACH TO COMMON GERIATRIC SYNDROMES

As a nurse practicing in long-term care, you need to consider whether a resident's presenting symptom is related to multiple factors that initially may appear unrelated. For example, there are several factors that may be contributing to urinary incontinence outside of the genitourinary system. Moderate to severe cognitive impairment may make it difficult for the resident to recognize the sensations of a full bladder and then to locate and recognize the bathroom or commode. A resident who is fearful of falling may postpone walking to the bathroom and experience incontinence. Arthritic fingers may make it difficult for the resident to lower pants and undergarments in a timely manner. Taking a diuretic may result in greater urine output and urinary urgency that may result in incontinence. The resident may also have an underlying genitourinary disorder; however, if your assessment and the intervention is exclusively focused on the organ system and is not inclusive of other factors that influence the urinary incontinence, then symptomatic improvement or resolution of the geriatric syndrome is less likely.

Several risk factors are associated with the development of geriatric syndromes:

- Advanced age
- Multimorbidity
- Advanced cognitive impairment
- Impaired mobility
- Functional impairment

While geriatric syndromes are common in older adults, they are not a normal part of aging. For example, symptoms of memory loss and disorientation should not be attributed to advanced age. You should explore alternative explanations, such as early symptoms of dementia or an acute delirium caused by an adverse effect of medication(s) and/or an acute medical condition. Even though geriatric syndromes can have a negative impact on functional ability, quality of life, rehabilitation potential, and life expectancy of older adults in post-acute and long-term care (PA-LTC) settings, unfortunately, they remain under-recognized (Bell et al., 2016).

Screening for Geriatric Syndromes

The St. Louis University Rapid Geriatric Assessment is a straightforward screening instrument that assesses the four common geriatric syndromes: cognitive impairment, nutritional deficits, frailty, and loss of muscle, also called *sarcopenia* (Sanford et al., 2020). It can be completed with the resident or an informant who knows the resident well, such as a family member or a nursing assistant. The assessment is freely available (see https://www.slu.edu/medicine/internal-medicine/geriatric-medicine/aging-successfully/assessment-tools/index.php) and can be completed on paper or may be embedded into an electronic medical record as part of a resident's admission assessment into PA-LTC. The assessment quantifies several geriatric syndromes in one brief instrument, and there are several screening and assessment tools that are specific to each individual geriatric syndrome.

Medications Associated With Geriatric Syndromes

While medication may be helpful in treating many medical conditions, an adverse effect of prescribed medication may frequently exacerbate geriatric syndromes. For example, a nursing home resident with an unsteady gait and poor safety awareness is prescribed two antihypertensive medications; a few weeks later, he experiences episodes of hypotension that result in repeated falls. Consultant pharmacists in PA-LTC settings frequently help the interdisciplinary team to identify and consider the impact of drug-drug interactions and drug-disease interactions on resident health and well-being. It is also important for you to consider the impact of medications on geriatric syndromes in a nursing home population.

Drug interactions are particularly common contributors to the following three geriatric syndromes: falls, delirium (an acute confusional state), and urinary incontinence (Onder et al., 2018). Table 6.1 describes medication classes that are associated with geriatric syndromes. Among nursing home residents, opioids and psychotropic medications, such as antipsychotics, antidepressants, and benzodiazepines, are most likely to be associated with multiple geriatric syndromes, and their use may be inappropriate among some older adults (American Geriatrics Society Beers Criteria Update Expert Panel, 2019).

TABLE 6.1 Medication Classes Associated With Geriatric Syndromes

GERIATRIC SYNDROME	MEDICATION CLASSES	
Cognitive impairment (delirium)	Anticholinergics Antihistamines Antiparkinsonian agents Antipsychotics Benzodiazepines	Digoxin H2 receptor antagonists Muscle relaxants Sedative hypnotics Steroids
Poor appetite and weight loss	Acetyl cholinesterase inhibitors Antibiotics Anticonvulsants	Antidepressants • Selective serotonin reuptake inhibitors • Serotonin and norepinephrine reuptake inhibitors GLP-1 agonists for diabetes Opioids
Falls	Anticonvulsants Antidepressants • Selective serotonin reuptake inhibitors • Tricyclics	Antihypertensives Antipsychotics Benzodiazepines Opioids Sedative-hypnotics
Urinary incontinence	ACE inhibitors Alpha blockers Anticholinergic drugs Antipsychotics	Calcium channel blockers Diuretics Sedative hypnotics

Atypical Presentation of Illness Among Nursing Home Residents

Atypical presentation of an acute illness or exacerbation of a chronic disease is common among older adults. Subtle and mild changes in a nursing home resident's status may reflect a significant health concern due to decreased physiologic reserve and responsiveness. For example, a resident who has pneumonia may not present with classic symptoms such as a cough, high fever, and elevated white blood cell count. The resident may have a low-grade fever, fatigue, acute confusion, and functional decline. This atypical presentation makes accurate diagnosis and treatment more complicated. Nursing assistants who are familiar with the resident and family members may report that the resident "isn't acting like herself today." These alerts need to be taken seriously and should prompt you to gather additional history of the presenting problem and change from baseline, conduct a physical examination of the resident, provide ongoing monitoring of any symptoms, and report your findings to the physician or advanced practice provider if you have evidence of a change in the resident's health status.

Characteristics of Nursing Home Residents

Approximately 1.3 million individuals are residents of nursing homes in the United States (Sengupta et al., 2022). Long-stay nursing home residents are functionally dependent, and many require supervision or physical assistance with dressing, bathing, transferring, toileting, and eating. Very few nursing home residents are able to ambulate independently without supervision or assistance. Dementia, depression, and multimorbidity are common among nursing home residents. Older age, white race, multiple medical comorbidities, cognitive impairment, depression, behavioral and psychological symptoms of dementia, incontinence, and pressure injuries were associated with a new admission to PA-LTC following a hospitalization (Middleton et al., 2018). There is significant overlap between the risk factors for geriatric syndromes and risk factors for nursing home admission.

While geriatric syndromes are associated with negative health outcomes for nursing home residents, you have an important role to play in early identification and treatment of geriatric syndromes. The complexity and subtlety of changes in condition in nursing home residents require nurses to have well-developed assessment skills, as they are frequently the key healthcare professional to detect, understand, and communicate these changes to the healthcare team.

Most geriatric syndromes do respond to a combination of nonpharmacological interventions and medical treatments or deprescribing. By recognizing and addressing common geriatric syndromes, such as cognitive impairment, nutritional deficits, frailty, falls, and incontinence, you will help residents minimize disability and optimize quality of life. The remainder of this chapter will define and describe common geriatric syndromes, including prevalence and risk factors and strategies for assessment and treatment.

COGNITIVE IMPAIRMENT

An individual with cognitive impairment has a decline in mental functioning and may show symptoms of memory loss, disorientation, impaired reasoning, decreased attention, language, and perceptual impairments. Cognitive impairment is not an illness by itself but is a geriatric syndrome that reflects an underlying condition or disease process. Cognitive impairment can occur suddenly or may occur insidiously and progress slowly. The two major causes of cognitive impairment in nursing home residents are dementia and delirium.

Dementia

Dementia or *neurocognitive disorders* are global terms to indicate that an individual has a significant decline in cognitive functioning from the previous baseline in one or more areas, including attention, executive functioning, learning, memory, language, perceptual abilities, learned motor skills, and/or social interaction (American Psychiatric Association, 2013). The symptoms of cognitive decline need to be severe enough to impair the individual's day-to-day function, and the diagnosis can only be made outside the context of an acute change in mental status (delirium) when the resident's cognitive baseline is not known.

There are several different types of dementia, with Alzheimer's disease being the most common cause. Other causes of dementia include vascular dementia, frontotemporal dementia, Lewy body dementia, and Parkinson's disease dementia. The Alzheimer's Association (2022) provides resources that describe the different types of dementia, their pathophysiology, and differentiating symptoms. Approximately half of all PA-LTC residents have dementia (Sengupta et al., 2022). The prevalence of dementia is less common among short-stay residents (36%) versus long-stay nursing home residents (58%; Alzheimer's Association, 2022).

The nursing assessment of a nursing home resident with dementia should focus on identifying changes in cognition, function, and behavior.

The progression of dementia is gradual and progressive and occurs over several years. More sudden changes in cognition, function, and behavior are more likely to reflect an acute problem such as an exacerbation of a chronic illness or an adverse response to medication and should not be attributed to normal progression of dementia.

In nursing homes, the Minimum Data Set (MDS) 3.0 is a standardized assessment instrument that provides data about residents' cognition, physical function, and medical and psychosocial conditions. The MDS 3.0 is utilized to evaluate resident status and quality of care outcomes at least on a quarterly basis or more frequently depending on the resident's status. The MDS 3.0 provides valuable information regarding a resident's status; however, you may want to utilize additional assessment tools in your clinical practice in PA-LTC settings.

The following list briefly describes various tools to be used for cognitive assessment:

- The MDS 3.0 assesses cognition using a performance measure, the Brief Inventory of Mental Status (BIMS; Saliba et al., 2012). The instrument assesses registration, orientation, and recall, and scores range from 0–15. Scores of 12 or below indicate cognitive impairment that may reflect dementia.
- Additional instruments that you can use to more comprehensively assess cognition include the St. Louis University Mental Status Exam (Tariq et al., 2006) and the Montreal Cognitive Assessment (Nasreddine et al., 2005). These instruments are more useful in identifying individuals with minor cognitive impairment or mild dementia than the BIMS, but they take longer to complete.
- The Mini-Cog (Borson et al., 2003) is a freely available, quick screening test of cognition that includes clock drawing and three item recall. Even though it is brief, it assesses multiple cognitive domains such as memory, executive function, receptive language, and visual motor skills.
- The AD-8 (Galvin et al., 2005) is a brief informant-based screening tool that assesses memory, orientation, judgment, and function. It can be helpful to identify individuals with dementia at the time of admission to the nursing home when done with a reliable informant (Hendry et al., 2019).

To perform a functional assessment, tools are available to help you assess a resident's physical capabilities, but observing a resident's ability to perform various functions is also important, as described in this list:

- Individuals with dementia experience gradual decline in functional abilities primarily due to motor apraxia (impairment in learned motor skills), which affects the resident's ability to engage in activities of daily living such as dressing, grooming, toileting, bathing, mobility, and eating.
- The ability to engage in self-feeding and eating is often the most well-preserved activity of daily living among nursing home residents living with dementia.

- While asking a family member, care partner, or staff member about the resident's functional ability may be helpful, the best method of functional assessment is to assess what the resident can do based on their actual performance.
- If a resident is unable to perform an activity independently or with verbal cueing, you should attempt to role-model what you want the resident to do and assess the ability of the resident to engage in the activity.
- The Physical Capability Measure (Resnick et al., 2013, 2014) helps assess the resident's underlying physical and cognitive abilities and can be used to plan functional care goals for the resident.
- The Tinetti Gait and Balance assessment (Tinetti et al., 1986) is a performance measure that you can use to assess a resident's ability to stand safely.

Finally, this list summarizes behavioral symptoms, information on assessing these symptoms, and a couple tools to help you do so:

- Behavioral and psychological symptoms of dementia include physical and verbal aggression, changes in mood, psychotic symptoms, agitation, and resistiveness to care. These symptoms are commonly experienced by nursing home residents with dementia and are a primary factor that leads to nursing home admission.
- Expression of these behaviors may be related to an unmet need that the resident is unable to communicate verbally, such as untreated pain, boredom, or hunger.
- Sudden changes in behavioral symptoms may also indicate a possible episode of delirium, which is more likely to be related to medications, acute illness, or significant environmental changes.
- While behavioral symptoms are assessed by the MDS 3.0, you may also consider using instruments such as the Neuropsychiatric Inventory Nursing Home Version (Wood et al., 2000) or the Cohen-Mansfield Agitation Inventory (Cohen-Mansfield, 1991; Cohen-Mansfield et al., 1989).

Delirium

Delirium is an acute change in mental status and level of consciousness that develops suddenly, indicates a change from baseline in attention and awareness, and has a fluctuating and changing course throughout the day (American Psychiatric Association, 2013). These changes are also accompanied by abrupt changes in cognition such as memory impairment, disorientation, impaired perception, and language difficulties. The prevalence of delirium varies by setting but ranges from 4% up to 70% when subsyndromal delirium is included (Flaherty & Morley, 2013; Komici et al., 2022).

Risk factors for delirium are similar to the risk factors for geriatric syndromes and are outlined in Table 6.2. Common causes of delirium in nursing home residents include fluid and electrolyte disturbance such as dehydration or hyponatremia, other metabolic disorders such as hypoxia and hypo/hyperglycemia, infection, medications, blood loss, trauma, stroke, cardiac abnormalities, and exposure to temperature extremes (hypo/hyperthermia).

TABLE 6.2 Risk Factors for Delirium

UNMODIFIABLE RISK FACTORS	POTENTIALLY MODIFIABLE RISK FACTORS
Advanced dementia	Polypharmacy (particularly psychotropic medications and opioids)
Multiple medical co-morbidities	Use of general anesthesia for surgical procedure
Advanced age	Sensory deficit (hearing or vision loss)
Functional impairment	Tethering (urinary catheters, restraints, intravenous lines)
Past delirious episodes	Malnutrition

Delirium can be hyperactive, hypoactive, or mixed:

- *Hyperactive delirium* typically presents with agitation and restlessness and may be accompanied by psychotic symptoms. Hyperactive delirium is easier to recognize but occurs less frequently.
- *Hypoactive delirium* is more common and presents with symptoms of lethargy, sedation, apathy, and a rapid decline in function. Hypoactive delirium is frequently under-recognized due to the quiet nature of the symptoms.
- *Mixed delirium* includes elements of both hyperactive and hypoactive delirium. A resident who typically has a normal sleep-wake pattern who suddenly is sleeping more during the day and is awake intermittently at night should be promptly screened for delirium.

It is important for you to be able to differentiate delirium from dementia and to identify when delirium is superimposed on a resident who has previously been diagnosed with dementia. Delay in the recognition of delirium has an increased risk of morbidity and mortality.

There are several screening tools for delirium including the Confusion Assessment Method (CAM; Inouye et al., 1990), which is an observational measure, and the Delirium Rating Scale (Rockwood et al., 1996; Trzepacz et al., 2001), which is an informant-based survey. The CAM (Inouye et al., 1990) assesses for the following four symptoms of delirium:

1. Acute change in mental status with a fluctuating course
2. Inattention and distractibility
3. Disorganized or incoherent thinking or conversation
4. Altered level of consciousness (unarousable, lethargic, hypervigilant)

To screen positive for delirium on the CAM, the resident must have at least three symptoms. Items 1 and 2 must be present. Subsyndromal delirium may be present when two or more features are present.

Nursing Interventions for Cognitive Impairment

The majority of nursing interventions for dementia and delirium are overlapping and include the following:

- Provide structure and predictable routine for the resident when feasible. Facilitate care interactions provided by consistent caregivers who know that resident well and can incorporate personal preferences into care routines.
- Promote a regular sleep-wake cycle and avoid long or frequent daytime napping.
- Provide adequate nutrition and hydration.
- Optimize resident engagement in physical and functional activities. Perform care “with the resident” rather than “for the resident.” See this website for freely available video coaching: https://functionfocusedcare.wordpress.com/video-coaching/

- Prevent and recognize acute illnesses or unstable chronic illnesses and refer the resident for treatment.
- Optimize sensory input by encouraging residents to wear their glasses and hearing aids.
- Provide familiar and personally meaningful objects in the resident's room.
- Encourage opportunities for socialization and interaction with other residents, family, and staff as tolerated.
- Be aware of and modulate the environmental press, such as extremes with noise, temperature, and interpersonal stimulation.
- Avoid correcting residents or saying words such as "no, stop, don't, can't."
- Consistently implement nonpharmacological interventions to address behavioral symptoms of distress such as personalized music, sensory stimulation, distraction, recreational activities, validation, physical activity, and interventions designed to improve person-centered caregiver interaction with residents. The Nursing Home Toolkit is an evidence-based repository of nonpharmacological interventions designed to promote positive behavioral health for nursing home residents with dementia: http://www.nursinghometoolkit.com/
- Limit requests for psychoactive medications to manage behavioral symptoms when feasible. Monitor for and report side effects of medications such as sedation, gait changes, increased confusion, weight loss, and functional decline, particularly for residents who are prescribed antidepressants, antipsychotics, benzodiazepines, mood stabilizers/anticonvulsants, and/or sedative/hypnotics.

MALNUTRITION

Malnutrition is common among nursing home residents and is associated with negative health outcomes such as frailty, functional decline, pressure injuries, hospitalization, increased healthcare costs, morbidity, and mortality (Norman et al., 2021; van den Berg et al., 2021). In a recent study of almost 12,000 nursing home residents who were 65 years of age or older, 10.5% of the non-malnourished residents developed malnutrition after six months (Torbahn et al., 2022). Malnutrition occurs when a resident lacks adequate caloric energy and/or nutrients to maintain optimal health.

While malnutrition is typically identified through unexplained weight loss of 5%–10% over six months or a low body mass index, malnutrition also can occur in residents who are overweight or obese. Malnutrition is associated with other geriatric syndromes such as cognitive impairment, frailty, and falls (Azzolino et al., 2021; Liu et al., 2020; Torbahn et al., 2022).

Risk factors for malnutrition among nursing home residents include:

- Severe cognitive impairment
- Older age
- Immobility
- Depression
- Poor oral health including dental and gum disease
- Multimorbidity
- Social isolation
- Polypharmacy
- Dysphagia

Assessment of nutritional status includes measures of body composition such as weight, body mass index, skin fold measurement to estimate body fat, and measurement of upper arm circumference to assess lean body mass. Serum albumin less than 3.5 g/dl is associated with malnutrition; however, results may be skewed in the presence of hepatic impairment. The serologic measure of pre-albumin is a more sensitive test for identifying malnutrition but also is significantly more costly. Food intake by observed plate assessment is also utilized in the MDS as an assessment of nutrition. The Simplified Nutritional Assessment Questionnaire (Wilson et al., 2005) is a brief survey measure that you can use with nursing home residents who can reliably report information about their oral intake. A score of less than or equal to 14 suggests a significant risk of malnutrition within the next six months.

Nursing Interventions for Malnutrition

Nursing interventions for malnutrition include the following:

- Facilitate referral to dietitian.
- Liberalize diet to include food preferences with input from the resident and family.
- Optimize eating performance through setup, cueing, and role-modeling during mealtime.
- For residents with cognitive impairment, simplify meal presentation, provide finger foods, or utilize careful hand feeding using hand-under-hand technique.
- Provide good oral care and refer to a dental professional if needed.
- Administer supplements as ordered.
- Provide pleasant environmental modifications to support oral intake (soft music, socialization, comfortable seating).
- There are no pharmacological treatments that have a Food and Drug Administration approved use for the treatment of unintended weight loss among older adults. The off-label use of megestrol acetate and mirtazapine has been used to treat unintentional weight loss among older adults; however, this has not been well studied, and any potential benefit needs to be weighed against the risk of adverse side effects associated with these medications.

FRAILTY

Frailty is a state of physiologic vulnerability to stressors that carries increased susceptibility to negative health outcomes in older adults, such as acute illness, falls, functional decline, physical dependency, and death (Fried et al., 2001). Frailty is not a normal or expected consequence of aging; rather, it is considered a geriatric syndrome in which some factors are preventable and/or reversible.

Characteristics of frailty include unexplained weight loss, fatigue, decreased muscle strength, slow walking speed, and decreased physical activity (Fried et al., 2001). Approximately half of nursing home residents are frail (Veronese et al., 2021). Frailty is highly associated with malnutrition (Medeiros et al., 2020) and loss of muscle mass (sarcopenia).

There are several ways to assess frailty among older adults. Performance measures such as gait speed and grip strength can be utilized to measure frailty. Additionally, frailty indexes such as the Program of Research to Integrate the Services for Maintenance of Autonomy 7 (Raîche et al., 2008) and the Simple FRAIL Questionnaire (Morley et al., 2013) both provide rapid screening using physical markers of decline and/or accumulation of deficits.

Frailty can be addressed by encouraging nursing home residents to engage in resistance or strengthening exercises. Resistance exercises can be against gravity or using elastic bands or small free weights. Sit to stand exercises, which can be incorporated into care activities such as toileting or transferring, may help decrease functional decline in nursing home residents (Grönstedt et al., 2020; Slaughter et al., 2014). Combining nutritional supplementation, particularly protein intake that is spread throughout the day, has been beneficial to older adults when combined with resistance exercise (Liao et al., 2019).

CASE STUDY Resident Showing Symptoms of Frailty

Mrs. Jackson is an 84-year-old woman with atrial fibrillation, hypertension, hypothyroidism, osteoarthritis of her knees, and dementia—probably Alzheimer's disease. She is admitted to the nursing home for continuing care following the sudden death of her husband. Prior to her admission to the nursing home, she had lost 20 pounds over the past year. Her husband had been cooking all the meals, encouraging her to eat and assisting her with bathing, dressing, and medication administration. Her closest relative is a niece who lives three hours away.

Mrs. Jackson is admitted to the nursing home following a brief hospitalization for treatment of dehydration and stabilization of her atrial fibrillation because she had not been taking her medications routinely. She is accompanied by her niece, who until recently hadn't seen Mrs. Jackson in one year. Her niece expresses concern to you, as the admitting nurse, about the progression of Mrs. Jackson's cognitive decline, weight loss, and slowed gait speed. "My aunt has really declined in the past year. She can't remember much and doesn't recognize me sometimes. She seems unaware that her husband has died. She isn't interested in eating and just moves the food around on her plate. She used to be so active cooking and cleaning the house, but today she had trouble opening a bottle of juice. She seems weak and walks slowly."

Mrs. Jackson has no known allergies. Her medications include:

- Apixaban 5 mg PO BID
- Metoprolol 25 mg PO BID
- Synthroid 100 mcg PO Q Day
- HCTZ 25 mg PO Q Day
- Lisinopril 5 mg PO Q Day
- Acetaminophen 650 mg PO BID
- Donepezil 10 mg PO QHS

Mrs. Jackson's physical exam elicits the following:

- 97.9, 64, 16, 124/86, weight 117 pounds, height 5'7"
- An alert, pleasant, thin woman in no apparent distress.
- She wears glasses for reading but examination of her head, eyes, ears, nose, and throat is otherwise unremarkable.
- Her lungs are clear with vesicular breath sounds.
- Her heart rate is irregular.
- Her abdomen is soft and nontender, with active bowel sounds in all four quadrants and no hepatosplenomegaly.
- She has no lower extremity edema.
- Her gait is wide-based and slow but appears steady.

Mrs. Jackson is cooperative and appropriately dressed for the season and weather. Her clothes appear large on her. Her eye contact is good. Her speech is spontaneous with a regular rate, rhythm, and volume. She has some word-finding difficulties. Her mood is euthymic with good vital sense and self-attitude and no suicidality, delusions, or hallucinations. Her insight regarding her cognitive deficits is limited, and her Mini Mental Status Examination score is 10/30.

Geriatric Syndromes Related to the Case Study

As the nurse, you recognize that Mrs. Jackson is impacted by three interrelated geriatric syndromes: cognitive impairment, malnutrition, and frailty. She has symptoms of dementia including memory loss, language impairment, impaired insight into her cognitive deficits, perceptual impairment, and functional decline. She does not appear to exhibit symptoms of delirium, as she is alert and has no deficits in attention or distractibility. Her cognitive deficits seem to have progressed slowly over the past year. Given her recent hospitalization, diagnosis of dementia, and change in environment, you recognize that she is at risk for delirium and plan to develop a consistent care routine, make sure that she wears her glasses, and screen for delirium using the CAM.

Nursing Interventions Related to the Case Study

Mrs. Jackson's BMI is 18.3, which is underweight. She has lost 20 pounds in the past year, and her appetite is limited. As Mrs. Jackson's nurse, you recognize that one of her prescription medications, donepezil, has a side effect of gastrointestinal upset and anorexia, and you will alert the interdisciplinary team. You also will learn about her favorite foods and preferences related to mealtimes. You will collaborate with the dietitian and conduct an oral assessment to see if a referral to a dentist is needed.

To address Mrs. Jackson's frailty, you will assess her serum albumin and notify the physician or advanced practice provider if it is low, work in collaboration with her physical and occupational therapists to integrate resistive exercise into her routine, and encourage favorite foods high in protein such as lean meats, milk, eggs, cottage cheese, and beans that are integrated into her meals.

FALLS

Falls are common and have a significant negative impact on nursing home residents with increases in morbidity and mortality. Approximately 50% to 75% of all nursing home residents will fall at least once every year, and approximately 10% of falls result in serious injuries such as severe contusions, dislocation, fractures, and head trauma (Centers for Disease Control and Prevention, 2023). Falls in nursing homes are under-reported (Sanghavi et al., 2020).

According to the Centers for Medicare & Medicaid Services (2023, p. 325), a *fall* "refers to unintentionally coming to rest on the ground, floor, or other lower level, but not as a result of an overwhelming external force (e.g., resident pushes another resident). An episode where a resident lost his/her balance and would have fallen, if not for staff intervention, is considered a fall." Falls that occur in nursing homes are multifactorial in nature and consist of complex interactions among demographic, medical, medication, cognitive, behavioral, and environmental factors.

Table 6.3 describes common contributors to falls among nursing home residents that can be incorporated into a comprehensive nursing assessment.

TABLE 6.3 Common Contributors to Fall Risk in Nursing Home Residents

FALL RISK CONTRIBUTORS	COMMON EXAMPLES	
Demographic	Advanced age Female sex	White race
Age-associated changes	Sensory (decreased visual acuity, slower light and dark adaptation, decreased visual fields, impaired depth perception, vestibular system impairment) Cardiac (decreased cardiac output, decline in baroreflex sensitivity)	Musculoskeletal (decreased muscle strength) Neurological (decreased proprioception, delayed reaction time, decreased postural control)
Medical	Cardiovascular disease Cerebellar disease Foot deformities Hypotension Dementia Diabetes Dehydration Osteoarthritis	Parkinsonism Peripheral neuropathy Sarcopenia Seizure disorder Stroke Urinary incontinence Vestibular disease Vitamin D deficiency
Medication	Anticonvulsants Antidepressants Antihypertensives Antipsychotics Benzodiazepines	Insulin Muscle relaxants Opioids Sedative-hypnotics

(continues)

TABLE 6.3 *(continued)*

FALL RISK CONTRIBUTORS	COMMON EXAMPLES	
Cognitive	Memory impairment Poor judgment	Poor safety awareness
Behavioral	Risk-taking behavior Fear of falling	Improper use of assistive device
Environmental	New or unfamiliar environment Inadequate lighting Lack of proper footwear Lack of person-environment fit for bed, chair toilet height	Clutter/tripping hazards Unsafe furniture

Assessment

It is beyond the scope of this chapter to provide a review of the screening instruments designed to assess for fall risk. Many fall-prevention screening instruments were developed and tested in populations of community-dwelling older adults. When survey and performance fall risk measures that were designed for community-dwelling older adults are utilized in a nursing home setting, due to a lack of discrimination of many of the instruments, almost all nursing home residents will score as high risk for falls. The Mobility Interaction Fall Chart (Lundin-Olsson et al., 2000) and the Morse Fall Scale (Morse et al., 1989) were both developed for use in PA-LTC or acute-care settings and have some evidence of predictive value of falls in these settings (Kehinde, 2009). Some fall risk scientists support that a nursing evaluation of fall risk based on history, physical assessment, and resident observation is more likely to be predictive of fall risk compared to a screening instrument (Glass et al., 2020; Haines et al., 2007).

A fall-related injury risk algorithm for nursing home residents using relevant data from the MDS 3.0 was recently developed and may prove useful in predicting fall risk that results in serious injury (Duprey et al., 2023). The investigators proposed a short clinical tool, the INJURE-Nursing Home-short form, to predict fall risk with serious injury over two years using five variables from the MDS 3.0, including activity of daily living score, recent fall, hospitalization in the past year, ability to walk in a room, and history of a non-hip fracture (Duprey et al., 2023). For newly admitted nursing home residents, the addition of disorganized thinking and visual impairment to the previous five items increased the predictive power of the instrument.

You will frequently be called upon to assess a resident who has fallen. In many instances, the fall may be unwitnessed by staff, and the resident will be found on the floor. In your assessment of the resident who has fallen, you will need to conduct a thorough history of the fall, investigate contributing factors, conduct a physical examination to determine the extent of injury and possible cause of the fall, and identify any patterns that may help to prevent future falls. For a resident who has fallen, it is important to conduct an examination that includes the following elements:

1. Vital signs (including orthostatic blood pressure and pulse)
2. Skin and head for signs of trauma
3. Pupil size and reactivity
4. Neck injury/range of motion
5. Cardiac assessment (rate and rhythm)
6. Musculoskeletal (range of motion of extremities, strength, pain with movement of joints, contusions, lacerations, fracture)
7. Neurologic (change in level of consciousness, pupillary size and reactivity, weakness)

Nursing Interventions for Fall Prevention

Because falls among nursing home residents are predominately multifactorial, your nursing interventions will be guided by your risk assessment. The Agency for Healthcare Research and Quality (AHRQ) provides online resources to reduce the risk of falls that were designed for implementation in nursing homes. AHRQ's Safety Program for Nursing Homes: On-Time Falls Prevention (https://www.ahrq.gov/patient-safety/settings/long-term-care/resource/ontime/fallspx/assess.html) and the Falls Management Program: A Quality Improvement Initiative for Nursing Facilities (https://www.ahrq.gov/patient-safety/settings/long-term-care/resource/injuries/fallspx.html) are freely available and are designed for use by the interdisciplinary team in nursing homes.

Table 6.4 describes the nursing management for nursing home residents with gait instability and/or a history of falls. As a nurse, one of the most important things that you can do is to provide residents who are at risk for falls the opportunity to engage in exercise and physical activity. Multiple research studies have demonstrated the significant impact of exercise and physical activity in preventing and reducing the risk of falls even among residents living with dementia (Cordes et al., 2021; Courel-Ibáñez et al., 2022; Galik et al., 2014; Gulka et al., 2020).

TABLE 6.4 Nursing Management of Instability and/or History of Falls

FALL RISK CONTRIBUTORS	NURSING MANAGEMENT
Gait instability and muscle weakness	Encourage sit to stand exercises in the presence of staff to build strength Refer to physical or occupational therapy Integrate opportunities for accompanied ambulation into care (walk to dine, walk to the bathroom) Encourage use of floor pedal bike
Medical comorbidities	Monitor and report changes in medical conditions to physician or advanced practice provider
Medications	Assess orthostatic blood pressure and pulse for residents taking medications associated with increased fall risk Identify and report any changes in gait and balance after starting on a new medication Collaborate with consultant pharmacist, physician, and advanced practice provider to support efforts in deprescribing high-risk medications
Cognitive impairment	Supervise residents in common areas Provide intermittent rest periods with distracting activities for residents who wander
Behavioral hazards	Toilet resident in the morning, after meals, and before bed Provide opportunities for residents to ambulate with staff to decrease the fear of falling Reinforce proper us of assistive device
Environmental hazards	Optimize lighting Well-fitting, supportive shoes Bed, chair, and toilet height that is appropriate for the height of the resident Minimize clutter or tripping hazards Encourage the use of handrails and grab bars

CASE STUDY Resident at Risk for Falls

One of the nursing assistants shares with you that Mrs. Jackson has not been acting like her usual self over the past two days. Mrs. Jackson seems more confused and tires easily. She typically enjoys walking around the unit but has been spending more time in her room. You find Mrs. Jackson dozing off in a chair in the dining room and walk with her back to her room to examine her. You notice that she becomes short of breath and is unsteady. In your assessment, you notice that she is afebrile, and her respiratory rate is 22. Her lungs are clear to auscultation, and her heart rate is irregular with a rate of 120. You wait a few minutes and recheck her heart rate, which is now 116. Her attention and eye contact are poor, and she has difficulty following simple directions. You are concerned about atrial fibrillation with an uncontrolled rate with mental status changes and contact the physician on call to report the results of your assessment. Her metoprolol is increased to 50 mg PO BID, and a potential hospitalization is avoided.

URINARY INCONTINENCE

Urinary incontinence, the involuntary loss of urine, is common among nursing home residents. It is estimated that 77%–90% of nursing home residents experience urinary incontinence (Batmani et al., 2021). Older adults may be hesitant to discuss their symptoms of incontinence with you due to embarrassment or belief that their symptoms cannot be helped. Therefore, it is important for you to ask residents about their bladder control.

Urinary incontinence may result in residents avoiding activities, limiting trips out of the nursing home, and may also impact their ability to sleep well at night. It is no surprise that urinary incontinence is often associated with decreased quality of life among nursing home residents (Jachan et al., 2019).

There are four primary types of urinary incontinence:

1. **Stress:** An involuntary loss of urine that is caused by weakness of the muscles in the pelvic floor.
2. **Urge:** Urine leakage that results when the individual is unable to delay voiding after the bladder fullness is identified.

3. **Overflow:** Urine leakage from an overdistended bladder; incomplete bladder emptying.
4. **Functional:** Loss of urine due to the inability to get to the toilet due to cognitive impairment or physical disability.

Potentially modifiable contributors to urinary incontinence include:

- Decreased mobility
- Acute delirium
- Infection
- Uncontrolled diabetes that results in polyuria
- Medication side effects (diuretics, anticholinergics, psychotropics, narcotics, cholinesterase inhibitors)
- Alcohol and/or caffeine intake

Assessment

Screening for urinary incontinence should be conducted annually because most older adults will not disclose that they have urinary incontinence unless they are asked. Screening questions include:

- Do you have any difficulty controlling your bladder?
- Do you ever experience urine leakage?

The majority of residents in nursing homes do experience urinary incontinence. When a history of urinary incontinence is known, the nurse should ask about onset, frequency, volume, factors that decrease incontinence, and factors that increase incontinence. Additionally, it is helpful to ask about typical fluid intake, type of fluids, and any new medications.

Nursing Interventions for Urinary Incontinence in the Nursing Home

Nursing interventions for urinary incontinence include the following:

- Residents who are cognitively intact and experience stress or urge incontinence may benefit from engaging in Kegel/pelvic floor muscle exercises.

A simple way of teaching Kegel exercises is to have the resident practice stopping their urine stream while the resident is voiding. This method will help the resident engage the pelvic floor muscles. Work with the resident to have them practice Kegel exercises by contracting the pelvic floor muscles for three to five seconds and then relaxing. Encourage the resident to gradually increase the number and frequency of Kegel exercises until the resident reaches 10 repetitions three times a day.

- Scheduled toileting programs works well to decrease incontinence episodes for nursing home residents, even those with cognitive impairment. You can attempt to adapt the resident's toileting schedule based on their patterns of voiding, or you can set a routine schedule such as after waking up, following each meal, and before bed.
- Utilize incontinence products such as pads or adult briefs as appropriate.

SUMMARY

Nurses in PA-LTC settings play an important role in the early identification and treatment of geriatric syndromes including cognitive impairment, nutritional deficits, frailty, falls, and urinary incontinence. Geriatric syndromes are not a normal part of aging but instead are atypical symptoms experienced by older adults that often have multiple causes and are not specific to one organ system. Geriatric syndromes require the nurse to serve as the eyes and ears of the interdisciplinary team by obtaining a history of subtle changes in cognition function and behavior, conducting a thorough physical assessment of the resident, and reporting findings to the treatment team.

REFERENCES

Alzheimer's Association. (2022). 2022 Alzheimer's disease facts and figures. *Alzheimer's & Dementia: The Journal of the Alzheimer's Association, 18*(4), 700–789. https://doi.org/10.1002/alz.12638

American Geriatrics Society Beers Criteria Update Expert Panel. (2019). American Geriatrics Society 2019 updated AGS Beers Criteria for potentially inappropriate medication use in older adults. *Journal of the American Geriatrics Society, 67*(4), 674–694. https://doi.org/10.1111/jgs.15767

American Psychiatric Association. (2013). *Diagnostic and statistical manual of mental disorders.* Author.

Azzolino, D., Marzetti, E., Proietti, M., Calvani, R., de Souto Barreto, P., Rolland, Y., & Cesari, M. (2021). Lack of energy is associated with malnutrition in nursing home residents: Results from the INCUR study. *Journal of the American Geriatrics Society, 69*(11), 3242–3248. https://doi.org/10.1111/jgs.17393

Batmani, S., Jalali, R., Mohammadi, M., & Bokaee, S. (2021). Prevalence and factors related to urinary incontinence in older adults women worldwide: A comprehensive systematic review and meta-analysis of observational studies. *BMC Geriatrics, 21*(1), 212. https://doi.org/10.1186/s12877-021-02135-8

Bell, S. P., Vasilevskis, E. E., Saraf, A. A., Jacobsen, J. M. L., Kripalani, S., Mixon, A. S., Schnelle, J. F., & Simmons, S. F. (2016). Geriatric syndromes in hospitalized older adults discharged to skilled nursing facilities. *Journal of the American Geriatrics Society, 64*(4), 715–722. https://doi.org/10.1111/jgs.14035

Borson, S., Scanlan, J. M., Chen, P., & Ganguli, M. (2003). The Mini-Cog as a screen for dementia: Validation in a population-based sample. *Journal of the American Geriatrics Society, 51*(10), 1451–1454.

Centers for Disease Control and Prevention. (2023). *Web-based Injury Statistics Query and Reporting System (WISQARS).* https://www.cdc.gov/injury/wisqars/index.html

Centers for Medicare & Medicaid Services. (2023). *State Operations Manual Appendix PP: Guidance to Surveyors for Long Term Care Facilities.* https://www.cms.gov/medicare/provider-enrollment-and-certification/guidanceforlawsandregulations/downloads/appendix-pp-state-operations-manual.pdf

Cohen-Mansfield, J. (1991). *Instruction manual for the Cohen-Mansfield Agitation Inventory.* The Research Institute of the Hebrew Home of Greater Washington. https://www.dementiaresearch.org.au/wp-content/uploads/2016/06/CMAI_Manual.pdf

Cohen-Mansfield, J., Marx, M., & Rosenthal, A. (1989). A description of agitation in a nursing home. *Journal of Gerontology, 44,* M77–M84.

Cordes, T., Schoene, D., Kemmler, W., & Wollesen, B. (2021). Chair-based exercise interventions for nursing home residents: A systematic review. *Journal of the American Medical Directors Association, 22*(4), 733–740. https://doi.org/10.1016/j.jamda.2020.09.042

Courel-Ibáñez, J., Buendía-Romero, Á., Pallarés, J. G., García-Conesa, S., Martínez-Cava, A., & Izquierdo, M. (2022). Impact of tailored multicomponent exercise for preventing weakness and falls on nursing home residents' functional capacity. *Journal of the American Medical Directors Association, 23*(1), 98–104.e3. https://doi.org/10.1016/j.jamda.2021.05.037

Duprey, M. S., Zullo, A. R., Gouskova, N. A., Lee, Y., Capuano, A., Kiel, D. P., Daiello, L. A., Kim, D. H., & Berry, S. D. (2023). Development and validation of the Fall-Related Injury Risk in Nursing Homes (INJURE-NH) prediction tool. *Journal of the American Geriatrics Society, 71*(6), 1851–1860. https://doi.org/10.1111/jgs.18277

Flaherty, J. H., & Morley, J. E. (2013). Delirium in the nursing home. *Journal of the American Medical Directors Association, 14*(9), 632–634. https://doi.org/10.1016/j.jamda.2013.06.009

Fried, L. P., Tangen, C. M., Walston, J., Newman, A. B., Hirsch, C., Gottdiener, J., Seeman, T., Tracy, R., Kop, W. J., Burke, G., McBurnie, M. A., & Cardiovascular Health Study Collaborative Research Group. (2001). Frailty in older adults: Evidence for a phenotype. *The Journals of Gerontology: Series A, Biological Sciences and Medical Sciences, 56*(3), M146–156. https://doi.org/10.1093/gerona/56.3.m146

Galik, E., Resnick, B., Hammersla, M., & Brightwater, J. (2014). Optimizing function and physical activity among nursing home residents with dementia: Testing the impact of function-focused care. *The Gerontologist, 54*(6), 930–943. https://doi.org/10.1093/geront/gnt108

Galvin, J. E., Roe, C. M., Powlishta, K. K., Coats, M. A., Muich, S. J., Grant, E., Miller, J. P., Storandt, M., & Morris, J. C. (2005). The AD8: A brief informant interview to detect dementia. *Neurology, 65*(4), 559–564. https://doi.org/10.1212/01.wnl.0000172958.95282.2a

Glass, A., Mendelson, G., & Ben Natan, M. (2020). Comparison of two fall-risk assessment tools used in a long-term care facility. *International Journal of Health Care Quality Assurance, 33*(3), 237–246. https://doi.org/10.1108/IJHCQA-03-2019-0065

Grönstedt, H., Vikström, S., Cederholm, T., Franzén, E., Luiking, Y. C., Seiger, Å., Wimo, A., Faxén-Irving, G., & Boström, A.-M. (2020). Effect of sit-to-stand exercises combined with protein-rich oral supplementation in older persons: The older person's exercise and nutrition study. *Journal of the American Medical Directors Association, 21*(9), 1229–1237. https://doi.org/10.1016/j.jamda.2020.03.030

Gulka, H. J., Patel, V., Arora, T., McArthur, C., & Iaboni, A. (2020). Efficacy and generalizability of falls prevention interventions in nursing homes: A systematic review and meta-analysis. *Journal of the American Medical Directors Association, 21*(8), 1024–1035.e4. https://doi.org/10.1016/j.jamda.2019.11.012

Haines, T. P., Hill, K., Walsh, W., & Osborne, R. (2007). Design-related bias in hospital fall risk screening tool predictive accuracy evaluations: Systematic review and meta-analysis. *The Journals of Gerontology: Series A, Biological Sciences and Medical Sciences, 62*(6), 664–672. https://doi.org/10.1093/gerona/62.6.664

Hendry, K., Green, C., McShane, R., Noel-Storr, A. H., Stott, D. J., Anwer, S., Sutton, A. J., Burton, J. K., & Quinn, T. J. (2019). AD-8 for detection of dementia across a variety of healthcare settings. *The Cochrane Database of Systematic Reviews, 3*(3), CD011121. https://doi.org/10.1002/14651858.CD011121.pub2

Inouye, S. K., van Dyck, C. H., Alessi, C. A., Balkin, S., Siegal, A. P., & Horwitz, R. I. (1990). Clarifying confusion: The confusion assessment method. A new method for detection of delirium. *Annals of Internal Medicine, 113*(12), 941–948. https://doi.org/10.7326/0003-4819-113-12-941

Jachan, D. E., Müller-Werdan, U., & Lahmann, N. A. (2019). Impaired mobility and urinary incontinence in nursing home residents: A multicenter study. *Journal of Wound, Ostomy, and Continence Nursing, 46*(6), 524–529. https://doi.org/10.1097/WON.0000000000000580

Kehinde, J. O. (2009). Instruments for measuring fall risk in older adults living in long-term care facilities: An integrative review. *Journal of Gerontological Nursing, 35*(10), 46–55. https://doi.org/10.3928/00989134-20090902-01

Komici, K., Guerra, G., Addona, F., & Fantini, C. (2022). Delirium in nursing home residents: A narrative review. *Healthcare (Basel, Switzerland), 10*(8), 1544. https://doi.org/10.3390/healthcare10081544

Liao, C.-D., Chen, H.-C., Huang, S.-W., & Liou, T.-H. (2019). The role of muscle mass gain following protein supplementation plus exercise therapy in older adults with sarcopenia and frailty risks: A systematic review and meta-regression analysis of randomized trials. *Nutrients, 11*(8), 1713. https://doi.org/10.3390/nu11081713

Liu, W., Chen, S., Jiang, F., Zhou, C., & Tang, S. (2020). Malnutrition and physical frailty among nursing home residents: A cross-sectional study in China. *The Journal of Nutrition, Health & Aging, 24*(5), 500–506. https://doi.org/10.1007/s12603-020-1348-x

Lundin-Olsson, L., Nyberg, L., & Gustafson, Y. (2000). The mobility interaction fall chart. *Physiotherapy Research International: The Journal for Researchers and Clinicians in Physical Therapy, 5*(3), 190–201. https://doi.org/10.1002/pri.198

Medeiros, M. M. D. de, Figueredo, O. M. C. de, Pinheiro, M. A., Oliveira, L. F. S. de, Wanderley, R. L., Cavalcanti, Y. W., & Rodrigues Garcia, R. C. M. (2020). Factors associated with the overlap of frailty and nutrition in institutionalized older adults: A multicenter study. *Archives of Gerontology and Geriatrics, 90*, 104150. https://doi.org/10.1016/j.archger.2020.104150

Middleton, A., Li, S., Kuo, Y.-F., Ottenbacher, K. J., & Goodwin, J. S. (2018). New institutionalization in long-term care after hospital discharge to skilled nursing facility. *Journal of the American Geriatrics Society, 66*(1), 56–63. https://doi.org/10.1111/jgs.15131

Morley, J. E., Vellas, B., van Kan, G. A., Anker, S. D., Bauer, J. M., Bernabei, R., Cesari, M., Chumlea, W. C., Doehner, W., Evans, J., Fried, L. P., Guralnik, J. M., Katz, P. R., Malmstrom, T. K., McCarter, R. J., Gutierrez Robledo, L. M., Rockwood, K., von Haehling, S., Vandewoude, M. F., & Walston, J. (2013). Frailty consensus: A call to action. *Journal of the American Medical Directors Association, 14*(6), 392–397. https://doi.org/10.1016/j.jamda.2013.03.022

Morse, J. M., Morse, R. M., & Tylko, S. J. (1989). Development of a scale to identify the fall-prone patient. *Canadian Journal on Aging, 8*(4), 366–377. https://doi.org/10.1017/S0714980800008576

Nasreddine, Z. S., Phillips, N. A., Bédirian, V., Charbonneau, S., Whitehead, V., Collin, I., Cummings, J. L., & Chertkow, H. (2005). The Montreal Cognitive Assessment, MoCA: A brief screening tool for mild cognitive impairment. *Journal of the American Geriatrics Society, 53*(4), 695–699. https://doi.org/10.1111/j.1532-5415.2005.53221.x

Norman, K., Haß, U., & Pirlich, M. (2021). Malnutrition in older adults: Recent advances and remaining challenges. *Nutrients, 13*(8), 2764. https://doi.org/10.3390/nu13082764

Onder, G., Giovannini, S., Sganga, F., Manes-Gravina, E., Topinkova, E., Finne-Soveri, H., Garms-Homolová, V., Declercq, A., van der Roest, H. G., Jónsson, P. V., van Hout, H., & Bernabei, R. (2018). Interactions between drugs and geriatric syndromes in nursing home and home care: Results from Shelter and IBenC projects. *Aging Clinical and Experimental Research, 30*(9), 1015–1021. https://doi.org/10.1007/s40520-018-0893-1

Raîche, M., Hébert, R., & Dubois, M.-F. (2008). PRISMA-7: A case-finding tool to identify older adults with moderate to severe disabilities. *Archives of Gerontology and Geriatrics, 47*(1), 9–18. https://doi.org/10.1016/j.archger.2007.06.004

Resnick, B., Boltz, M., Galik, E., & Wells, C. (2013). Physical capability scale: Psychometric testing. *Clinical Nursing Research, 22*(1), 7–29. https://doi.org/10.1177/1054773812447943

Resnick, B., Galik, E., & Boltz, M. (2014). Basic physical capability scale: Psychometric testing with cognitively impaired older adults. *American Journal of Alzheimer's Disease and Other Dementias, 29*(4), 326–332. https://doi.org/10.1177/1533317513517039

Rockwood, K., Goodman, J., Flynn, M., & Stolee, P. (1996). Cross-validation of the Delirium Rating Scale in older patients. *Journal of the American Geriatrics Society, 44*(7), 839–842. https://doi.org/10.1111/j.1532-5415.1996.tb03745.x

Saliba, D., Buchanan, J., Edelen, M. O., Streim, J., Ouslander, J., Berlowitz, D., & Chodosh, J. (2012). MDS 3.0: Brief interview for mental status. *Journal of the American Medical Directors Association, 13*(7), 611–617. https://doi.org/10.1016/j.jamda.2012.06.004

Sanford, A. M., Morley, J. E., Berg-Weger, M., Lundy, J., Little, M. O., Leonard, K., & Malmstrom, T. K. (2020). High prevalence of geriatric syndromes in older adults. *PloS One, 15*(6), e0233857. https://doi.org/10.1371/journal.pone.0233857

Sanghavi, P., Pan, S., & Caudry, D. (2020). Assessment of nursing home reporting of major injury falls for quality measurement on nursing home compare. *Health Services Research, 55*(2), 201–210. https://doi.org/10.1111/1475-6773.13247

Sengupta, M., Lendon, J. P., Caffrey, C., Melekin, A., & Singh, P. (2022). Post-acute and long-term care providers and services users in the United States, 2017–2018. *Vital & Health Statistics: Series 3, Analytical and Epidemiological Studies, 47*, 1–93.

Slaughter, S. E., Wagg, A. S., Jones, C. A., Schopflocher, D., Ickert, C., Bampton, E., Jantz, A., Milke, D., Schalm, C., Lycar, C., & Estabrooks, C. A. (2014). Mobility of Vulnerable Elders Study: Effect of the sit-to-stand activity on mobility, function, and quality of life. *Journal of the American Medical Directors Association, 16*(2), 138–143. https://doi.org/10.1016/j.jamda.2014.07.020

Tariq, S. H., Tumosa, N., Chibnall, J. T., Perry, M. H., & Morley, J. E. (2006). Comparison of the Saint Louis University Mental Status Examination and the Mini-Mental State Examination for detecting dementia and mild neurocognitive disorder—A pilot study. *The American Journal of Geriatric Psychiatry, 14*(11), 900–910. https://doi.org/10.1097/01.JGP.0000221510.33817.86

Tinetti, M. E., Williams, T. F., & Mayewski, R. (1986). Fall risk index for elderly patients based on number of chronic disabilities. *The American Journal of Medicine, 80*(3), 429–434. https://doi.org/10.1016/0002-9343(86)90717-5

Torbahn, G., Sulz, I., Großhauser, F., Hiesmayr, M. J., Kiesswetter, E., Schindler, K., Sieber, C. C., Visser, M., Weber, J., & Volkert, D. (2022). Predictors of incident malnutrition: A nutrition day analysis in 11,923 nursing home residents. *European Journal of Clinical Nutrition, 76*(3), 382–388. https://doi.org/10.1038/s41430-021-00964-9

Trzepacz, P. T., Mittal, D., Torres, R., Kanary, K., Norton, J., & Jimerson, N. (2001). Validation of the Delirium Rating Scale-Revised-98: Comparison with the Delirium Rating Scale and the Cognitive Test for Delirium. *The Journal of Neuropsychiatry and Clinical Neurosciences, 13*(2), 229–242. https://doi.org/10.1176/jnp.13.2.229

van den Berg, G. H., Huisman-de Waal, G. G. J., Vermeulen, H., & de van der Schueren, M. A. E. (2021). Effects of nursing nutrition interventions on outcomes in malnourished hospital inpatients and nursing home residents: A systematic review. *International Journal of Nursing Studies, 117*, 103888. https://doi.org/10.1016/j.ijnurstu.2021.103888

Veronese, N., Custodero, C., Cella, A., Demurtas, J., Zora, S., Maggi, S., Barbagallo, M., Sabbà, C., Ferrucci, L., & Pilotto, A. (2021). Prevalence of multidimensional frailty and pre-frailty in older people in different settings: A systematic review and meta-analysis. *Ageing Research Reviews, 72*, 101498. https://doi.org/10.1016/j.arr.2021.101498

Wilson, M.-M. G., Thomas, D. R., Rubenstein, L. Z., Chibnall, J. T., Anderson, S., Baxi, A., Diebold, M. R., & Morley, J. E. (2005). Appetite assessment: Simple appetite questionnaire predicts weight loss in community-dwelling adults and nursing home residents. *The American Journal of Clinical Nutrition, 82*(5), 1074–1081. https://doi.org/10.1093/ajcn/82.5.1074

Wood, S., Cummings, J. L., Hsu, M. A., Barclay, T., Wheatley, M. V., Yarema, K. T., & Schnelle, J. F. (2000). The use of the neuropsychiatric inventory in nursing home residents: Characterization and measurement. *The American Journal of Geriatric Psychiatry, 8*(1), 75–83. https://doi.org/10.1097/00019442-200002000-00010

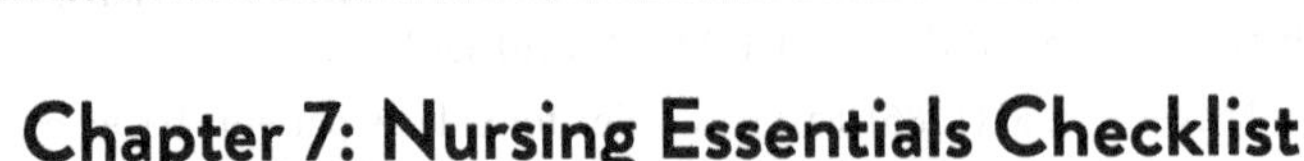

Chapter 7: Nursing Essentials Checklist

SPHERES OF CARE

Nursing occurs within four spheres of care, ranging from prevention to supportive care and all the areas in between. This chapter is relevant to the following spheres of care:

- ☐ Disease Prevention/Health Promotion
- ☑ Chronic Disease Care
- ☑ Regenerative or Restorative Care
- ☐ Hospice/Palliative/Supportive Care

DOMAINS OF PRACTICE

The American Association of Colleges of Nursing has identified 10 broad domains of practice for nursing. Students are expected to master these domains of practice across the spheres of care. This chapter addresses:

- ☑ Knowledge for Nursing Practice (Nursing and Other Disciplines)
- ☐ Person-Centered Care
- ☐ Population Health
- ☑ Scholarship for Practice
- ☐ Quality and Safety
- ☑ Interprofessional Partnerships
- ☑ Systems-Based Care
- ☐ Information & Healthcare Technologies
- ☑ Professionalism
- ☑ Personal, Professional, Leadership Development

CONCEPTS FOR PRACTICE

Integrated across the domains of practice are eight concepts which the student is expected to master across the spheres of care and across the domains of practice. This chapter addresses:

- ☑ Clinical Judgment
- ☑ Communication
- ☐ Compassionate Care
- ☐ Diversity, Equity, Inclusion
- ☐ Ethics
- ☑ Evidence-Based Practice
- ☐ Health Policy
- ☐ Social Determinants of Health

CHAPTER 7

DEVELOPING THE WORKFORCE OF THE FUTURE

Maureen Saxon-Gioia, MSHSA, BSN, RN
Emily K. Franke, MSW, LSW
Elena O. Siegel, PhD
Flora Petillo, MSN, CRNP, CWS
Christine Mueller, PhD, RN, FGSA, FAAN
Joan Weiss, PhD, RN, CRNP, FAAN

OBJECTIVES

1. Describe key roles and positions for nurse staffing and leadership in nursing homes.
2. Examine nursing care models, scope, and practices that support collaborative care and professional development in nursing homes.
3. Discuss opportunities to enhance nurse preparation for practice in the nursing home setting: academic-practice partnerships and nurse residency programs.

INTRODUCTION

As you consider your nursing career, it is important to know about the care-delivery models and the professional nursing opportunities in nursing homes. As the name implies, *nursing* homes are intended to provide nursing care to persons who are there for long-term care or transitional/subacute care. This chapter outlines positions for nurse staffing and leadership in nursing homes and provides details about each of the key positions: the director of nursing, licensed nurses (registered nurses and licensed practical/vocational nurses), unlicensed nursing staff (commonly referred to as certified nursing assistants or nurse aides), and advanced practice registered nurses. The first section discusses some of the key factors that reflect the nurse practice work environment (care-delivery models and metrics for quality of care). When making employment decisions, you can use this information to identify the right nursing home, along with how nurses can positively impact care delivery. Opportunities for career advancement and professional growth are explored. The chapter concludes with an overview of two key opportunities to enhance nurse preparation for practice in the nursing home setting: academic-practice partnerships and nurse residency programs.

NURSING POSITIONS IN NURSING HOMES

The Centers for Medicare & Medicaid Services (CMS) regulations require a director of nursing (DON) in all nursing homes. The DON serves as a member of the top leadership team, collaborating with the licensed nursing home administrator (NHA) and medical director (MD). While not a CMS requirement, some nursing homes also employ or contract with advanced practice registered nurses (APRNs)—primarily nurse practitioners (NPs) and clinical nurse specialists (CNSs).

Nurse staffing in nursing homes reflects a mix of licensed nurses (registered nurses [RNs] and licensed practical/vocational nurses [LPNs/LVNs]) and unlicensed nursing staff (certified nursing assistants or nurse aides). CMS requires a licensed nurse (either an RN or LPN/LVN) to be present 24 hours a day, 7 days a week, and an RN must be present in the nursing home for eight of those hours (CMS, 2022).

Director of Nursing

The nursing home DON—sometimes referred to as director of nursing services—serves as a link between other members of the leadership team and the full breadth of nursing care and staff. Most commonly, the DON reports to the facility's licensed NHA, a position responsible for oversight of all nursing home operations. In some larger multi-facility organizations, the DON may also report to a regional-level nursing director. Traditionally, many nursing homes are characterized by a flat organizational chart, with relatively few or no levels of middle management between the executives and the point-of-care staff, with the DON serving as the highest-level nurse leader with day-to-day responsibilities for the nursing department. In this position, the DON oversees all nursing personnel, including associate or assistant DONs, nurse managers, supervisors, and nursing staff who may report directly or indirectly to the DON.

Scope of the DON Position

The DON position is required by CMS, but the regulations are not prescriptive about the scope of the DON position and specific responsibilities. Absent a standardized job description, various professional nursing organizations that specifically support nursing home DONs offer important guidance about the position domains and foundational knowledge requirements and competencies of a DON. A list of these professional resources can be found in Table 7.1.

TABLE 7.1 Professional Resources That Provide Guidance About the DON Position

RESOURCE	WEBSITE	ROLE INFORMATION AND PROFESSIONAL DEVELOPMENT OPPORTUNITIES
National Association of Directors of Nursing Administration in Long Term Care	https://nadona.org/	Educational resources Director of Nursing Certification Executive Fellows Leadership Academy
American Association of Post-Acute Care Nursing	https://www.aapacn.org/	Educational resources Director of Nursing Services Certification
American Organization for Nursing Leadership	https://www.aonl.org/	Educational resources Executive Nursing Practice and Nurse Manager/Leader Certifications Fellowship programs Nurse Executive Competencies: Pos-Acute Care
American Nurses Association	https://www.nursingworld.org/	American Nurses Credentialing Center Nurse Executive Certification Educational resources, including *Nursing Administration: Scope and Standards of Practice*, 2nd Edition

Broadly speaking, the DON is positioned to lead and improve the quality and efficiency of nursing services and work environments for nursing staff. The scope of the DON role includes advocating for initiatives and resources that improve quality and efficiency of various aspects of nursing services and the work environment, and establishing clinical and administrative systems and processes to ensure nursing services and practices align with:

- RN and LPN/LVN scope of practice as set forth by state boards of nursing and configuration of team nursing approaches that optimizes the capacity of all nursing team members, including nursing assistants
- Care models and practices that support scopes of practice and collaborative care
- Nursing home regulations set forth by CMS and other agencies
- Successful implementation of evidence-based best practices in geriatric nursing care, including person-centered approaches and high-quality work environments

Preparation for the DON Position

RN licensure is the only regulatory requirement for the DON position set forth by CMS. Yet, RN licensure alone is inadequate preparation to meet DON role demands. The DON has a pivotal role in leadership and management in nursing homes. Understanding the breadth and depth of this critical nursing leadership position is the first step in preparing for the DON role and recognizing that on-the-job training is not sufficient to effectively carry out the sophisticated roles and responsibilities of the DON.

The need for DON role-specific preparation is well-established by industry experts and nursing home researchers (Kolanowski et al., 2021; Siegel et al., 2010); however, there is no universal requirement or consensus about the requisite formal training and education DONs need to successfully lead and manage nursing services and effectively address role responsibilities. To fill this gap, some nursing home organizations offer internal nursing leadership training programs for DONs and nurses in other leadership positions. Additionally, many resources and individual professional development opportunities, including professional certifications, are available (refer to Table 7.1). DONs may benefit from peer networks and mentorship to support them in effectively navigating role responsibilities. Peer networks and mentorship opportunities are also available through professional organizations.

Important Questions to Ask When Considering a DON Position

When speaking with potential employers about a DON position, it's important to consider the concept of person-job fit (Kristof-Brown et al., 2005) and recognize that the role responsibilities required and role resources available in one facility might be quite different from another based on a variety of facility-level factors.

Examples of facility-level factors that contribute to DON role responsibilities include:

- Quality metrics (i.e., quality measures and survey inspection results)
- Nurse staffing data (e.g., numbers and mix of RNs, LPN/LVNs, nursing assistants)

Other facility-level factors to consider include rates of job turnover among nursing staff and leadership, workforce satisfaction, and nursing care model and practices that support RN scope of practice and collaborative care. A detailed discussion of quality metrics and nurse practice models is covered in the later section "Key Factors That Reflect the Nurse Practice Environment in Nursing Homes."

Examples of facility-level factors that contribute to DON role resources include internal mentorship opportunities for the DON and resource allocations for formal role training/education.

Understanding facility-level differences in DON role demands and role resources provides opportunity to make intentional choices about the environment best suited for a new DON's transition into the role. Additionally, seeking perspectives of current and previous DONs provides important insights into ways DONs execute their role, resources they identify to enhance their role performance, and their strategies and recommendations for role success.

Role Rewards and Challenges

The DON position includes both rewards and challenges that are important to consider when making a career decision to seek out this role. Rewards are intrinsically tied to individual values and motivations for a nursing career in leadership and administrative roles, including an inclination to apply your nursing competencies through a systems-level lens, in contrast to engaging in direct nursing care. The rewards are an opportunity to create effective nursing teams and establish systems, processes, and work environments that ensure nursing home residents receive high-quality, person-centered care and the staff working in these settings thrive.

Common role challenges are rooted in long-standing gaps in the quality of care and quality of the work environments, limited resources compared to other healthcare settings, adequacy of RN staffing (refer to the later section "Nurse Staffing"), and high job turnover across the nursing staff and leadership teams. To effectively address these challenges, DONs require strong competencies in leading quality improvement initiatives across clinical and administrative/workforce domains and high-level expertise in the federal and state regulations that serve as a backdrop for care-delivery practices.

Together, DON role rewards and challenges underscore the importance of DONs receiving formal training and education to navigate and effectively enact this critically important nursing leadership position, and strong professional and peer networks to support ongoing role development.

Licensed Nursing Staff

Both RNs and LPNs function as licensed nurses in nursing homes, roles that should be complementary and collaborative and ensure scope of practice integrity. The scopes of practice for RNs and LPNs are not the same; however, it is not uncommon in nursing homes for the RN and LPN roles to look the same, especially when the RN and LPN are implementing tasks that require a licensed nurse, such as medication administration and treatments. By considering the two roles as interchangeable, LPNs are at risk for practicing outside of their legal scope of practice, and RNs are at risk for not practicing to their full scope of practice (Mueller et al., 2012; Mueller et al., 2018).

Registered Nurses

Assessment, care planning, evaluation of the care plan, surveillance, and monitoring are what RNs bring to the care of residents in nursing homes. RNs, by virtue of their license and scope of practice, are accountable for ensuring that residents are receiving the care to meet their needs. RNs provide coverage 24/7 to ensure that the residents' needs met by the RN's scope of practice are addressed. Supervision of nursing staff, monitoring and surveillance of residents, and evaluating resident care outcomes in the context of their care plan are all examples of how RNs enact accountability.

The RN's professional nursing role extends well beyond that of the LPN/LVN, and includes, for example:

- Ensuring that a resident with chronic congestive heart failure is well managed through ongoing assessment and monitoring
- Supporting a resident who is adjusting to a move into the nursing home after experiencing the loss of a spouse
- Working in collaboration with the resident's NP to develop and implement a pain management plan
- Monitoring for side effects and intended effects of a new medication recently prescribed to a resident
- Assessing the progress of wound healing and signs of infection

The role of the RN in nursing homes has been characterized as playing four roles that support person-centered care for residents (Mueller, 2022):

- **Care role model:** As a care role model, the RN role-models person-centered care by addressing the holistic needs of residents and partnering with residents and their families in determining their plan of care.
- **Gerontological nurse:** The RN has expertise in care of older adults as a gerontological nurse and uses evidence-based assessments and interventions to provide individualized care for residents.
- **Care partner:** As a care partner, the RN partners with other members of the healthcare team to ensure care is coordinated and with good exchange of information about the residents.
- **Mentor:** RNs mentor nursing staff through teaching, guiding, and developing their skills and knowledge to provide person-centered, quality care for residents.

Roles and Career Advancement Opportunities for RNs in Nursing Homes

There are multiple opportunities for career advancement for RNs in nursing homes. These roles are in the areas of nursing administration, infection control and prevention, staff development, quality assurance and improvement, and coordination of assessment and care planning. The DON role was described earlier in this chapter.

Other management or administrative roles held by RNs include a nurse manager or nurse supervisor of one or more nursing units. Other roles are briefly outlined in Table 7.2.

TABLE 7.2 Roles of RNs in Nursing Homes

ROLE	DESCRIPTION OF ROLE	REGULATIONS ABOUT ROLE*
Infection Preventionist	Assess, develop, implement, monitor, and manage the infection prevention and control program.	Primary professional training in nursing, medical technology, microbiology, epidemiology, or another related field Qualified by education, training, experience, or certification Work at least part time at the facility Completed specialized training in infection prevention and control
Coordinator of Quality Assurance and Performance Improvement	Coordinate the facility's required Quality Assurance and Performance Improvement (QAPI).	While there are no regulations specifically requiring someone in this role, most nursing homes will designate a nurse to oversee and coordinate the required QAPI program.
Director of Staff Development	Develop, plan, and implement a staff development program for all nursing home staff that also includes compliance with required trainings and assuring the competencies of nursing home staff. Provide an orientation program for new employees.	While there are no regulations specifically requiring someone in this role, most nursing homes will designate a nurse to oversee and coordinate staff development activities to address compliance.
Nurse Assessment Coordinator	Ensure all residents have completed accurate and timely assessments and care plans as required by regulations.	The facility must conduct initially and periodically a comprehensive, accurate, standardized, reproducible assessment of each resident's functional capacity. An RN must conduct or coordinate each assessment with the appropriate participation of health professionals.

**From CMS, 2022*

Licensed Practical/Vocational Nurses

LPNs/LVNs provide about 70% of the licensed nursing care in nursing homes (Corazzini et al., 2013). They usually complete a 12–15-month education program in a technical school and take a national examination to be licensed as an LPN/LVN. Their scope of practice is defined by their education and the state board of nursing's nurse practice act. They practice under the supervision of an RN. LPNs/LVNs function collaboratively with RNs and are supported in their scope of practice with a supportive DON and enough RNs (Mueller et al., 2012).

Nursing Assistants

Nursing assistants are vital to the care and support provided to nursing home residents. In fact, they provide the majority of direct care to residents by assisting them with daily functions including mobility, eating, dressing, bathing, personal hygiene, and toileting. Nursing assistants get to know the residents and their preferences because they spend the most time with the residents on a daily basis. RNs rely on nursing assistants to notice and report a change in a resident's condition. As an important member of the care team, nursing assistants provide valuable information to inform residents' care plans as well as revisions to the care plans.

Federal regulations specify a minimum of 75 hours of training; all nursing assistants are required to complete 16 hours of supervised clinical training to be employed in a nursing home. The required topics in the nursing assistant training curriculum include basic nursing, communication and interpersonal activities, care of cognitively impaired residents, basic restorative care, mental health and social services activities, and resident rights.

Nursing assistants are required to pass a written or oral examination and a performance examination at the completion of their training. At that time, they have the title of certified nursing assistant (CNA). Regulations also require nursing assistants to have 12 hours of continuing education annually. Nursing assistants can receive additional training to function as a medication aide that allows them to administer medications under the supervision of a licensed nurse.

Nursing homes that have adopted the small house model often have reconfigured the role of the nursing assistant to have a broader scope of responsibility and duties to maintain a home-like environment for residents. For example, in the small house model where there may be 10 to 12 residents, nursing assistants prepare and serve the meals, do the residents' personal laundry, and perform light housekeeping, in addition to providing personal care for the residents. In this model, nursing assistants have autonomy in determining how and when the work is done.

Career Advancement for Nursing Assistants

LPNs/LVNs and RNs have commonly started their nursing career as a nursing assistant. Thus, one of the more obvious opportunities for career advancement of nursing assistants is completing the education requirements to become an LPN/LVN or RN. However, organizations have also developed career advancement options for nursing assistants that provide more responsibility and require additional competencies. Some nursing homes have lead nursing assistants or a nursing assistant that assists with the training of other nursing assistants. The National Institute of CNA Excellence (n.d.) provides a variety of education opportunities for nursing assistants on topics such as leadership, communication, and team-building.

Advanced Nursing Practice

You may choose to further your nursing practice by seeking graduate education. The nursing home setting is both an excellent place to garner valuable experience before seeking further education and a valuable place to practice once you have achieved it. APRNs, which include NPs, CNSs, certified nurse anesthetists, and certified nurse midwives, are a vital part of the healthcare workforce in the United States.

The publication *The National Imperative to Improve Nursing Home Quality: Honoring Our Commitment to Residents, Families, and Staff* (National Academies of Sciences, Engineering, and Medicine [NASEM], 2022) describes the various roles that APRNS have held in nursing homes, including diagnosing, prescribing, and treating patients' acute and chronic conditions; staff development and education; and infection control. The report illustrates the positive impacts that APRNs have on clinical outcomes, family, and staff satisfaction, specifically noting that medical directors report "high effectiveness of and high satisfaction with nurse practitioners" (p. 236).

Positive impacts that NPs have on delivering medically necessary care to nursing home residents include the following (NASEM, 2022):

- Improved management of chronic illnesses
- Improved functional and health status

- Improved quality of life
- Reduced or equivalent mortality and hospital admissions
- Improved self-care
- Reduced emergency department use and transfers
- Lower costs
- Increased time spent with residents
- Increased resident, family, and staff satisfaction

The Role of the Nurse Practitioner in Nursing Homes

Patients and residents in nursing homes are medically complex and require the expertise of an interprofessional team. Approaching the care of patients in nursing homes through the nursing lens enables the NP to develop a holistic plan of care that is resident-centered and addresses the individualized needs of the whole person. This requires a collaborative relationship with the resident, their family, and the interprofessional team, including the DON, RNs, LPNs/LVNs, nursing assistants, social services, dietitians, and rehabilitation specialists.

In nursing homes, changes in the health status of patients may manifest with only subtle changes from baseline. At other times, residents may decompensate quickly. In either scenario, an immediate and skilled assessment by an NP can make the difference between successfully treating in place or transferring the patient to acute care that places older adults at risk for "hazards of hospitalization," which include delirium, malnutrition, new incontinence, pressure injuries, falls, restraint use, infection, functional decline, adverse drug effects, and death (Fernandez et al., 2008; Mudge et al., 2019).

Every resident encounter is an opportunity for discussion among colleagues of different disciplines and with varying scopes of practice. Working together as an interprofessional team to address a broad spectrum of clinical issues presents opportunities for APRNs to model critical nursing practices including infection control, physical assessment and risk identification, procedural skills, patient education, and discussion of goals of care.

These discussions impart knowledge and build the competence and confidence of the nursing staff and other members of the interprofessional team. Further, NPs can support new graduate nurses as they master technical skills and develop confidence by mentoring them both formally and informally. These skills and opportunities to collaborate among a diverse clinical team will improve clinical outcomes for patients and the quality measure outcomes for the facility.

Preparation for the Advanced Nursing Role in Nursing Homes

The core nursing skills of physical assessment, clear written and oral communication, ability to recognize and investigate changes from baseline, and prioritizing based on need are the basis for providing safe, effective, compassionate care and are carried through all aspects of a nurse's career. The experience of working as an RN in a nursing home will prepare you to seek this career advancement, but there are other requirements to becoming an NP (American Association of Nurse Practitioners, 2020):

- Master's or doctoral degree in nursing
- National certification (common certifications for working in a nursing home setting include family, adult-gerontology primary or acute care, and psychiatric/mental health)
- Licensed as an RN or APRN (depends on the state board of nursing)

KEY FACTORS THAT REFLECT THE NURSE PRACTICE ENVIRONMENT IN NURSING HOMES

When you are considering a nursing position at a nursing home, it is important to understand the practice environment in which RNs work. Nurse practice models and metrics that reflect quality care, including staffing, are two foundational considerations when deciding about employment options and broadly differentiating one facility from another. Nursing practice models vary across facilities, and asking about care models and practices that support the RN scope of practice and collaborative care is critically important to fully enacting the RN role in a nursing home setting. Additionally, useful information about a facility's staffing, quality measures, and inspections—available at NursingHome Compare (www.medicare.gov/care-compare/?providerType=NursingHome)—offers important insights into a facility's foundational structures and processes available to support minimum standards for quality.

Nursing Care-Delivery Models

As you consider the care-delivery models used in nursing homes, pay close attention to the following components:

- Decision-making about resident care
- Strategies to ensure continuity of information about residents
- Strategies to support residents having consistent nursing staff caring for them
- The accountability of the RN

All these components contribute to quality care and life for residents (Mueller, 2022; Mueller & Savik, 2010). See Table 7.3 for examples of these important care-delivery model components.

TABLE 7.3 Components of Care-Delivery Models

COMPONENT	EXAMPLE
Decision-making about resident care	Nursing practice council made up of licensed nurses who deliberate on identifying and implementing geriatric-focused evidence-based practices and identify priorities for quality improvement in the nursing home
Continuity of information	Use of huddles as check-ins with all nursing staff caring for residents to communicate information about residents that was observed or requires action
Consistent nursing staff	Scheduling that reflects the same nursing assistants and licensed nursing staff, when they are scheduled to work, regularly assigned to the same residents. Both research evidence and best practice substantiates the use of consistent assignments as contributing to higher quality of care and life for residents (Castle, 2011, 2013).
Accountability	RN supervision of nursing staff, monitoring and surveillance of residents, and evaluating resident care outcomes in the context of their care plan

A professional nurse practice model in nursing homes supports the RN's accountability and decision-making about the delivery of nursing care for nursing home residents. The assumptions about implementing professional practice models in nursing homes include the following (Lyons et al., 2008):

- RN practice is based on specialized knowledge.
- RNs lead assisting staff (CNAs and LPNs) in the delivery of care.

- Each RN has a caseload of persons for whom she/he is accountable for nursing care over an extended period of time.
- RNs are accountable for the nursing care delegated and/or assigned to assisting nursing staff.
- RNs have licensed authority to define the scope of nursing practice, standards that will be used to evaluate the quality of practice, qualifications of the nursing staff, and knowledge needed by all nursing staff to deliver care that meets the standards of practice.
- RNs are accountable for the quality of care, including quality improvement.
- RNs are accountable for the translation and dissemination of new and existing knowledge for quality nursing.
- RNs perform activities for which they are educated and licensed.

Implementing professional practice models in nursing homes can increase RN satisfaction, recruitment, and retention and result in overall improved quality of care and life for residents.

NursingHome Compare

Every nurse should aspire to the highest quality care delivery and practice environment and will benefit from understanding, implementing, and leading quality efforts in healthcare. Information about nurse staffing in nursing homes, quality measures, and survey inspection results (both current and trends) is available at NursingHome Compare (www.medicare.gov/care-compare/?providerType=NursingHome).

As a composite measure of this information, a 5-star rating system is used to reflect an overall quality rating for each nursing home. The ratings, ranging from 5 (the highest rating) to 1 (the lowest), offer a comparative sense of the quality of care across different facilities; these ratings are one aspect to consider when seeking a nursing home conducive to practicing to the top of your nursing license. Reviewing this information prior to an interview will provide you with a basis for asking meaningful questions throughout the hiring process and will serve to prepare you in your nursing practice. Refer to Chapter 12 to learn more about quality measures.

Nurse Staffing

CMS issued a report in 2001 with findings that inadequate nurse staffing is the primary root cause for serious negative resident outcomes (e.g., dehydration, pressure sores, abuse, neglect, etc.; Feuerberg, 2001). The adequacy of RN staffing in nursing homes has been called into question for decades; ongoing efforts to mandate RN staffing standards in nursing homes have had limited success to date. There have been numerous studies on the relationship between quality care and RN staffing in nursing homes, with the majority of evidence pointing to higher RN staffing associated with better quality outcomes for residents (Castle, 2008; Dellefield et al., 2015; Spilsbury et al., 2011). Some states have specific RN staffing standards; however, the federal RN staffing standard has remained the same since 1987, when the US Congress passed the Nursing Home Reform Act (100th US Congress, 1987).

The data for nurse staffing are submitted electronically through the Payroll Based Journal system, developed by CMS, which provides actual paid hours worked by nursing home personnel (see https://www.cms.gov/medicare/quality-initiatives-patient-assessment-instruments/nursinghomequalityinits/staffing-data-submission-pbj). The staffing data are also conveniently summarized each quarter on the Long Term Care Community Coalition website (https://nursinghome411.org/data/staffing/).

Attending to the professional nursing care needs of residents in a nursing home setting is essential to the residents' quality of care and life. Defining those professional nursing needs is important to ensure RN staffing is adequate to meet resident needs. CMS is currently conducting a large study to inform future nurse staffing standards for nursing homes (Karikari-Martin & Ingram, 2022).

Factors to Consider in Selecting a Nursing Home as a Place of Employment

When families or individuals are considering whom to trust with the care of their loved one, they are encouraged to complete due diligence by looking at a number of factors and asking a number of questions about the physical facility, the quality of the care provided, the staffing and leadership models, and the ownership of the facility. Medicare.gov and NursingHome Compare are great resources for much of this information.

Interestingly, as a potential employee, you should consider these questions for yourself as well. Once you have made the decision to work in a nursing home (whether immediately after graduation or later in your nursing career), you should complete your own due diligence to make sure you know the working conditions you will face and whether this is the right place for you to work, contribute, and grow in your career. Consider these questions:

- Is the nursing home's location convenient (for transportation, in case of emergency, culturally compatible)?
- Does the nursing home offer a range of services to match current and changing resident needs and staff skill sets? How do these services align with your skill sets and career goals?
- What referral relationships does this nursing home have in case residents need acute care, rehabilitation, hospice, home care, pharmacy care, physician, or specialty care?
- Is the nursing home in good physical condition?
- What is the quality and regulatory compliance record of the nursing home? Has it changed over time? For the better? For worse? What is the reputation in the community—both local and in the healthcare community?
- What are the nursing home's identified quality priorities?
- Is the nursing home adequately staffed? Does it have necessary specialty staff? What is its rate of turnover? Does it have consistent staffing, or does it rely on agency staff? How are staffed trained?
- What is the leadership of the nursing home like? Has there been turnover in recent periods?
- Is the staff of the facility a part of a union? How does that align with your work culture beliefs?
- Who owns the nursing home? Is it part of a large national organization or a stand-alone, privately owned facility? Does it operate as a for-profit or nonprofit nursing home? Is it faith-based?

The answer to some of these questions are nice to know so that you understand what to expect in your work life. Some are need-to-know to understand if the organization you are joining matches your personal mission and nursing career goals.

According to the 2022 report from NASEM, *The National Imperative to Improve Nursing Home Quality: Honoring Our Commitment to Residents, Families, and Staff,* most nursing homes have been for-profit for decades; 69.3% of homes are for-profit entities, and nearly 60% are affiliated with companies that own or operate more than one nursing home (Harris-Kojetin et al., 2019; NASEM, 2022). That report goes on to state that for-profit status is associated with lower levels of quality and resident satisfaction, generally (NASEM, 2022).

These findings do not automatically mean that all for-profit nursing homes are bad and all nonprofit homes are good. There are variations in each category. Just as you will be counted on to use your critical thinking and judgment on every shift on the job in the care your provide, you should apply a high level of critical thinking when it comes to exercising your judgment about where you will work, and then once hired, how you will use your judgment and your voice to advocate for the highest standards of quality for yourself, your fellow team members, and on behalf of the residents you serve.

Opportunities to Enhance the Role of RNs in the Nursing Home Setting

Two exemplars for enhancing the role of RNs in nursing homes include academic-practice partnerships (APPs) and nurse residency programs (NRPs). APPs offer nursing students exemplary clinical learning experiences where they can apply skills learned in the classroom directly to the nursing home clinical setting and opportunities to collaborate with nursing academia to conduct research, implement evidence-based practices, and implement a structure to support the autonomy and accountability of the RN role. NRPs offer new graduates and RNs new to the nursing home setting longitudinal formal orientation and training opportunities tailored to the unique aspects of providing nursing care in the nursing home setting.

Academic-Practice Partnerships

APPs are strategic relationships between educational settings and clinical practice settings (Halili et al., 2022). Traditionally, APPs have been between hospitals and schools of nursing. With the number of nursing home residents projected to increase to over 3 million by 2030, the pressure is mounting to ensure nursing students in BSN programs are prepared to practice in nursing homes. The use of nursing homes as sites for clinical and leadership skill application for students will contribute to that need. Nursing homes offer significant opportunities for nursing students to develop clinical judgment and the application of evidence-based gerontological nursing interventions. The use of nursing homes in APPs allows for a synergy between students and the nursing home staff that can result in improvement in resident outcomes. The American Association of Colleges of Nursing (AACN, n.d.) recommends that APPs serve as a mechanism in strengthening the nursing role in clinical practice and preparing future nurses to be leaders. Nursing students can develop a wide range of clinical skills in nursing homes, ranging from palliative, hospice, and wound care to infection control protocols and care planning. Nursing homes also offer a unique opportunity to explore various nursing leadership roles (Mezey et al., 2008).

Teaching Nursing Homes (akin to teaching hospitals) have seven key characteristics that make APPs successful (Mezey et al., 2008):

- Shared accountability to quality of care and quality of life for residents
- Commitment to a collaborative learning environment
- Opportunity for sharing resources
- Culture that values, supports, and disseminates best practices
- Reciprocity in learning opportunities
- Research opportunities
- Commitment to transparency and quality improvement

CASE STUDY of Academic-Practice Partnership in Action: Revisiting the Teaching Nursing Home

In the 1980s, Teaching Nursing Homes were established and demonstrated significant benefits to nursing students and nursing homes in the collaboration between schools and nursing homes. Students engaged in the program left nursing home clinicals more knowledgeable about geriatric care, and nursing home residents experienced improved health outcomes (Mezey et al., 2008). Unlike hospital settings, nursing homes provide students with access to a continuum of diverse acute and long-term services including hospice, short-term rehabilitation, dementia care, and supportive services for residents with differing levels of functional ability. Given that patients are having shorter lengths of stay in acute-care settings, a clinical experience in a nursing home can provide an opportunity to apply assessments and clinical tools more thoroughly.

Following the initial efforts in the 1980s, the schools that engaged in the Teaching Nursing Homes model continued to have a leadership role in gerontologic education as demonstrated by the courses they require and the programs they offer that prepare nurses at both the undergraduate and graduate level (Mezey et al., 1997). In the decades following, nursing students across the country continued to engage with nursing homes as a site for clinical learning. However, in 2020, as COVID-19 impacted the workforce and residents in nursing homes in profound ways, it also complicated the process of engaging students in clinical placements.

The Revisiting the Teaching Nursing Home initiative began in 2021 to support nursing homes and schools of nursing through this period that saw unprecedented devastation across the healthcare continuum. Revisiting the Teaching Nursing Home aimed to engage nursing students in meaningful clinical experiences at nursing homes with the long-term goal of enhancing university faculty and student knowledge regarding nursing home care, improving resident outcomes, and enriching clinical skills of the nursing home workforce to promote retention.

As part of the initiative, schools of nursing and nursing homes partnered and tailored student placements, allowing students to practice clinical skills and observe nurse autonomy in the nursing home. These revamped clinical placements expanded student learning from theory to practice by engaging students in quality improvement projects, applying evidence-based geriatric assessment tools, participating in care planning for residents, and developing leadership skills.

The Revisiting the Teaching Nursing Home initiative underscored the breadth of the learning opportunities that are available to students in a nursing home. These skills translate to all settings that employ nurses, making nursing homes a universally beneficial learning experience for student nurses.

(continues)

(continued)

Skills Learned Through the Revisiting the Teaching Nursing Home Initiative

SKILLS DEVELOPED THROUGH NURSING HOME CLINICAL PLACEMENT	SKILLS TRANSLATED TO RESUMÉ BUILDERS
Leadership skills	Shadowed nurse leadership
Chronic illness management and care planning	Rounded with interprofessional team
Complex wound care	Designed quality improvement project
Hospice care	Participated in huddles with interprofessional team
Discharge planning and transitions of care	Provided resident-centered care to those living with chronic illnesses
Quality improvement strategies	
Medication optimization and deprescribing	

Nurse Residency Programs in Nursing Homes

The demand for RNs in nursing homes has increased as hospital stays have decreased and care has moved into community and residential settings. NRPs are designed to support RNs who are new to the nursing home setting and/or new graduates. The goal of these programs is to orient novice RNs and RNs who are new to nursing homes to this unique work setting, address transition-to-practice challenges, and promote retention. Many graduate nurses and RNs new to nursing homes have inadequate preparation in care of older adults, communication with older adults, clinical leadership, and experience working with interdisciplinary teams. These skills are necessary to care for older adults residing in nursing homes.

NRPs in nursing homes are an effective way to increase competency in gerontological nursing, leadership, and communication skills of new nurse graduates and RNs new to nursing homes. They also help to improve the nurse resident's confidence, clinical practice, and personal satisfaction. As a result of these programs, nurse retention has increased, turnover has decreased, and patient outcomes and safety have improved (Cadmus et al., 2016; Salmond et al., 2017). NRPs offer opportunities for nursing home leadership to implement strategies that ensure a positive workplace environment with shared decision-making and educational and promotional opportunities for staff (Cadmus et al., 2016; Neller et al., 2021; Salmond et al., 2017). An added benefit of some NRPs is that they provide contact hours to enable nurses completing an NRP to take the American Nurses Credentialing Center Gerontological Nursing certification examination.

Important components of NRPs in nursing homes include the following:

- Geriatric care competency-based education
- Adequate length to ensure that nurse residents have the necessary knowledge and skills to provide care
- Integration into educational content of resilience building and strategies for mitigation of burnout
- Mentors for the nurse residents and a mentoring program to support preceptors
- Commitment by the nursing home to ensure nurse residents do not fill in for staffing needs but that they can be fully engaged in learning

While there are few NRPs in nursing homes compared to approximately 600 NRPs in hospitals and health systems nationwide (AACN, 2022), there are several successful programs developed to support NRPs in nursing homes. The following three programs exemplify best practices for NRPs in preparing nurse residents for practice and to support new RNs in nursing homes.

A one-year program in New Jersey was developed to address retention and turnover concerns among RNs in nursing homes. By the end of the first year, the program significantly increased the retention rate, to 86%, and nurse residents reported an increase in their confidence and skills providing care for older adults (Cadmus et al., 2016; Salmond et al., 2017):

- Geriatric care competency-based education (problem solving, communication, knowledge enhancement, and confidence building)
- Preceptor development (fosters the development of mentor knowledge, skills, and attitudes to support new nurse residents)

- Nurse resident development (educational sessions including case studies, active learning exercises, role-playing, standardized patients, and other teaching strategies to reinforce content and serve as a basis for application and critical reflection)
- Joint preceptor/nurse resident collaboration (monthly guest speakers and breakout sessions)

The University of Wisconsin-Madison School of Nursing established an online program to address the transition-to-practice gap. This program fully identified exemplars of NRPs in nursing homes including (University of Wisconsin-Madison School of Nursing, n.d.):

- Geriatric care competency-based education (clinical geriatric best practices, problem-solving techniques, and communication strategies)
- Intentional design to improve nurse residents' knowledge, confidence, and job satisfaction

And finally, the University of Utah developed a nine-month, distance-based NRP for RNs with less than a year of experience in nursing homes. This program utilized similar principles as those programs developed to support nursing students and other nurse residents. The NRP intended to increase nurse residents' gerontological nursing competencies to enable them to provide quality care to older adults, while improving the nurse residents' intent to stay in the nursing home setting. In addition to those elements utilized by other NRPs, this program also established the following as exemplars of NRPs in nursing homes (Neller et al., 2021):

- Utilization of distance-based, asynchronous and synchronous formats allowing rural and urban access to educational content
- Core competencies (leadership, coaching, communication, client assessment, and geriatrics expertise)
- Support for RN resilience embedded in curriculum
- Quality improvement project is completed in the nurse resident's home facility
- Mentorship available for clinical support and quality improvement activities

SUMMARY

This chapter highlights the potential for career advancement and professional growth within the nursing home setting. It does so by exploring staff and leadership positions available to nurses within nursing homes through care delivery models and metrics, which shape the nursing home practice environment. This, along with the various educational opportunities discussed in this chapter, supports nurse competency in geriatric clinical care and provides valuable insights for nurses interested in nursing home practice.

Further, two exceptional educational opportunities, academic-practice partnerships and nurse residency programs, are discussed in the context of skill development for nurses. Academic-practice partnerships are examined from the perspective of how nursing students may engage to bolster their geriatric care competency through research collaboration and application of clinical skills during a nursing degree program. Nurse residency program benefits are discussed for nursing students, new graduates, or nurses transitioning to a new specialty through confidence building and refinement of clinical skills.

Understanding the professional and educational opportunities available in nursing homes enables informed decision-making by nurses seeking employment and serves to strengthen nursing practice in this specialty of care.

REFERENCES

American Association of Colleges of Nursing. (n.d.). *The guiding principles for academic-practice partnerships.* https://www.aacnnursing.org/our-initiatives/education-practice/academic-practice-partnerships/the-guiding-principles-for-academic-practice-partnerships

American Association of Colleges of Nursing. (2022). *Vizient/AACN nurse residency program.* https://www.aacnnursing.org/our-initiatives/education-practice/nurse-residency-program

American Association of Nurse Practitioners. (2020). *The path to becoming a nurse practitioner (NP).* https://www.aanp.org/news-feed/explore-the-variety-of-career-paths-for-nurse-practitioners

Cadmus, E., Salmond, S. W., Hassler, L. J., Black, K., & Bohnarczyk, N. (2016, May 1). Creating a long-term care new nurse residency model. *The Journal of Continuing Education in Nursing, 47*(5), 234–240. https://doi.org/10.3928/00220124-20160419-10

Castle, N. G. (2008). Nursing home caregiver staffing levels and quality of care: A literature review. *Journal of Applied Gerontology, 27*(4), 375–405. https://doi.org/10.1177/0733464808321596

Castle, N. G. (2011). The influence of consistent assignment on nursing home deficiency citations. *The Gerontologist, 51*(6), 750–760. https://doi.org/10.1093/geront/gnr068

Castle, N. G. (2013). Consistent assignment of nurse aides: Association with turnover and absenteeism. *Journal of Aging and Social Policy, 25*(1), 48–64. https://doi.org/10.1080/08959420.2012.705647

Centers for Medicare & Medicaid Services. (2022). *State operations manual appendix PP – Guidance to surveyors for long term care facilities.* https://www.cms.gov/medicare/provider-enrollment-and-certification/guidanceforlawsandregulations/downloads/appendix-pp-state-operations-manual.pdf

Corazzini, K. N., Anderson, R. A., Mueller, C., Thorpe, J. M., & McConnell, E. S. (2013). Licensed practical nurse scope of practice and quality of nursing home care. *Nursing Research, 62*(5), 315–324. https://doi.org/10.1097/NNR.0b013e31829eba00

Dellefield, M. E., Castle, N. G., McGilton, K. S., & Spilsbury, K. (2015). The relationship between registered nurses and nursing home quality: An integrative review (2008–2014). *Nursing Economics, 33*(2), 95–108, 116.

Fernandez, H. M., Callahan, K. E., Likourezos, A., & Leipzig, R. M. (2008). House staff member awareness of older inpatients' risks for hazards of hospitalization. *Archives of Internal Medicine, 168*(4), 390–396. https://doi.org/10.1001/archinternmed.2007.87

Feuerberg, M. (2001). *Appropriateness of minimum nurse staffing ratios in nursing homes report to Congress: Phase II final, volume 1.* Centers for Medicare & Medicaid Services. https://theconsumervoice.org/uploads/files/issues/CMS-Staffing-Study-Phase-II.pdf

Halili, X., Välimäki, M., Li, Z., Tang, S., Wang, H., & Chen, Q. (2022, Sept. 22). Academic-practice partnerships in evidence-based nursing practice: A scoping review protocol. *BMJ Open, 12*(9), e065049. https://doi.org/10.1136/bmjopen-2022-065049

Harris-Kojetin, L., Sengupta, M., Lendon, J., Rome, V., Valverde, R., & Caffrey, C. (2019). Long-term care providers and services users in the United States, 2015–2016. *National Center for Health Statistics. Vital and Health Statistics, 3*(43). https://www.cdc.gov/nchs/data/series/sr_03/sr03_43-508.pdf

Karikari-Martin, P., & Ingram, C. (2022). *Centers for Medicare & Medicaid Services staffing study to inform minimum staffing requirements for nursing homes.* https://www.cms.gov/blog/centers-medicare-medicaid-services-staffing-study-inform-minimum-staffing-requirements-nursing-homes

Kolanowski, A., Cortes, T. A., Mueller, C., Bowers, B., Boltz, M., Bakerjian, D., Harrington, C., Popejoy, L., Vogelsmeier, A., Wallhagen, M., Fick, D., Batchelor, M., Harris, M., Palan-Lopez, R., Dellefield, M., Mayo, A., Woods, D. L., Horgas, A., Cacchione, P. Z., Carter, D., Tabloski, P., & Gerdner, L. (2021, March 1). A call to the CMS: Mandate adequate professional nurse staffing in nursing homes. *American Journal of Nursing, 121*(3), 24–27. https://doi.org/10.1097/01.NAJ.0000737292.96068.18

Kristof-Brown, A., Zimmerman, R., & Johnson, E. (2005). Consequences of individuals' fit at work: A meta-analysis of person–job, person–organization, person–group, and person–supervisor fit. *Personnel Psychology, 58*(2), 281–342. https://doi.org/https://doi.org/10.1111/j.1744-6570.2005.00672.x

Lyons, S. S., Specht, J. P., Karlman, S. E., & Maas, M. L. (2008, July). Everyday excellence: A framework for professional nursing practice in long-term care. *Research in Gerontological Nursing, 1*(3), 217–228. https://doi.org/10.3928/19404921-20080701-08

Mezey, M. D., Mitty, E. L., & Bottrell, M. (1997). The Teaching Nursing Home Program: Enduring educational outcomes. *Nursing Outlook, 45*(3), 133–140. https://doi.org/10.1016/s0029-6554(97)90044-0

Mezey, M. D., Mitty, E. L., & Burger, S. G. (2008, February). Rethinking Teaching Nursing Homes: Potential for improving long-term care. *The Gerontologist, 48*(1), 8–15. https://doi.org/10.1093/geront/48.1.8

Mudge, A. M., McRae, P., Hubbard, R. E., Peel, N. M., Lim, W. K., Barnett, A. G., & Inouye, S. K. (2019, February). Hospital-associated complications of older people: A proposed multicomponent outcome for acute care. *Journal of the American Geriatrics Society, 67*(2), 352–356. https://doi.org/10.1111/jgs.15662

Mueller, C. (2022, June). Multidimensional aspects of nurse staffing in nursing homes. *Nursing Clinics of North America, 57*(2), 179–189. https://doi.org/10.1016/j.cnur.2022.02.001

Mueller, C., Anderson, R. A., McConnell, E. S., & Corazzini, K. (2012). Licensed nurse responsibilities in nursing homes: A scope-of-practice issue. *Journal of Nursing Regulation, 3*(1), 13–20. https://doi.org/10.1016/S2155-8256(15)30229-5

Mueller, C., Duan, Y., Vogelsmeier, A., Anderson, R., McConnell, E., & Corazzini, K. (2018, November). Interchangeability of licensed nurses in nursing homes: Perspectives of directors of nursing. *Nursing Outlook, 66*(6), 560–569. https://doi.org/10.1016/j.outlook.2018.09.004

Mueller, C., & Savik, K. (2010, October). Identifying and validating the components of nursing practice models for long-term care facilities. *Research in Gerontological Nursing, 3*(4), 270–281. https://doi.org/10.3928/19404921-20091207-97

National Academies of Sciences, Engineering, and Medicine. (2022). *The national imperative to improve nursing home quality: Honoring our commitment to residents, families, and staff.* National Academies Press. https://doi.org/doi:10.17226/26526

National Institute of CNA Excellence. (n.d.). *About NICE!* https://www.nicecna.org/about-nice/

Neller, S., Beynon, C., McLeskey, N., Madden, C., & Edelman, L. S. (2021, Feb. 1). Development of a long-term care nurse residency program. *Journal of Gerontological Nursing, 47*(2), 37–43. https://doi.org/10.3928/00989134-20210113-03

100th US Congress. (1987). *42 CFR Part 483 requirements for states and long-term care facilities.* Omnibus Budget Reconciliation Act.

Salmond, S. W., Cadmus, E., Black, K. K., Bohnarczyk, N., & Hassler, L. (2017, Oct. 1). Long-term care nurse residency program: Evaluation of new nurse experiences and lessons learned. *The Journal of Continuing Education in Nursing, 48*(10), 474–484. https://doi.org/10.3928/00220124-20170918-09

Siegel, E. O., Mueller, C., Anderson, K. L., & Dellefield, M. E. (2010). The pivotal role of the director of nursing in nursing homes. *Nursing Administration Quarterly, 34*(2), 110–121. https://doi.org/10.1097/NAQ.0b013e3181d91813

Spilsbury, K., Hewitt, C., Stirk, L., & Bowman, C. (2011, June). The relationship between nurse staffing and quality of care in nursing homes: A systematic review. *International Journal of Nursing Studies, 48*(6), 732–750. https://doi.org/10.1016/j.ijnurstu.2011.02.014

University of Wisconsin-Madison School of Nursing. (n.d.). *Geri-Res: A transition-to-practice residency program for the long term care nurse.* https://gerires.nursing.wisc.edu/

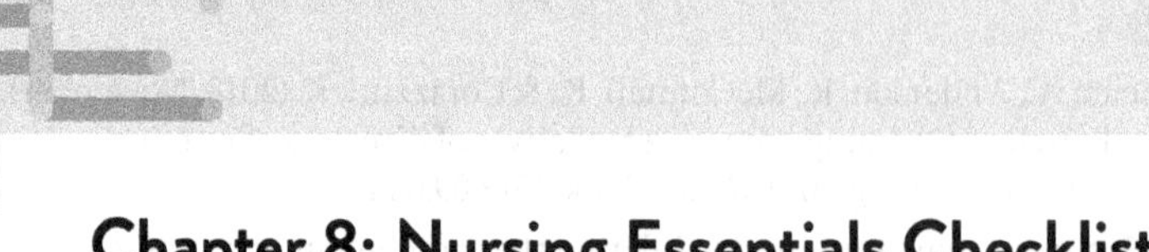

Chapter 8: Nursing Essentials Checklist

SPHERES OF CARE

Nursing occurs within four spheres of care, ranging from prevention to supportive care and all the areas in between. This chapter is relevant to the following spheres of care:

- ☑ Disease Prevention/Health Promotion
- ☑ Chronic Disease Care
- ☑ Regenerative or Restorative Care
- ☑ Hospice/Palliative/Supportive Care

DOMAINS OF PRACTICE

The American Association of Colleges of Nursing has identified 10 broad domains of practice for nursing. Students are expected to master these domains of practice across the spheres of care. This chapter addresses:

- ☑ Knowledge for Nursing Practice (Nursing and Other Disciplines)
- ☐ Person-Centered Care
- ☐ Population Health
- ☐ Scholarship for Practice
- ☑ Quality and Safety
- ☐ Interprofessional Partnerships
- ☐ Systems-Based Care
- ☐ Information & Healthcare Technologies
- ☑ Professionalism
- ☑ Personal, Professional, Leadership Development

CONCEPTS FOR PRACTICE

Integrated across the domains of practice are eight concepts which the student is expected to master across the spheres of care and across the domains of practice. This chapter addresses:

- ☑ Clinical Judgment
- ☐ Communication
- ☐ Compassionate Care
- ☐ Diversity, Equity, Inclusion
- ☐ Ethics
- ☐ Evidence-Based Practice
- ☑ Health Policy
- ☐ Social Determinants of Health

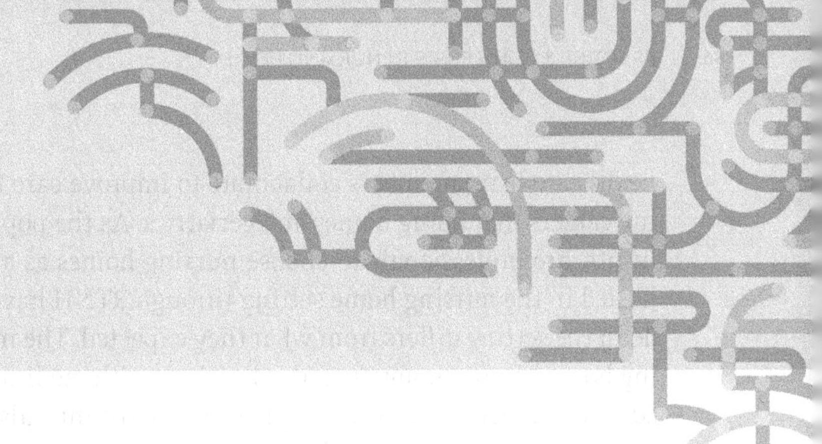

CHAPTER 8

STAFF DEVELOPMENT AND TRAINING

Tara A. Cortes, PhD, RN, FAAN, FGSA
Taylor McMahon, RN, CNDLTC
Amy Stewart, MSN, RN, RAC-MT, RAC-MTA, DNS-MT, QCP-MT
Marianne Shaughnessy, PhD, AGPCNP-BC, GS-C, FAAN

OBJECTIVES

1. Describe staff training and development in the context of the nursing home environment.
2. Explain the importance and elements of staff performance evaluation.
3. List methods for staff training and development.

INTRODUCTION

This chapter describes professional nursing practice in long-term care and gives an overview of the structure and organization of the nursing team. It provides insights into expected nurse competencies and highlights the relationship of those competencies to performance evaluation. Different components of staff education are presented, and the processes used for delivering educational resources are described. The importance of self-care and resilience for a high-functioning team are also discussed.

REVISITING THE TEACHING NURSING HOME

As presented in Chapters 2 and 7, the Revisiting the Teaching Nursing Home (RTNH) initiative establishes a "teaching" environment where students, nursing faculty, and healthcare team members collaborate to improve care for residents and foster nursing careers in nursing homes and geriatrics. As the population is aging, the need for healthcare professionals to choose nursing homes as a career is essential. Students hosted in the nursing home setting through RTNH have noted that the work nurses do in the setting differs from what they expected. The nurse who practices in a nursing home has autonomy to make decisions with medical team members (physicians, advanced practice nurses, and physician assistants, also referred to as "providers") that directly affect quality of life.

Students can see this work through an interdisciplinary approach such as Quality Assurance and Performance Improvement. This regulatory, facility-based structure looks at factors that directly impact the older adult's quality of life through the collection and review of past and current data and determines measures to improve quality of services delivered in this setting. The nursing student in this collaboration participates with the nursing home quality committee to promote quality assurance, directly impacting the life of the older adult. Age-Friendly Health Systems also set a framework of quality and evidence-based measures to provide holistic, person-centered care to the long-term care setting.

The collaboration of nursing homes and schools of nursing yielded independent studies in the nursing home that looked at older adults as individuals and what mattered to them. It aligned their medication, mentation, and mobility with a human-centered approach. Students that presented on this model of care felt that it was impactful and meaningful work. An undergraduate from the University of Pittsburgh School of Nursing stated, "I really enjoyed being able to spend time getting to know the residents and being able to learn about their lives, families, hobbies and interests, and beliefs."

Providing staff and nursing students with time to spend with the older adult is essential for clinical management and engagement in this work. To know the older adult on a very personal level and what is important to them often guides the care in this setting, which may differ from acute care. Standard clinical experiences in the nursing home often center around activities of daily living (ADL) care in the early semesters of associate degree training. While providing ADL care is a component of nursing care, this focus does not entail the entirety of professional nursing practice in this setting. Although these standard clinicals give insight to the work that a certified nursing assistant (CNA) may provide, they do not encapsulate the top-of-license critical thinking skills, collaboration, and autonomous work that the long-term care professional nurse provides on a day-to-day basis.

With independent studies or clinicals in a more advanced semester, the nursing home is able to provide the student with substantial learning in the areas of nurse leadership and interdisciplinary team collaboration. Geriatric nursing organically promotes meaningful moments, and resident advocacy provides the ability to build relationships with residents, patients, and their families.

The engagement of students in nursing homes is critical for the continuum of care for older adults. Nursing students can see the value of choosing geriatrics as a specialty and engage with seniors on an intimate level and utilize their critical thinking skills. The student can learn about the vast opportunities for leadership advancement and provide the resident with compassionate, person-centered care.

PROFESSIONAL PRACTICE IN LONG-TERM CARE

The Professional Nurse Practice model (PNP) drives quality resident/patient-centered care in long-term care. The fundamental tenet of this model is that care is guided, coordinated, and delivered by clinically competent professional nurses. The elements that characterize the PNP include:

- Leadership
- Interdisciplinary collaboration
- Research and evidence-based practice
- Professional standards
- Shared governance
- Continuing professional growth and development

It is well documented that this model improves staff recruitment and retention and improves the quality of care delivered (Porter-O'Grady, 2019).

The nursing department in long-term care includes CNAs, registered nurses (RNs), and licensed practical nurses (LPNs). CNAs comprise about 70% of the nursing care staff and provide most of the direct care to residents. CNAs are valuable team members, as they are often the "eyes and ears" of residents because they are so well-acquainted with them. They are responsible for the day-to-day care of residents, including bathing and feeding as necessary, transferring from bed to chair, taking vital signs, and completing required documentation.

Some states have passed legislation allowing CNAs to be trained to distribute medications as well. Federal regulations require CNAs to have 75 hours of training to be certified. States have the option to require additional hours. Each state has its own requirement for annual continuing education for CNAs. This most often includes topics on the care of people with dementia and infection control practices.

Nurses are responsible for directing resident care in long-term-care. The Centers for Medicare & Medicaid Services (CMS, 2013) requires that skilled nursing facilities provide 24-hour licensed nursing services by an LPN or RN. In addition, it requires that an RN be on the premises for eight consecutive hours a day, seven days a week (more than 40 hours a week), and that there be an RN designated as director of nursing on a full-time basis (Coffman et al., 2015). However, these requirements can be waived under certain circumstances. Most commonly this waiver is granted when a nursing home can show it has made diligent efforts to recruit appropriate personnel but has been unable to do so. These waivers are provided by the state if it can determine the health and safety of the resident in the home is not imperiled.

Educational preparation of nurses in long-term care is variable. In urban areas there may be nurses with advanced degrees, although most often RNs in long-term care are prepared at the bachelor's or associate degree level. Although an RN is preferred in long-term care, LPNs, who attend a one-year licensure program, comprise the largest portion of licensed nurses in most long-term care facilities. The RNs and LPNs are responsible for overseeing the quality of care provided in the facility. They provide care that is specific to their scope of practice such as completing the initial assessment and care plan, the management of controlled substances, distribution of medications, and provision of certain treatments such as wound care and enteral feedings.

Nursing homes and long-term care facilities are the largest employer of LPNs, with more than one-third of LPNs working in that setting. The presumed interchangeability of the RN and LPN roles is due to the fact that the recruitment of RNs to long-term care is difficult. However, while overlapping somewhat, the scope of practice for these two roles is different, and the LPN cannot fulfill the same scope as the RN.

Pre-licensure associate and bachelor's degree nursing programs offer very little clinical experience in long-term care, and graduates are often not comfortable going into an area where they have had little or no practice. However, there is an emerging need to increase the number of RNs in long-term care, as the care needed in these settings is some of the most complex care nurses can administer. Most of these residents have several chronic conditions and very often also have dementia. While there are evidence-based standard protocols for some aspects of care delivery (e.g., delirium assessment, dementia care, wound assessment, and falls risk), each resident is unique and requires a tailored, person-centered plan of care.

Nursing homes therefore need professional nurses who can make clinical decisions based on research and evidence, assess resident outcomes, and adjust care plans accordingly. The emerging role of professional nurses in this environment demands leadership skills to ensure a culture that is person-centered and values respect, collaboration, inclusion, and high-quality care. It also requires nurses to have excellent clinical skills and to make informed clinical decisions (see Figure 8.1).

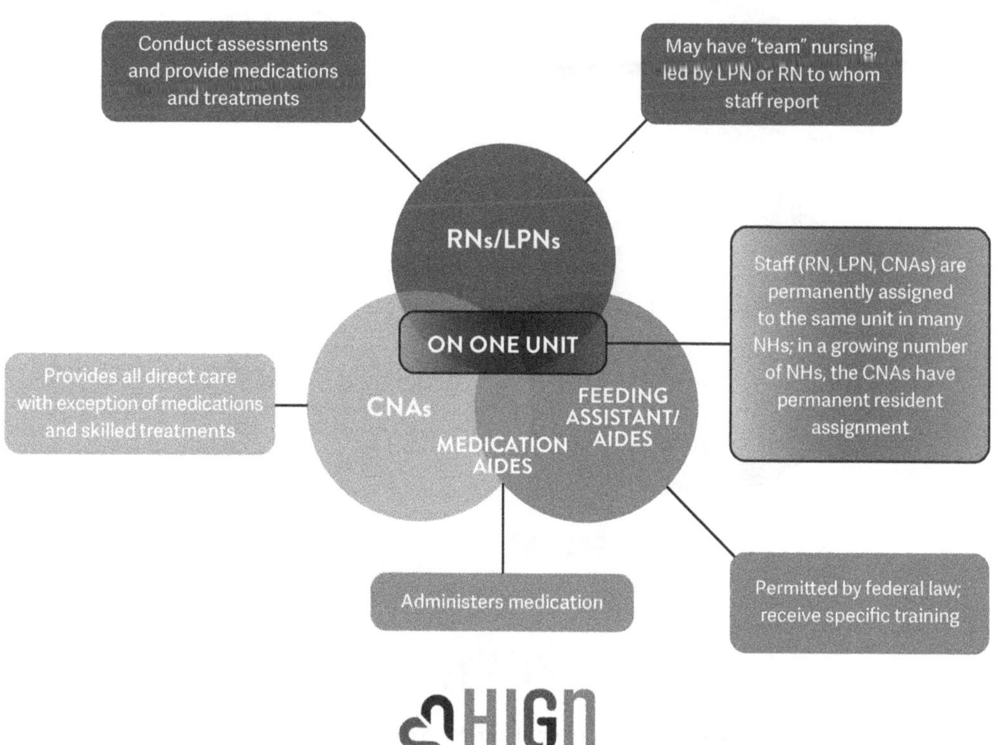

FIGURE 8.1 Roles of nursing care staff.

Advanced Nursing Roles in Long-Term Care

Advanced practice nurses are also providers of care in skilled nursing facilities. Most often these are nurse practitioners (NPs), although they may be clinical nurse specialists (CNSs). These nurses have master's or doctoral degrees and are certified in a particular area of practice. NPs serve as primary care providers to residents, manage chronic diseases, and respond to emergencies. CNSs are most often wound care specialists. Although these nurses may be employed by a facility, they are often contracted employees through a specialty agency or a primary care practice.

Organizational Structure

The director of nursing services, an RN, is responsible for the overall care of residents and any nurses or CNAs on the staff. Organizational nurse leadership includes RN or LPN supervisors and RN or LPN nurse managers (see Figure 8.2). Additional nursing leadership positions include a nurse educator, an infection control nurse, and a

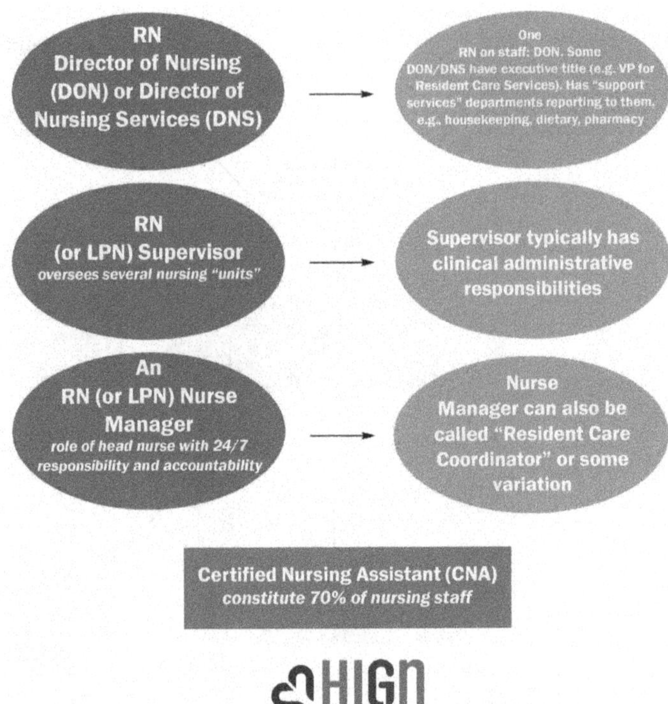

FIGURE 8.2 Nursing hierarchy in nursing homes.

nurse assessment coordinator who is responsible for the Minimum Data Set (MDS), a required standardized clinical assessment, along with oversight of care-planning processes. Nursing homes also have a nursing home administrator (NHA) who is responsible for the business and regulatory aspects of the nursing home. While a nursing degree is not a requirement to obtain an NHA license, many NHAs do possess this preparation. The qualifications for obtaining an NHA license vary, but most states require at least a baccalaureate degree and supervised training.

LEADERSHIP, MANAGEMENT, AND MENTORSHIP

Although management and leadership are often used interchangeably, they are not the same thing. Ideally, leaders inspire people to leave their comfort zone and try new ways of practice to become a better person and a better nurse. Nurses providing care in the long-term care environment should look to leaders for furthering the organizational mission and enabling a culture that encourages personal and professional growth, integrity, and respect for all staff as well as residents.

Managers create and hold team members accountable to systems, infrastructure, and policies to bring patterns and equity to programs of residents' care. Managers provide clear goals and expectations for performance, organize the provision of resident care so that it reflects standards of excellence, and create open channels of communication to ensure that all staff are heard and have input into decisions that may affect their workday. In long-term care, the director of nursing provides both leadership and management of clinical programs and the nursing team.

Mentorship is important to the development of any professional nurse, regardless of whether they are a beginner or expert. A mentor can be a person who is proficient in an area in which a nurse is trying to grow and develop. Nurses working in long-term care should identify a mentor who values professional and personal growth and understands the importance of a long-term care environment that practices person-centered care and shared decision-making. This person may be in the same organization or not. Good mentorship should benefit both the mentor and mentee, as good mentors are open to listening and learning from those they mentor, while mentees are transparent in sharing situations in which they do not have the level of confidence needed to be successful. To be successful in this relationship, it is important to identify short-term and long-term benchmarks and celebrate their achievement.

PERFORMANCE EVALUATION AND FEEDBACK

Performance evaluation (PE) should be based on standards, scope of practice, and the job description. It is a process that involves not only a written document evaluating performance but also a dialogue between the manager and the nurse that highlights satisfactory practice and offers ways to improve work areas. The domains of the PE usually include resident care outcomes, evidence of knowledge and skills and their application to practice, and other behaviors stated in the job description such as communication skills, decision-making, and conflict resolution (Resnick & Mitty, 2008).

The PE measurement should be shared with a new nurse at the time of hire so there is clear understanding of the expectations. It is important to set short-term and long-term goals with staff members so that there are established benchmarks for personal and professional growth. Progress toward the goals should be reviewed with the nurse periodically, not just at the time of the annual PE. New hires should ask how the facility or organization will support them in their development.

COMPETENCY-BASED EDUCATION

To provide competent care, nurses must demonstrate they have the knowledge, skills, and ability to care for the patient population they serve. Nursing education programs use competency-based education to prepare nursing students for the ever-changing demands in healthcare. *Competency-based education* is "a system of instruction, assessment, feedback, self-reflection, and academic reporting that is based on students demonstrating that they have learned the knowledge, attitudes, motivations, self-perceptions, and skills expected of them as they progress through their education" (American Association of Colleges of Nursing, n.d., para. 1). Building one's competency doesn't end at graduation. Nurses need ongoing education to keep their knowledge current about standards of practice and advances in technology. Throughout a nurse's career, that ongoing education benefits the patients by equipping nurses with the competence they need to care for complex medical needs in a holistic manner.

In long-term care facilities, nursing leadership and regulatory requirements often determine what competency-based education staff will receive. This may differ from acute-care settings, where acuity and evidence-based practice are more likely to drive education.

"Competence (ability) is a premise for developing competency (behavioral characteristics)" (Fukada, 2018, p. 1). In other words, knowledge is a base to build on, but knowledge alone is not competency. To become competent in an area, one must gain information and apply that education to change or improve current practice. This approach allows for individualized learning plans designed to achieve mastery or competency (Lewis et al., 2022). This may include education related to the use of new technology, specific skills, or advances in practice. In addition, new employee orientation often includes competency-based education to ensure a new hire has a minimum level of knowledge before they begin working independently.

Competency-based education allows a healthcare organization to examine the current knowledge, skills, and capabilities of its staff members and help them identify gaps, provide education, and improve outcomes for both patients and the organization. For example, as wound care techniques advance, competency-based education can enhance nurses' ability to assess and treat wounds. Or, if an organization has a high volume of acquired pressure injuries, educating staff about pressure injury prevention can help transition the organization into the future state, one with a lower number of pressure ulcers.

Nursing homes must abide by federal requirements regarding competency-based education and staffing. The requirement states that nursing homes "must have sufficient staff with the appropriate competencies and skill sets to provide nursing and related services to assure resident safety and attain or maintain the highest practicable physical, mental, and psychosocial well-being of each resident" (CMS, 2023, p. 478). The regulation goes on to state that the facility "must ensure that licensed nurses have the specific competencies and skill sets necessary for residents' needs, as identified through resident assessments and described in the plan of care" (CMS, 2023, p. 478). CMS's intent for this regulation is "to assure that all nursing staff possess the competencies and skill sets necessary to provide nursing and related services to meet the residents' needs safely and in a manner that promotes each resident's rights, physical, mental and psychosocial well-being" (CMS, 2023, p. 478).

According to the State Operations Manual, Appendix PP, "nursing leadership with input from the Medical Director should delineate the competencies required for all nursing staff to deliver, individualize, and provide safe care for the facility's residents. There should also be a process to evaluate staff skill levels, and to develop individualized competency-based training, that ensures resident safety and quality of care and service being delivered" (CMS, 2023, p. 481). As nursing home facilities complete their facility assessments, many aspects of facility operations can help identify competency needs. For example, the facility assessment may identify several residents from a specific culture. Facility leaders will want to address cultural competencies as part of the ongoing competency-based education. Cultural competencies help staff communicate and provide care for the residents in a manner that is appropriate to the culture and the individual (CMS, 2023).

An Example of Competency-Based Education in Action

A skilled nursing facility is preparing to offer dialysis services to residents, so leadership is updating the facility assessment as part of the planning. The facility assessment identified that the change in acuity and addition of a specialized service require nurses who will be assigned to administer the dialysis as well as those who will care for residents pre- and post-dialysis. The nurses completing the MDS and developing care plans will need to learn new competencies to ensure timely and accurate data collection.

Competency-based education provides a measurable method of education delivery that requires a change in behavior from the current state to what will be. Each facility must determine what types of education are necessary to meet the needs of the unique patient population. Continued competency requires ongoing assessment of needs and continual education to meet the constantly shifting demands in healthcare.

To comply with regulations and provide the care residents need, nurse leaders must identify the necessary competencies nurses must have. The skill sets needed will vary depending on the needs of the resident population served. For example, if a facility offers memory care, it will utilize competency-based education to strengthen the staff's ability to communicate with individuals who have dementia. Or nurses may need to enhance their competence to assess residents experiencing a change in condition, as those with impaired communication may not be able to clearly communicate their symptoms.

ACUITY AS AN INDICATOR OF EDUCATION NEEDS

Nursing homes care predominantly for the aging population, although a smaller portion may care for younger residents with disabilities. The ongoing education needed differs greatly between these two populations, but both require competency and skills to meet the needs of the patient population. The trend to care for higher acuity patients continues, and many nursing homes are expanding services to offer highly specialized care such as dialysis and cardiac rehabilitation. Patient care needs differ based on resident acuity.

Several factors determine acuity in long-term care. One source is the resident assessment instrument MDS and the resulting care plans. The MDS identifies a patient's needs, strengths, goals, functional and health status, life history, and preferences. These, in turn, inform the development of a comprehensive care plan, outlining individualized resident care needs. For example, MDS data that reveal several residents with tube feedings may signal to nursing leadership that competency-based education on tube feedings is necessary.

Additionally, in 2019, CMS implemented a new Medicare reimbursement methodology, the Patient Driven Payment Model (PDPM), that categorizes nursing home patients based on resident characteristics that drive resource utilization. PDPM was designed to support Medicare reimbursement for short-term patients admitted for skilled care. It classifies residents into 25 nursing groups within six nursing categories:

- Extensive Services
- Special Care High
- Special Care Low
- Clinically Complex
- Behavior Symptoms and Impaired Cognition
- Reduced Physical Function

Facilities can use these six basic nursing acuity levels, listed from highest to lowest, to identify acuity needs. These categories identify both the nursing and certified nurse aide care needs (Harrington et al., 2020). Understanding patient acuity assists with staffing planning and ensures sufficient resources in number of nurses, skill mix, education, or expertise (Juve-Udina et al., 2020).

Finally, in 2016, CMS implemented federal regulations that require nursing facilities to conduct a facility-wide assessment. One purpose of the facility assessment is to determine what resources and staff are needed to meet the needs of the patients. This analysis must consider the "number, acuity, and diagnoses of the facility's resident population" (CMS, 2023, p. 471) and must be updated at least annually.

CERTIFICATION

Nursing certification "is the formal recognition of the specialized knowledge, skills, and experience demonstrated by the achievement of standards identified by a nursing specialty to promote optimal health outcomes" (American Board of Nursing Specialties, n.d., Our History). Whereas *nursing licensure* is based on minimal state requirements, certification denotes a higher level of knowledge and skill (Altman, 2011). To attain certification in a specialty area, a nurse must develop a level of expertise that reflects that higher level of practice. The certifying agency establishes standards that demonstrate advanced competency in a specific area or discipline of nursing.

Nurses who want to obtain the certification must show that they meet the standards; they then may take an exam that verifies their advanced knowledge. Upon passing, an individual becomes certified and earns the use of credentials. Certifications continue for a certain number of years before an individual must renew, demonstrating that their knowledge and skills remain current. This process, with formal benchmarks for greater knowledge, skills, and competency, is oriented around achieving a higher level of nursing practice.

Long-term care nurses have multiple certification options. Certifications can be topic-specific, such as wound or dementia certification, or population-specific, such as geriatrics or rehabilitation. In addition, certifications for specific roles in long-term care emphasize one's expertise in positions such as the director of nursing services or nurse assessment coordinator (the individual responsible for the MDS). The various nurse certifications involve different benefits and barriers.

Benefits

Certified nurses have worked over a period of time to gain knowledge and skills that prepare them to become certified. Often, working with a certified nurse will prompt others to seek the advanced knowledge that certification recognizes. While this knowledge requires ongoing maintenance, the learning itself is rewarding, both for the certified nurse and new graduate nurses that the certified nurse inspires, guides, or mentors.

Certification in a specialty or subspecialty area also conveys personal benefits like confidence, credibility, and a feeling of personal accomplishment. Professional benefits include employee recognition, increased consumer confidence, and increased salary (Van Wicklin et al., 2020). And because certifications prioritize knowledge that promotes optimal health outcomes, certified nurses can know that they are delivering a higher quality of patient care.

Employers benefit from having nurses with an advanced skill level, so to encourage certification, some employers offer certification incentives, such as a pay increase or reimbursement for the cost of the examination. Staff specialization and a higher level of knowledge and skill may influence patient choice when selecting a provider. An organization that has several nurses on staff with certification in specialty areas, therefore, can inform patients that its staff holds this expertise. When considering a potential employer's benefits, inquire about professional development opportunities the employer offers that may enable the newly licensed nurse to progress toward a level of practice expertise necessary for certification.

Many long-term care organizations include certifications as a part of a career ladder. Making progress toward and eventually attaining certification can be key milestones for career advancement. Moreover, certifications are often required for or part of the ongoing professional development expectations for certain roles. The director of nursing and nurse assessment coordinator, for example, are two roles that often hold certifications.

Nurses working in long-term care who hold certifications report that their advanced knowledge and skills help them better navigate the unique population of patients they care for. For example, a nurse who is dementia certified has gained skills to better communicate with patients and reduce dementia-related behaviors (Alzheimer's Association, 2023).

Barriers

There can be multiple barriers to the achievement of certification. The cost of purchasing study guides or an online certification review course, attending a workshop, or sitting for the examination can be a substantial barrier. Personal barriers, such as the time commitment required to prepare for certification and the fear of failing, can also challenge would-be participants. Yet the first step in mitigating individual barriers is identifying them.

Employers' assistance can help to offset the cost of certification. In addition to the certification incentives previously discussed, some long-term care organizations host workshops or offer certification preparation courses through their online learning system. Some organizations may allow nurses to take these courses during work hours to help increase the number of certified staff.

The time required to develop into a nurse eligible for certification can be a daunting yet vital part of the process. As a new graduate, it will take time and experience to progress from a brand-new nurse to one who is qualified at a higher level of practice. Certification is about more than passing a test. It requires expert-level knowledge that one can use in practice to improve quality of care and outcomes. Successfully achieving certification requires time and effort on the part of the individual.

Having a solid base of knowledge and skill regarding the topic can better prepare one for certification and help to overcome individual barriers. To overcome fear of failing, nurses can seek out other certified individuals who have successfully completed the certification. Mentorship by someone who has been through the process can better prepare one for certification.

THE ROLE OF EDUCATOR

The nurse educator role in long-term care varies from facility to facility. This role may carry other important responsibilities but must have a key focus on clinical and regulatory education. The long-term care nurse educator is typically a registered nurse with several years of experience in the clinical field (Graham Gibson, 2011). The role may be blended with other job duties such as care management, assistant director, quality, or another specialty that the facility decided.

The nurse educator's role in long-term care is essential for orienting new employees and providing annual skills fairs or care-simulation sessions. The nurse educator must also collaborate with the interdisciplinary team to understand the needs the team has to care for a medically complex population.

The nurse educator is an essential role that aids in the growth and development of CNAs and long-term care nurses, which ultimately promotes quality processes and outcomes of geriatric care. During new hire orientation, the nurse educator plays an important role to ensure the team members understand person-centered care, regulatory compliance, policy/procedure, and familiarity with the facility to aid in retention. Nursing homes often host nursing students in their facilities that aid in clinical training for geriatrics. This focused clinical specialty aids in development of the next generation of geriatric nursing, as this rewarding experience shows the appreciation that older adults often give to their caregivers. The nursing home's focus on person-centered care enables the student to get to know their patient/resident to provide meaningful, individualized care.

Responsibilities of the educator include developing, planning, implementing, and tracking staff training, as well as growth and development opportunities needed to ensure the provision of quality care. The educator will stimulate personal/professional growth and assure completion of employees' required core competencies. It is important for the nurse educator to keep records of staff training to ensure regulatory compliance and aid in staff accountability. The nurse educator is also responsible for development and implementation of training modules across the continuum of care. The educator then must evaluate training events and educational processes to make continuous improvements due to the changes that are occurring in the workforce in long-term care.

METHODS OF TRAINING

Methods for delivering staff training vary from facility to facility but focus on core clinical competencies and regulatory compliance. This focus includes but is not limited to:

- Person-centered care
- Resident rights and abuse
- Chronic and acute disease management
- Palliative care, regulatory compliance
- Policy and procedure
- A range of clinical skills

Nurse leaders/supervisors use various approaches to develop and train staff, including utilization of staff meetings, on-unit huddles, learning circles, and "just in time" learning sessions that aid in the development of skills and understanding for the knowledge-based clinical competencies needed to care for older adults. Virtual learning also aids in the required or optional methods to engage clinical staff in educational sessions. This method of training includes identification of learning objectives to build leadership and clinical skill sets and CNA/nurse knowledge so team members have greater resilience to thrive in our ever-changing environment.

Long-term care facilities often have programs to promote growth and development of nursing team members. These programs may include, but are not limited to, tuition reimbursement, flex scheduling for student schedules, partnerships with schools of nursing for team member enrollment, CNA career ladders, and educational sessions on opportunities for promotions.

ENGAGING STAFF IN EFFECTIVE AND EFFICIENT CARE DELIVERY

Process improvement and quality control are essential components of nursing home care. It is important to engage the frontline team members in improving work-related processes. This aids in sustainability and dissemination of best practices. One method of process improvement that has a high focus in healthcare is the team huddle, which is an effective way of reviewing problems systematically to cultivate change and team member engagement.

Nursing home leaders must be resourceful to address the ongoing staffing shortages across care settings throughout the nation. Leaders must be creative to maximize the staff that they have and create a culture of identifying value to those that they serve by removing the waste in the work so that they can deliver better services to the end customers. Supporting daily continuous improvement is implemented through problem identification and the application of the scientific method to solve problems through small tests of change that lead to data-based results yielding positive outcomes. Best practices are then sustainable, and frontline team members feel empowered and engaged in their work.

Nurse leaders in long-term care must commit to this level of engagement by being involved in team meetings and rounding with their team to understand barriers that they face and celebrate wins that they achieve. Throughout the COVID-19 pandemic, transparency and communication were key for nursing homes to survive. The nation watched as nursing homes were epicenters of the grim, adverse outcomes of the virus. Huddles or nurse meetings surrounding new infection control guidelines, changing regulations, and internal outbreaks were essential for frontline team members to be successful in a fearful time.

Reflective practice is an important aspect of geriatric care. In nursing homes, family dynamics surrounding progressive illness, death, and dying may conflict with staff members' views, creating ethical dilemmas. Reflecting on one's own beliefs and feelings is important to ensure that the patient's wishes are being followed and not influenced. This may pose a personal dilemma at times, but understanding reflective practice and core principles surrounding this may be helpful. Several models of care explored with reflective practice include self-awareness, description, critical analysis, synthesis, and evaluation (Ingham-Broomfield, 2021).

Often, nursing school curriculum and experience take place in acute-care settings where the focus is medical treatment, whereas in the nursing home, the focus may more appropriately be palliative care (symptom management), not curative care. It is important that the nurse in this setting has self-awareness to alleviate stressors related to end of life and to maintain advocacy for the patient.

Considering the nature of the population living and receiving care in nursing homes, training programs should include core competencies related to palliative care, end-of-life care, death and dying, and bereavement. Families are often appreciative of the care that the nurse/nurse aide provides at a difficult time in this journey of life and inevitable outcome of aging.

AVOIDING BURNOUT AND PRACTICING SELF-CARE

Long-term care is among the most challenging and also rewarding environments in which nurses practice. Professionals from multiple healthcare disciplines and service areas must work together to prioritize the physical, social, mental, and emotional needs of residents with complex medical problems. The nurse at the center of all this activity must possess exceptional interpersonal, organizational, and communication skills, along with patience and compassion.

Nurses in long-term care settings coordinate team activity to provide care to persons at the most vulnerable times in their lives, when functional and/or cognitive independence have waned. Whether temporary or permanent, the loss of independence can profoundly change how residents view and interact with the world around them. Restorative or rehabilitative care can sometimes help restore or maintain some level of independence, but teams are challenged every day to face these challenges along with their residents. When communication is impaired, the challenges become even greater for residents to maintain their identities as individuals and be active participants in their own lives.

Burnout

Working in long-term care can be very rewarding, allowing for the development of close relationships among residents, their families, and coworkers. Members of high-functioning teams effectively rely on each other to understand and perform their roles and achieve results. However, short staffing, ambiguity in role expectations, and lack of management support can lead to frustration and stress, which can manifest in unhealthy habits and a lack of self-care that can ultimately lead to burnout. *Burnout* is a syndrome conceptualized as resulting from chronic workplace stress and is characterized by three dimensions (World Health Organization, 2023, para. 1):

1. Feelings of energy depletion or exhaustion
2. Increased mental distance from one's job, or feelings of negativism or cynicism related to one's job
3. A sense of ineffectiveness and lack of accomplishment

Research into the risk factors for burnout points to both organizational and personal factors. Organizational risk factors may include high workload, value incongruence, low control over the job, low decision-making authority, poor social climate/social support, and low rewards as predictors of burnout (Dall'Ora et al., 2020). Personal risk factors for burnout include lack of sleep, inadequate breaks, unhealthy diet, and lack of regular exercise; lack of access to social or mental health support and role overload may also contribute to burnout (Dall'Ora et al., 2020).

Nurses working in long-term care settings may not be able to control many organizational factors, but interventions such as workload and/or schedule rotation, self-scheduling, team-building, and stress management training are all options that can be explored. Nurse leaders should pay careful attention to team dynamics; increasing staff decisional responsibility for workload, care management, and time management can alleviate stress for all members.

Self-Care

According to the World Health Organization (n.d.), *self-care* is defined as actions people take for themselves to establish and maintain health and prevent/manage illness with or without the support of a healthcare provider and is critical for maintaining well-being, particularly when working in potentially high-stress environments.

Making self-care part of the work culture normalizes and encourages self-care behaviors that can lessen the impacts of stress on the individual:

- Yoga, Tai-Chi, meditation, and mindfulness activities may benefit staff and residents alike.
- Breaks should be interrupted only in case of an emergency.
- Schedules should allow for sufficient rest between shifts.
- Nurses as team leaders can role-model and encourage others on the team to address their own identified personal risk factors and engage in self-care behaviors on a regular basis.

Nurses in long-term care settings can build long-standing and fulfilling relationships with members of the care team and residents alike. Awareness of responsibilities to self, each other, and residents and attention to the needs of each are critical to long-term success.

The following case study illustrates some of the important aspects long-term care nurses have demonstrated for the need for further training.

CASE STUDY VHA/National Hartford Center of Gerontological Nursing Excellence

Nurse Manager

Leadership Training Program

The Veterans Health Administration (VHA), the largest integrated health system in the US, and the National Hartford Center of Gerontological Nursing Excellence (NHCGNE), an organization of schools of nursing with extensive geriatric expertise, partnered to develop and deliver a training course for new nurse managers in the VHA's long-term care settings known as Community Living Centers (CLCs).

As in the community at-large, VHA nurse managers in long-term care generally come from acute-care backgrounds and have little to no experience with a long-term care population or setting. Many are placed into CLC management positions without knowledge of geriatric care principles and no experience in long-term care leadership. Consequently, when acute care-based positions become available,

(continues)

(continued)

nurse managers tend to move back to more familiar practice settings, leaving a perpetual vacuum of nurse leadership in long-term care.

Interviews with new nurse managers revealed the need for content about geriatric multimorbidity as well as information regarding long-term care regulations, philosophy of care (cultural transformation), managing staff shortages, and building teams. To address these issues, a brief seven-module course was designed to give new nurse managers foundations in basic geriatric care, long-term care regulations, and leadership. Each module contained content on both geriatric care and leadership skills as well as breakout sessions for smaller group discussions and networking. Seven synchronous online "classes" ran for three hours every three to four weeks. Fourteen new nurse managers enrolled in the pilot offering, which ran from January to June 2019. Attendance at the classes averaged 12 per class.

At the conclusion of the program, 11 participants agreed to interviews about their experience. Most were glad they had participated, but while some had protected time to attend the classes, a few did not, and these respondents reported feeling overwhelmed with trying to attend class while juggling normal work responsibilities. Most found the online delivery of the program through videoconferencing to be an effective means of making connections with the faculty and each other, and many reported the breakout sessions for discussion and networking as especially high value. Feedback on the availability of faculty was very positive, as participants often contacted them outside of class while working on assignments. The content of the modules was reported to be relevant to their practice, but the leadership content was especially valued by students. Nearly all reported they would recommend the course to other new nurse managers.

Overall, the NHCGNE program was well received by CLC nurse managers in this pilot program. Suggestions for future offerings included shortening the classes and offering them more frequently, as well as adding more VHA-specific content and adding modules related to the survey process, hospice, rehabilitation, managing staffing ratios/shortages, staff management (especially discipline and team relationships), and quality measures.

SUMMARY

Professional nursing practice in long-term care is characterized by strong leadership, engagement in interdisciplinary collaboration, use of research and evidence-based practice, implementation of professional standards, shared governance with staff, and promotion of staff development. When the professional nurse demonstrates these qualities, there is evidence that residents experience better quality of life, staff deliver better quality of care, and the nursing home has a better track record of recruitment and retention. Within long-term care settings, a major responsibility of the professional nurse is to ensure that all members of the nursing team (CNAs, LPNs, and newly hired RNs) have the necessary competencies (knowledge and skills) to function at a high level of performance. Timely and targeted education, mentorship, and evaluation are key to successful staff performance. The professional nurse should invest a significant amount of their time in nursing team development and their self-care to ensure that this valuable resource has the support it needs to function at a high level.

REFERENCES

Altman, M. (2011). Let's get certified: Best practices for nurse leaders to create a culture of certification. *AACN Advanced Critical Care, 22*(1), 68–75. https://doi.org/10.1097/NCI.0b013e3182057772

Alzheimer's Association. (2023). *Pathways to dementia care training and certification: Options for individuals and providers.* https://www.alz.org/professionals/professional-providers/dementia-care-training-certification

American Association of Colleges of Nursing. (n.d.). *What is competency-based education?* https://www.aacnnursing.org/Essentials/Definition-of-Competency-Based-Education

American Board of Nursing Specialties. (n.d.). *About us.* https://www.nursingcertification.org/About-ABNS

Centers for Medicare & Medicaid Services. (2013). *Manuals.* https://www.cms.gov/regulations-and-guidance/guidance/manuals

Centers for Medicare & Medicaid Services. (2023). *State operations manual appendix PP: Guidance to surveyors for long term care facilities.* https://www.cms.gov/medicare/provider-enrollment-and-certification/guidanceforlawsandregulations/downloads/appendix-pp-state-operations-manual.pdf

Coffman, J. M., Chan, K., & Bates, T. (2015). *Trends in licensed practical nurse/licensed vocational nurse education and licensure examinations, 1998 to 2013.* https://healthworkforce.ucsf.edu/sites/healthworkforce.ucsf.edu/files/Report-Trends_in_LPN-LVN_Education_and_Licensure_Examinations_1998-to-2013.pdf

Dall'Ora, C., Ball, J., Reinius, M., & Griffiths, P. (2020). Burnout in nursing: A theoretical review. *Human Resources for Health, 18*(1), 41. https://doi.org/10.1186/s12960-020-00469-9

Fukada, M. (2018, March). Nursing competency: Definition, structure and development. *Yonago Acta Medica, 61*(1), 1–7. https://doi.org/10.33160/yam.2018.03.001

Graham Gibson, C. (2011). Nurse educator roles and long-term care. *Journal for Nurses in Professional Development, 27*(6), 259–261. https://doi.org/10.1097/NND.0b013e3182371136

Harrington, C., Dellefield, M. E., Halifax, E., Fleming, M. L., & Bakerjian, D. (2020). Appropriate nurse staffing levels for U.S. nursing homes. *Health Services Insights, 13.*

Ingham-Broomfield, B. (2021). A nurses' guide to using models of reflection. *Australian Journal of Advanced Nursing, 38*(4). https://doi.org/https://doi.org/10.37464/2020.384.395

Juve-Udina, M. E., Gonzalez-Samartino, M., Lopez-Jimenez, M. M., Planas-Canals, M., Rodriguez-Fernandez, H., Batuecas Duelt, I. J., Tapia-Perez, M., Pons Prats, M., Jimenez-Martinez, E., Barbera Llorca, M. A., Asensio-Flores, S., Berbis-Morello, C., Zuriguel-Perez, E., Delgado-Hito, P., Rey Luque, O., Zabalegui, A., Fabrellas, N., & Adamuz, J. (2020, November). Acuity, nurse staffing and workforce, missed care and patient outcomes: A cluster-unit-level descriptive comparison. *Journal of Nursing Management, 28*(8), 2216–2229. https://doi.org/10.1111/jonm.13040

Lewis, L. S., Rebeschi, L. M., & Hunt, E. (2022). Nursing education practice update 2022: Competency-based education in nursing. *SAGE Open Nursing, 8*, 23779608221140774. https://doi.org/10.1177/23779608221140774

Porter-O'Grady, T. (2019, January). Principles for sustaining shared/professional governance in nursing. *Nursing Management, 50*(1), 36–41. https://doi.org/10.1097/01.NUMA.0000550448.17375.28

Resnick, B., & Mitty, E. (2008). *Assisted living nursing: A manual for management and practice.* Springer Publishing.

Van Wicklin, S. A., Leveling, M. E., & Stobinski, J. X. (2020, September). What is the perceived value of certification among registered nurses? A systematic review. *Journal of Nursing Scholarship, 52*(5), 536–543. https://doi.org/10.1111/jnu.12579

World Health Organization. (n.d.). *Self-care interventions for health.* https://www.who.int/health-topics/self-care#tab=tab_1

World Health Organization. (2023). *ICD-11 for mortality and morbidity statistics: QD85 burnout.* https://icd.who.int/browse11/l-m/en#/http://id.who.int/icd/entity/129180281

Chapter 9: Nursing Essentials Checklist

SPHERES OF CARE

Nursing occurs within four spheres of care, ranging from prevention to supportive care and all the areas in between. This chapter is relevant to the following spheres of care:

- ☑ Disease Prevention/Health Promotion
- ☑ Chronic Disease Care
- ☑ Regenerative or Restorative Care
- ☑ Hospice/Palliative/Supportive Care

DOMAINS OF PRACTICE

The American Association of Colleges of Nursing has identified 10 broad domains of practice for nursing. Students are expected to master these domains of practice across the spheres of care. This chapter addresses:

- ☑ Knowledge for Nursing Practice (Nursing and Other Disciplines)
- ☑ Person-Centered Care
- ☐ Population Health
- ☐ Scholarship for Practice
- ☑ Quality and Safety
- ☑ Interprofessional Partnerships
- ☐ Systems-Based Care
- ☐ Information & Healthcare Technologies
- ☑ Professionalism
- ☐ Personal, Professional, Leadership Development

CONCEPTS FOR PRACTICE

Integrated across the domains of practice are eight concepts which the student is expected to master across the spheres of care and across the domains of practice. This chapter addresses:

- ☐ Clinical Judgment
- ☑ Communication
- ☑ Compassionate Care
- ☐ Diversity, Equity, Inclusion
- ☐ Ethics
- ☑ Evidence-Based Practice
- ☐ Health Policy
- ☑ Social Determinants of Health

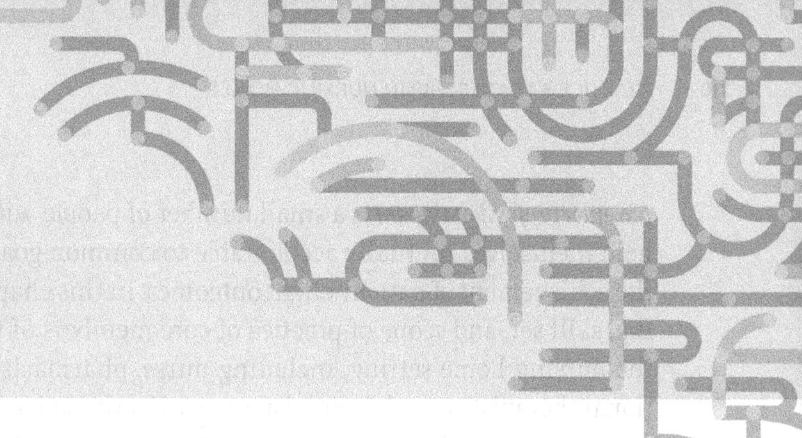

CHAPTER 9

THE INTERPROFESSIONAL TEAM AND COLLABORATIVE PRACTICE

Jennifer C. Sidelinker, DPT, PT
Bethany Sewell, MSW
Stacey E. Bergmann, MS, CTRS, ADC, CDP
Dawn Clayton Bieber, BS, OTR/L
Jeanne Copeland, MS, CCC-SLP, FNAP, RAC-CT
Nancy Munoz, DCN, MHA, RDN, FAND
Tara A. Cortes, PhD, RN, FAAN, FGSA
Noll L. Campbell, PharmD, MS

OBJECTIVES

1. **Describe principles of interprofessional practice in the nursing home setting.**
2. **Differentiate specialized areas of practice for each team member.**
3. **Apply an interprofessional practice model to the care of a resident with complex chronic illness.**

INTRODUCTION

As in other settings, person-centered, quality care in the nursing home environment is dependent on consistent and effective communication, collaboration, and coordination among a team of care providers with unique and specialized skill sets. Individuals living in nursing homes are complex, with a high prevalence of dementia and multiple comorbid conditions and chronic diseases (Luppa et al., 2010). As a result, it is even more critical to have high-functioning interprofessional care teams in this setting.

An *interprofessional team* is a small number of people with complementary skills who hold themselves mutually accountable to common goals and a unified approach for the achievement of patient/client outcomes. In this chapter, we will outline the training, skill set, and scope of practice of core members of the interprofessional team in the nursing home setting, including nurse, pharmacist, physical therapist, occupational therapist, speech therapist, recreation therapist, and social worker. (Note: The role of the nurse in long-term care (LTC) is described in more detail in other chapters in this text.) We will illustrate the application of these interprofessional roles for high-quality, integrated care planning and delivery, with frequent reference to the Age-Friendly Health Systems model focused on the 4Ms (What Matters, Medication, Mentation, and Mobility; Institute for Healthcare Improvement [IHI], 2022).

WHY NURSES NEED TO BE FAMILIAR WITH THE INTERPROFESSIONAL TEAM

The National Academies of Practice (NAP) defines *interprofessional collaborative practice* (IPCP) as multiple health workers from different professional backgrounds providing comprehensive services by working with patients/clients, their carers, and communities to deliver the highest quality of care across settings. IPCP is a model of team-based care that involves multiple health professionals working together to optimize the patient's care experience and health outcomes. It is characterized by shared decision-making and the assignment of specific roles and functions to each member according to their unique training, scope of practice, and skill set (NAP, 2022).

The focus of interprofessional team members is on the needs of the patient/client rather than on individual member contributions. For this reason, each team member is responsible for understanding not only their own role and expected contribution but also the unique role and expected contribution of each team member (NAP, 2022). To function effectively in their roles, nurses must have sufficient knowledge about each team member.

This is true regardless of how care is being delivered. Let's take a moment to discuss telehealth (covered at length in Chapter 13) in the LTC setting. It is estimated that 35% of the US population 65 years of age and older will need LTC services, while at the same time, the availability of healthcare personnel is limited (Administration for Community Living, 2021). There has been an increasing trend in the use of telehealth services to improve access to healthcare, patient management, and education

(Polinski et al., 2016). During the COVID-19 pandemic, the use of telemedicine in LTC facilities allowed for continuity of care and service as well as reducing exposure to the virus (Cormi et al., 2020).

In LTC, the use of telemedicine is at times thwarted by the disruption it causes in daily center operations and individuals' daily care routines. To promote the continued implementation and acceptance of telemedicine as a modality of care in LTC facilities, the awareness of its benefits must be highlighted (May et al., 2021).

NURSE

Licensed practical/vocational nurses (LPNs or LVNs) are typically educated through a 12–18-month program and, upon successful completion, the individual may sit for the National Council Licensure Examination-Practical Nurse (NCLEX-PN). The scope of practice for LPNs varies from state to state, but in any state, they must work under the supervision of a registered nurse or physician. Most states do not allow LPNs to perform functions that require assessment, care planning, critical thinking, or any very complex or high-risk procedures such as the management of central lines (Nursing Explorer, n.d.).

Registered professional nurses have graduated from a program from which they are eligible to sit for the National Council Licensure Examination-Registered Nurse (NCLEX-RN). An associate degree in nursing (ADN), most often granted through a community or junior college, is the minimal education for the RN licensure exam (Nursing Explorer, n.d.). A bachelor of science in nursing (BSN) is the preferred degree for entry into practice. Graduates from ADN and BSN programs sit for the same licensure exam (NCLEX), and both receive a license as a registered nurse (RN). Their scope of practice is the same and is defined by the state in which they are licensed and practice.

Nurses with BSNs have a broader education in social studies and sciences and thus have a greater capacity for leadership, independent decision-making, and applying evidence-based practice. These are all skills needed in LTC, as residents in this setting often have multiple comorbidities including dementia. Since the combination of chronic diseases and frailty make each resident unique, beyond the evidence-based care protocols that can be applied broadly, critical thinking and personalized care planning are essential.

The care of older adults is often termed a "team sport" because the care is very different and more complex than the care of younger adults. Nursing homes offer RNs the unique role of leading and coordinating the team of healthcare professionals and certified nursing assistants in providing person-centered care to drive quality outcomes. The RN has the education and skill to oversee the development and implementation of the care plan and conceptualize care around the 4Ms: What Matters, Medication, Mentation, and Mobility (IHI, 2022). Creative nurse leaders will develop teams to practice at a high level through engagement, shared decision-making, and providing continued opportunities for professional and personal growth.

PHARMACIST

As experts in the comprehensive management of pharmacologic treatment and prevention of disease, pharmacists have an important role in team-based care that includes the distribution, storage, administration, and monitoring of medications. Pharmacists supporting nursing homes are graduates of professional programs that may or may not require an undergraduate degree prior to admission. Thus, training is typically completed over a total of six or eight years (four years of a professional program that follow two or four years of an undergraduate bachelor's degree). While post-graduate specialty training exists for pharmacists in many practice areas and roles (e.g., clinical pharmacy services in ambulatory or hospital environments, cardiovascular, oncology, and geriatric specialties among several others), such training is not required for pharmacists working within nursing homes or LTC facilities at this time.

Central Pharmacy

Unlike acute-care settings, where pharmacies supporting medication supply and administration processes are located in the hospital and often directly on units, in nursing homes the pharmacy is independent of the nursing home. These pharmacies are most often centrally located to the nursing home's region and possess distribution capabilities to maintain medication supplies within each facility. Pharmacists in these locations maintain supplies at facility locations, with routine delivery at various intervals (weekly or biweekly as needed) and the ability for urgent distribution of supplies as needed in the event of a change in condition. These centrally located pharmacists are available for consultation and questions remotely, including support for payment or coverage of medications, but they do not have a routine physical presence within the nursing home environment. However, pharmacists are available to initiate and maintain medication storage, administration, and documentation procedures at each facility.

Consultant Pharmacist

Consultant pharmacists are also important members of the healthcare team and have a presence in each facility supporting the onsite storage, administration, selection, and destruction or removal of medications. Consultant pharmacists are required by law to visit facilities in person at least once monthly to review these procedures, monitor medication storage and supplies, and review medication administration records and medication regimens for appropriateness (US Government, 1987). During the process of review, pharmacists may also make recommendations to providers to adjust medications to align with goals of care, optimize symptom control or therapeutic targets, or minimize adverse events.

Most medication formulations administered in nursing home facilities are oral tablets or capsules; however, many facilities have some capacity for injectable medications (e.g., intramuscular or intravenous) in cases where antibiotics may be needed to prevent a hospitalization or when mobility may limit access to acute-care services or infusion centers. Pharmacists may also be helpful in recommending dosage forms such as delayed-release or liquid formulations to minimize frequency of administration or accommodate swallowing difficulties.

Because pharmacists and providers (including physicians, nurse practitioners, and physician assistants) are often not in the facilities at the same time, medication recommendations are often communicated through written or electronic messaging. While in the facilities, consultant pharmacists may engage with care-planning meetings and are available to provide medication education as desired by the facility staff.

Medication Management and Legal Requirements

Pharmacists are essential in integrating clinical decisions about medication management and legal requirements intended to optimize safety of medications in LTC environments. For example, psychotropic medications have been associated with harm in frail older adults, and as such, according to the Centers for Medicare & Medicaid Services (CMS, 2017), psychotropic medications must undergo an attempt to be withdrawn every six months. Pharmacists are expected to ensure that medication regimens are in compliance with this regulation, either through the monitored attempt at gradual dose reduction or by documenting why reduction or withdrawal is therapeutically inappropriate in a given patient.

In many states, pharmacists have authority to write orders to initiate or change medications when entering into a collaborative practice agreement with a supervising physician. Therefore, either through the authority established by the collaborative practice agreement or through an order agreed upon by a physician or advanced practitioner, pharmacists can initiate or change an existing medication order.

Consider a patient in a facility who has been using a psychotropic medication such as sertraline (Zoloft) for more than six months in the treatment of depression. Because 42 CFR § 483 (CMS, 2017) recognizes this as a psychotropic, a dose reduction or documentation of why reduction is clinically inappropriate is required. A pharmacist reviewing medications at monthly intervals will recognize this requirement and suggest a dose-reduction strategy if clinically appropriate. If a provider agrees, the pharmacist can write a legal medication order to not only reduce the dose of the psychotropic medication but also identify parameters to safely monitor the safety of that change.

Because visits by consultant pharmacists to nursing facilities may be no more frequent than once monthly, pharmacists require daily documentation or direct communication of clinical events, symptoms, and patterns from team members in the facility. The better the communication between pharmacists (consultant or central) and team members at each facility, the better the quality of care for residents. Pharmacists may have remote access to the nursing facility's electronic health records and medication administration records, which facilitates ongoing review and monitoring of the medication profile.

REHABILITATION SERVICES

It is important to note that physical, occupational, and speech therapy are often combined and referred to collectively as *rehabilitation services* or just *rehab.* This designation can be effective from an organizational structure standpoint, but it can be confounding from a care management standpoint, as each discipline is unique and has much to offer because of their highly specialized training, skills, and scope of practice. This must be understood and leveraged effectively by the full interprofessional team to optimize person-centered, value-based care delivery and meaningful, sustainable outcomes for the resident.

For a patient to qualify for direct care by a rehabilitation professional, and for that care to be reimbursed by a third party (such as Medicare or a Medicare Advantage insurance plan), the patient must demonstrate medical necessity, and the care provided by the rehabilitation professional must be considered skilled and reasonable to address needs identified through a comprehensive assessment and subsequent plan of care requiring the unique skills and training of that rehabilitation discipline. It is important to understand that at any given time, typically only a small percentage of the entire nursing home population will be on active caseload by one or more rehabilitation disciplines.

Physical Therapist

Physical therapists (PTs) are movement experts who focus on preserving, enhancing, and/or restoring movement and physical function impaired or threatened by disease, injury, or disability. They conduct comprehensive assessments and develop individualized treatment plans aimed at minimizing risk of negative outcomes such as falls and optimizing independence in functional mobility and quality of life.

Education Requirements and Licensure

To practice as a PT in the United States, an individual must earn a doctor of physical therapy (DPT) degree from an accredited professional PT education program and pass a state licensure exam. Prior to admission to a professional DPT program, one must obtain an undergraduate degree and meet pre-professional educational course requirements. The length of professional DPT programs is typically three years, and academic content includes coursework in areas such as anatomy, physiology, biomechanics, kinesiology, neuroscience, pharmacology, clinical reasoning, and evidence-based practice. Approximately 80% of the DPT curriculum is classroom (didactic) and lab study, and the remaining 20% (an average of 28 weeks, full time) is dedicated to clinical education, in which student PTs treat patients in a variety of practice settings under the supervision and direction of licensed PTs (American Physical Therapy Association [APTA], 2023).

Physical therapist assistants (PTAs) provide PT services under the direction and supervision of a PT, who is responsible for the services provided by the PTA. To work as a PTA in the US, one must graduate from an accredited PTA education program and pass a national exam to obtain state-specific licensure or certification. PTA education is typically an entry level, two-year associate degree program. Approximately 75% of the PTA curriculum is classroom and lab experiences, with the remaining 25% (an average of 16 weeks, full time) dedicated to clinical education in a variety of practice settings.

To maintain licensure to practice physical therapy, PTs and PTAs in most states must meet requirements for lifelong learning in the form of continuing education requirements. In addition, PTs may seek additional national board specialty certification in practice areas such as orthopedic, neurologic, and geriatric physical therapy (APTA, 2023).

Physical Therapy Interventions

PTs screen for mobility-related risk and perform comprehensive assessments that identify impairments contributing to functional activity limitations and life participation restrictions. Consistent with the Age-Friendly Health Systems framework (see Chapters 2 and 4), the PT must understand *What Matters* most to each patient to develop appropriate goals and a person-centered plan for mobility and care. When developing and executing the plan of care, the PT must consider and leverage all available resources to ensure that gains achieved during the physical therapy course of care are sustained in everyday life following discharge from physical therapy.

Areas of impairment commonly addressed by physical therapy intervention include but are not limited to strength, range of motion, balance, pain, coordination, aerobic capacity, and motor planning. Physical therapy treatment involves applying evidence-based techniques to optimize safety and functional capacity through restoration of normal performance if feasible. If full restoration is not possible, skilled physical therapy also entails training patients and their caregivers in adaptive strategies and techniques to safely compensate for lost abilities. Physical therapy services are provided in person or via telehealth. Modes of treatment delivery include one to one, concurrent (two people receiving physical therapy at the same time, with different treatment focus), or group (up to six people receiving physical therapy at the same time, with the same treatment focus; Academy of Geriatric Physical Therapy, 2022).

Physical therapy interventions are a critical component of a comprehensive approach to managing many of the most common geriatric syndromes including urinary incontinence, wounds, and falls.

Functional urinary incontinence

Functional urinary incontinence occurs when a person is unable to reach the toilet in time to urinate. Physical therapy interventions aimed at optimizing independence in mobility, whether at an ambulatory or wheelchair level, help to decrease functional incontinence. This includes not only direct interventions to improve the patient's mobility status but also recommendations for optimizing the safety and navigability of the environment in which the patient functions.

Wounds and falls

With respect to wound prevention and management, in addition to possessing the ability to provide direct wound care through application of specific techniques and modalities, the PT provides caregiver education, recommendations for positioning and offloading, assessment of surfaces and footwear, and the development and execution of patient-specific exercise and mobility plans with the patient and their care team (Academy of Geriatric Physical Therapy, 2022). Regarding falls, PTs are uniquely suited to lead the interprofessional team in addressing many modifiable risk factors most predictive of recurrent falls, including lower extremity weakness, decreased balance, unsteady gait, and fear of falling (Tinetti & Kumar, 2010).

Cognitive impairment

As introduced and discussed in prior chapters, there is a high prevalence of cognitive impairment in the nursing home population (Yuan et al., 2021). Individuals with cognitive impairment have physical therapy needs and can benefit from physical therapy intervention aimed at appropriate goals and integrating family members and other care team members to support carryover of gains made in the physical therapy course of care (Criss et al., 2022; Liu et al., 2022). PTs often rely on their occupational and/or speech therapy counterparts to assess the true level of cognitive impairment in an individual and inform the team of communication and facilitation strategies to promote optimal performance and active engagement.

Mobility

Mobility is one of the 4Ms in the framework of Age-Friendly healthcare (Cacchione, 2020). Specifically, the Mobility element of the 4M framework aims to ensure that older adults move safely every day to maintain function and do What Matters most to them. PTs working in nursing home settings have a responsibility to lead efforts for developing and sustaining a culture of mobility across the resident population. To understand how this might be feasible, one must first understand the basics of how physical therapy is typically provided and reimbursed in nursing home settings.

For physical therapy professionals to help create and sustain a culture of mobility, nursing home clinical and operational leaders must define the non-direct care roles expected of the physical therapy team and determine how the cost of that time is allocated and budgeted. In this model, PTs are expected to collaborate and participate in ongoing performance improvement efforts related to mobility and consult with and train team members to integrate mobility into everyday life at the center in a variety of ways. This enables the PT to serve as mobility-focused leaders in nursing homes, practicing at the top of their training, scope, and skill set and positively impacting the mobility efforts of the entire population at the center in an ongoing manner.

The active physical therapy caseload in a nursing home is typically a mix of short-stay patients and long-stay residents. In general, short-stay patients are recuperating from a recent hospitalization and have rehab goals aimed at returning home, and their physical therapy intervention is of high intensity and short duration. Conversely, LTC residents are typically referred to physical therapy due to a decline in their usual function, often because of a fall, illness, or exacerbation of an existing chronic condition. Physical therapy for these individuals tends to be of lower frequency and longer duration. An effective interprofessional collaborative team is an essential ingredient for optimizing the value of physical therapy care for the LTC resident. Other team members must be able to support continual application and integration of newly learned mobility skills into the resident's daily routine (e.g., a restorative nursing program).

In short, movement is medicine. PTs are uniquely suited to prescribe individually tailored movement prescriptions, administered in various ways with the support and assistance of many members of the interprofessional team. What this looks like in a nursing facility varies, depending on the needs of the population and the resources available. Ideally, there are a variety of opportunities for daily physical activity that meet the diverse needs of the nursing home population. Examples of what one might expect to see in a center with an active culture of mobility in which multiple options for mobility are supported and/or delivered by a variety of team members include:

- Daily presence of physical therapy staff, with active caseload of both short- and long-stay patients

- Recreation services programs regularly integrating movement
- Active restorative nursing and functional maintenance programs with elements such as "Walk to Dine"
- An environmental setup that encourages safe ambulatory mobility rather than defaulting to use of wheelchairs for all residents in all situations

Additional sources of integrated mobility with largely untapped potential due to real or perceived logistical and regulatory barriers include leveraging community-dwelling older adult volunteers, family members of residents, and community-based program providers.

Occupational Therapist

Occupational therapy enables people of all ages to participate in daily living by supporting engagement in meaningful tasks and activities that patients both want and need to do. Occupational therapists (OTs) and occupational therapy assistants are trained to deliver occupational therapy services to individuals across the life span.

In 2007, a master of occupational therapy was made the minimal degree requirement for all OTs, and occupational therapy assistants must complete an associate degree. Fieldwork education and training under the direction and supervision of an experienced practitioner are mandatory for successful completion of both degrees. Additional requirements include passing the national board certification examination and obtaining licensure in the state(s) in which one intends to practice.

OTs evaluate clients and collaboratively develop a plan of care that involves care team partners (physicians, nurses, nursing assistants, other therapy providers, etc.) and families and/or loved ones. Occupational therapy assistants work under the supervision of and in partnership with an OT and deliver services that have been outlined for them, providing regular feedback and updates to the therapist on clients' progress and status.

The Occupational Therapy Practice Framework

Domain and process (*American Journal of Occupational Therapy* [AOTA], 2020) states that occupational therapy practitioners use their knowledge of the transactional relationship among the client, their engagement in valuable occupations, and the context to design occupation-based intervention plans. Occupational therapy services are provided for habilitation, rehabilitation, and promotion of health and wellness for clients with disability- and non-disability-related needs.

Note that *occupation* does not just refer to one's work-related identity. In this context, occupations refer to the roles and activities that people have and do as individuals, in families, and with communities to occupy time and bring meaning and purpose to life. Occupations include the roles and tasks that people need to, want to, and are expected to do. Services promote acquisition and preservation of occupational identity for those who have—or are at risk for developing—an illness, injury, disease, disorder, condition, impairment, disability, activity limitation, or participation restriction (AOTA, 2020). Occupational therapy practitioners receive education in human anatomy and physiology that helps them understand the human body and how its systems function, including:

- Medical diagnoses
- Disease process
- Effects of and recovery from injuries
- Impact of aging
- Contributors to health and wellness

In the skilled nursing setting, occupational therapy services are ordered by a physician or other approved medical provider (e.g., nurse practitioner or physician assistant). Services are provided face to face or via telehealth. The occupational therapy evaluation process involves gathering the client history, routines, life experiences, and interests. This is referred to as the *occupational profile*, is unique to occupational therapy, and is grounded in the understanding that "only clients can identify the occupations that give meaning to their lives and select the goals and priorities that are important to them" (AOTA, 2020, p. 22). This occupational therapy focus also aligns with What Matters, one of the "4Ms" of Age-Friendly Health Systems, by ensuring that care and services are personalized and align with the unique goals and preferences of each individual.

If the client is unable to share this information directly, the OT will look to caregivers and others to gather and incorporate this crucial information into care. After additional assessment of the client is completed, an intervention plan and goals are developed based on the client's unique abilities and their assessed level of activities of daily living (ADLs) performance. Client goals and progress are reviewed regularly to ensure the interventions remain appropriate and client-centered.

The OT's involvement as an interprofessional team member and direct-care provider in the nursing home setting is vital and supports all four elements of the Age-Friendly Healthcare System 4M model (What Matters, Mentation, Medication, and Mobility) in various ways. The major areas of practice for occupational therapy professionals working in nursing homes are described in the following sections.

Activities of Daily Living

ADLs include bathing/showering, dressing, toileting (including routines/strategies and exercises for continence management), grooming, personal hygiene, leisure tasks, and eating. Proper seating and positioning that promotes the ability to participate in these activities is also considered and addressed. The setting/context, preferred habits and routines (What Matters), and cueing strategies needed during these activities is of great importance for optimal performance and engagement.

The term *cueing strategies* refers to actions provided by the therapist and intended to promote initiation, continuation, or termination of a task. Common cueing strategies include verbal, visual, and/or tactile cues. Occupational therapy interventions support clients with cognitive impairment due to a variety of conditions and diseases, such as dementia, traumatic brain injuries, and Parkinson's disease. OTs identify and employ techniques to aid in memory, concentration, and executive functioning (e.g., focused attention, planning and prioritizing). These skills are needed to support effective participation in and performance of ADLs (AOTA, n.d.).

Additional ADLs, known as instrumental activities of daily living, include homemaking, meal preparation, shopping, medication management (supporting the client's ability to take medications as prescribed, including strategies for memory, planning, and refills), driving, and money management.

Adaptive Equipment/Assistive Technology Identification and Recommendation

Occupational therapy providers recommend and train patients in the use of equipment such as tub/shower chairs, toilet seats/commodes, and specialty seating/wheelchairs/cushions and devices (e.g., reachers, sock aides, adapted utensils) to make performing the daily tasks easier. Additional areas may include identification and training in the use of technology that promotes independence in ADL performance or mobility such as voice-activated lights and other devices, emergency response devices, programmable medication dispensers for those with memory impairment, and vision or hearing-impaired assistive technology.

Caregiver and Family Training

Working together with the care team to develop and share strategies to optimize participation and independence is essential for successful carryover and long-term positive client outcomes, including mental well-being. Early identification and communication of changes in abilities/status help mitigate client decline. Occupational therapy practitioners also provide education to caregivers for maintaining their own health and wellness when caring for individuals in the nursing home setting. Stress-reduction strategies, maintaining proper body mechanics during care, and safe approaches to care to avoid injury and prevent negative responses or behaviors (especially for those caring for anyone with cognitive impairment) are areas commonly addressed.

Fall Prevention, Home Safety, and Accessibility

OTs provide education and training on health management, wellness routines, activity participation, environmental modification, equipment considerations that promote safety and independence, and aging in place for both short-term and long-term clients.

Contracture Management and Splinting

Occupational therapy provides intervention for musculoskeletal issues that benefit from splinting. Common goals for splinting include maintaining skin integrity, reducing pain, and promoting improved posture to support participation in ADLs, prevent further contractures, and promote functional use or protection of the impacted area.

Clients in skilled nursing facilities and nursing homes, whether short term or long term, are among those with the greatest need for occupational therapy services to improve participation, engagement, and performance in ADLs. Collaborative practice by occupational therapy practitioners with other care team members in this environment is critical to provide high-quality, client-centered care that optimizes functional independence and prevents decline.

Speech Therapist

Speech therapists are also known as *speech-language pathologists* (SLPs). SLPs working in nursing homes provide a broad range of services that can improve the safety and quality of life for both short-stay and long-term residents. Service delivery areas assessed and treated by SLPs include (American Speech-Language-Hearing Association [ASHA], 2016):

- Cognitive skills, including memory, attention, and problem-solving
- Receptive (listening/reading) and expressive (speaking/writing) language skills
- Intelligibility of speech
- Vocal quality and hygiene
- Tracheostomy management
- Augmentative and alternative communication
- Health literacy skills
- Communication and listening skills impacted by hearing loss

To learn these skills and prepare to practice, the minimum education requirement for SLPs is a master's degree from an accredited university program. Graduate students in speech-language pathology also gain practical experience with clients in a university clinic setting, as we discussed for PTs and OTs, while taking classes toward their degree and through supervised externship placements in a variety of settings. Upon graduation, licensed SLPs enter a mandatory clinical fellowship (CF) experience lasting approximately one year.

According to ASHA (n.d.), "The SLP CF is a mentored professional experience that begins after the completion of academic course work and clinical practicum. The goal of the CF is to allow the Clinical Fellow to transition between being a student enrolled in a communication sciences and disorders (CSD) program and being an independent provider of speech-language pathology clinical services" (para. 1).

As previously mentioned, dementia is highly prevalent in the nursing home population. Its management is supported by the SLP in collaboration with other team members. Changes in function that are assessed and treated within an SLP's scope are associated with many other chronic conditions experienced by short- and long-stay residents of nursing homes, including but not limited to chronic kidney disease (Murray, 2008; Pinto et al., 2016), chronic obstructive pulmonary disease (Drulia & Hodge, 2021), and diabetes (Saedi et al., 2016).

Speech-Language Pathologist Case Studies

The following three cases illustrate the diverse contributions of the speech therapist in the nursing home setting. These stories also highlight the importance of interprofessional collaborative practice in the LTC setting. Although we may take skills of communication, swallowing, voice, and cognition for granted, it is critical for SLPs to work in close partnership with other care team members to identify changes in function early and to collaborate to develop effective solutions. This is especially important for the LTC setting, where once skills are lost, they may never be regained. With mutual respect and an understanding of roles and responsibilities within each other's scopes of practice, healthcare professionals can work collaboratively to improve outcomes, optimize safety, and enhance the quality of life for nursing home residents.

SLP in Dysphagia Management

Resident: Randy

Focus: The role of the SLP in dysphagia management, and critical aspects of decision-making in complex illness and at end of life

I met Randy when I began working as an SLP in a skilled nursing facility near my hometown. Randy loved to laugh and could spit out a witty retort faster than you could snap your fingers. He had a history of mental health disorder with oral fixation, which led to either sucking on candy or smoking frequently throughout the day. Randy also had diagnoses of dementia, chronic obstructive pulmonary disease, and dysphagia, or difficulty swallowing. Due to his respiratory and swallowing status, he was prone to pneumonia. We worked together to treat his dysphagia and decrease his risk for recurrent pneumonia by improving the strength of muscles important for breathing and swallowing, and by identifying and learning strategies to compensate for his swallowing impairment.

SLPs working with individuals with dementia also assess their current ability to learn new information, along with the type and amount of cueing and support that may be required from caregivers. At that time, Randy was capable of learning new information using techniques such as repetition and errorless learning and benefited from intermittent verbal cues from caregivers to use swallowing strategies for improved safety and function. However, during one unfortunate hospitalization, Randy underwent a procedure to place a PEG, or percutaneous endoscopic gastrostomy tube. He returned from the hospital with an NPO status, meaning "nothing by mouth," and received all nutrition through his PEG tube.

Randy struggled to return to his life at the nursing home after his hospitalization when he received the PEG tube. He was no longer given his 20 pieces of candy per day and repeatedly asked for something to eat or drink. Randy's care team at the nursing home collaborated with the larger interprofessional team to explore alternative options, but the process takes time.

Randy began taking food and liquid from other sources, not fully understanding the rationale for his NPO status. Unfortunately, Randy passed away about a month following the PEG placement. Randy's story highlights dysphagia management, one area that SLPs often treat in a nursing home setting. In fact, the prevalence of oropharyngeal dysphagia in nursing homes is estimated to be 50.2% (Rivelsrud et al., 2023). This story also highlights the complexity of decision-making in complex illness and at end of life, where patient safety and patient autonomy often are in tension.

Short-Stay Versus Long-Term Nursing Home Residents
Resident: Charlie

Focus: Speech therapy treatment priorities and interprofessional collaboration needs when working with short-stay vs. long-term nursing home residents

Although SLPs' roles remain the same whether working with short-stay or long-term nursing home residents, what may change are the priorities of the treatment and the interprofessional collaboration needed to achieve sustainable outcomes. Let's consider Charlie, who came to the nursing home for a short-term stay following a stroke. He had a history of diabetes and lived alone. Charlie enjoyed eating apples, had an apple tree on his property, and knew that apples were a healthy food choice. However, Charlie began eating up to 12 apples a day, and sometimes this was all he ate in a day because he didn't enjoy cooking for himself. When Charlie went to the hospital with symptoms of a stroke, his blood sugar was over 300 mg/dL, and his care team discovered that he had not been managing his diabetes at home.

(continues)

(continued)

Charlie planned to return home alone, and although regaining his strength after the stroke was one component of his complex case, there were many other factors as well. To sustain his outcomes and reduce his risk for recurrent stroke and rehospitalization, Charlie also needed a high level of interprofessional collaboration to help him identify strategies for reducing his fall risk, to help manage chronic conditions (including his diabetes), for safe community mobility and re-integration, meal planning, and medication management. SLPs working with clients like Charlie will assess areas including swallowing function, cognitive-communication skills (which include memory, sequencing, problem-solving, and decision-making), receptive and expressive language skills, speech intelligibility, and voice, all of which may be affected by a stroke.

For Charlie, the main determinant for how quickly and safely he could return home proved to be his diabetes management. The dietitian helped Charlie identify information about protein, carbohydrates, and fats to plan meals and make food choices that would help him keep his blood sugar in a safe and appropriate range. The SLP then helped him to understand, remember, and apply this information while also working to improve his swallowing safety and efficiency. Charlie's physician and nursing team modified his diabetes medication regimen, and time was dedicated during speech therapy sessions to ensure he understood the sliding scale insulin dosage, as well as the sequence of steps for safe medication administration. Charlie was able to return home safely for a time, although eventually his condition progressed. He was later diagnosed with dementia and returned to the nursing home as a long-term resident.

Dementia

Resident: Jane

Focus: SLP role in optimizing cognition and communication in residents with dementia

When working with nursing home residents with dementia, the SLP's areas of assessment and treatment remain the same, although the tests, measures, and intervention strategies may change depending on client-specific factors. Up to a point within the dementia process, residents may still be able to learn new information such as finding their way to a new location or learning to use a walker to improve safety with ambulation. The SLP's assessment will help determine whether the resident is capable of learning new information, and the treatment may include specific strategies and techniques to enhance accuracy, safety, and generalization of the task. Although changes in language function are subtle in the early stages of dementia, as impairment progresses, SLPs play a critical role in helping the resident retain and enhance their ability to communicate with others.

To help understand communication changes during the dementia process and how that impacts function, let's discuss Jane. Jane's family cared for her at home late into her progression with dementia, until it became too much for them due to her combative behaviors and the overall complexity of care required. Jane would sometimes strike out at caregivers as they helped her to get dressed or brush her hair. Once Jane was sitting in a preferred location, she could be extremely resistant to standing. In the nursing home setting, it often required two caregivers to help her stand while Jane loudly voiced her displeasure and physically resisted the assistance, creating an unpleasant environment for other residents and increasing the risk for injury to herself and caregivers during the transfer.

In this situation, the SLP's role is to identify the cognitive and communication factors leading to the resident's behavior(s), and then to help caregivers understand how to modify their approach to better meet the needs of the person with dementia. As dementia progresses, changes occur in the person's ability to understand and interpret the visual information in their surroundings, especially in their visual periphery (Sheikh, 2022). Therefore, it is usually best to approach from the front, make eye contact with a friendly expression, and then communicate your message.

In Jane's case, the SLP identified that she could best understand instructions consisting of two or three words at a time, allowing for up to 30 seconds to process that single instruction without distractions of additional explanation. During those 30 seconds, she also benefited from nonverbal communication to support the message. To stand up, the caregivers' routine became to approach Jane from the front, smile and wave while saying her name, and use the three-word instruction, "Ready, stand up," as the caregiver performed a slow squat-to-stand while motioning with their hand in a "come with me" gesture. Using this technique, Jane could safely stand with minimal assistance from one person most of the time, and her verbal outbursts and physical resistance were greatly reduced.

The PT was able to utilize similar communication strategies to develop an exercise program for Jane to help maintain her strength and mobility, and the OT

(continues)

(continued)

incorporated the communication techniques into her daily routines to allow Jane to be as independent as possible. Jane had also withdrawn from previously preferred leisure activities due to increasing difficulty understanding others and expressing her thoughts, so the SLP worked with the life enhancement coordinator (sometimes called an activities or recreation therapy director) to apply the strategies during leisure activities to increase Jane's participation and enjoyment. Without these communication techniques applied throughout Jane's day by her caregivers, she was at increased risk for depression, decreased mobility, and accelerated physical and cognitive decline.

REGISTERED DIETITIAN/NUTRITIONIST

The registered dietitian/nutritionist (RDN) is one of the many members of the interprofessional team that works to maintain or improve the health status of older adults in LTC facilities. Specifically, RDNs work to maintain optimal standards of nutritional care for residents in LTC. Trained to manage the nutritional needs of many disease processes and allergies, RDNs work with the nursing facility's food service manager to coordinate menu planning and food preparation. RDNs assess patients' and residents' nutritional status, develop individualized interventions and plans of care, provide counseling and education to patients, help patients to manage therapeutic restrictions, and provide medical nutrition therapy.

RDN Education

The Commission on Dietetic Registration (2021, p. 30) defines an RDN as "an individual who has met current minimum academic requirements (baccalaureate degree granted by a US regionally accredited college or university or foreign equivalent) with successful completion of both specified didactic education and supervised-practice experiences through programs accredited by The Accreditation Council for Education in Nutrition and Dietetics (ACEND) of the Academy of Nutrition and Dietetics (The Academy), who has successfully completed the Registration Examination for Dietitians."

To maintain the RDN credential, the RDN must comply with the Professional Development Portfolio recertification requirements and accrue 75 units of approved continuing professional education every five years (Commission on Dietetic Registration, 2021). At the time of this writing, licensure is required in all states except Arizona and Michigan (ACEND, 2023). In addition, RDNs may be required to be licensed by the state in which they perform services.

RDN Role

In the nursing home setting, RDNs help to identify nutritional risk factors and recommend nutritional interventions based on each resident's medical condition, needs, preferences, and goals. Their scope of practice includes writing dietary orders, as delegated by the physician (CMS, 2023). This practice allows residents to have more frequent and timely adjustments to the nutrition therapy plan. The RDN can be either full time, part time, or a consultant, based on the needs of the facility. Their scope of practice focuses on food, nutrition, and dietetics practice, as well as related services developed, directed, and provided by the RDN to protect the public, community, and populations and enhance health and well-being of patients/clients and communities (Academy Quality Management Committee, 2018).

Food and dining are core components of quality of life and quality of care in the LTC setting. Older adults are at higher risk of developing malnutrition and its comorbidities, including increased dependency in performing ADLs (Cereda et al., 2016). Maintaining adequate nutritional status ensures that the nutrients needed to sustain critical metabolic processes and maintain and repair cells and organs—and the energy needed to support daily functioning—are available.

Impaired nutritional status is not part of the normal aging process. Older adults with compromised nutritional status have increased risk for impaired wound healing, dehydration, unplanned weight loss, and increased mortality. As part of the interprofessional team, the RDN performs the following:

- Assesses each resident's risk factors
- Analyzes the assessment data
- Develops and implements individualized nutritional approaches
- Monitors the effectiveness of the interventions
- Revises the plan with any changes in patient condition

Dietary restrictions such as therapeutic diets may help older adults in selected situations. In some instances, these restrictions can impair adequate nutrition and contribute to further decline in nutritional status, particularly in older adults already nutritionally compromised or at risk of malnutrition. When a resident is not eating well or is losing weight, the RDN is instrumental in evaluating the continued need for therapeutic restrictions and liberalizing the diet to improve the resident's food intake and stabilize their weight (CMS, 2023). The Academy of Nutrition and Dietetics (Dorner & Friedrich, 2018) supports that the nutritional status of older adults residing in LTC facilities may be enhanced by liberalization of diet prescriptions, providing greater autonomy to residents and enhancing their enjoyment of meals. RDNs are instrumental in assessing the risks versus benefits of liberalizing therapeutic diets.

RDN and Food Service Manager

RDNs must partner with the nutrition department food service manager to ensure that the meals served to LTC residents are enjoyable, palatable, culturally appropriate, and include a mechanism to promote resident choice while promoting quality of care. Food service managers in LTC must be certified as a dietary manager or have an associate level or higher degree in food service management or hospitality (CMS, 2023).

RECREATION THERAPIST

Recreational therapy (RT) or *therapeutic recreation* (TR) is a systematic process that utilizes recreation (leisure) and other activities as interventions to address the needs of individuals with illnesses and/or disabling conditions to achieve psychological and physical health, recovery, and being (American Therapeutic Recreation Association [ATRA], n.d.). TR is provided by recreation therapists (RTs) who are highly skilled and professionally trained.

Education Requirements and Certification

Recreation professionals are licensed in some but not all states, and requirements vary depending on the state (National Council for Therapeutic Recreation Certification [NCTRC], 2018). An RT has a bachelor's degree with certification as a certified therapeutic recreation specialist (CTRS) from the NCTRC. The CTRS must complete a degree that meets specific academic content in therapeutic recreation, an internship, and a certification exam. Certification is awarded for a five-year period; to renew certification, an individual must demonstrate experience in professional practice and evidence of appropriate professional continuing education (NCTRC, 2023).

Whereas RTs are focused on utilizing recreational services to achieve specific goals and outcomes, other "qualified individuals" such as activity directors certified (ADC) are trained to work in the field of geriatrics and provide meaningful, engaging activities for seniors. ADCs and their assistants use their knowledge to create person-centered programming for residents. The current requirements for ADCs include a minimum of a high school diploma/GED, working two years in the continuum of care with at least one year in an activities department, a 180-hour training program and exam, and ongoing relevant continuing education (National Certification Council for Activity Professionals, 2023).

RTs may be the sole provider of their specialized treatment in smaller settings, or they may collaborate in a department with other CTRSs, ADCs, and therapeutic recreation/activity assistants. RT assistants typically have completed an associate degree, diploma, or certification that prepares them to perform skilled work under the supervision of a licensed RT. RTs also supervise and instruct interns and volunteers to further enhance the well-being of nursing home residents and their families.

The regulatory requirements for leadership of a nursing home's activities department define qualified individuals as CTRSs, OTs or occupational therapy assistants, or persons with two years of experience in a social or recreational program within the last five years (one year must be in full-time employment) or who have completed a state approved training course (CMS, 2023).

Recreational Services

RTs are key members of interprofessional teams in many settings, actively collaborating on care plans and resident experience. In nursing homes, they provide essential goal-oriented interventions aimed at improving physical and mental health using specific, resident-centered approaches to restore, remediate, and rehabilitate an individual's level of functioning (ATRA, n.d.). Using recreation and leisure as a treatment modality is a highly effective way to motivate and engage residents. RTs provide enjoyable and purposeful tasks that address functional skills, using a variety of modalities such as arts and crafts, drama, music, dance, sports, games, and community outings to enhance an individual's psychosocial well-being (ATRA, n.d.). In addition to enhancing healthy engagement, RT interventions may also distract residents from secondary issues, such as pain, when they are engaged in meaningful activity (De Vries & Lake, 2005).

RTs gather assessment data regarding a resident's roles, routines, habits, preferences, strengths, and abilities as they relate to everyday participation in personally meaningful activities, then craft and adapt opportunities for individual and group engagement. Importantly, they seek to understand What Matters (IHI, 2022). Like nursing and other disciplines, RTs use the four-step systematic process of assessment, planning, implementation, and evaluation. They then utilize their assessment to adapt interventions—suggesting and utilizing adaptive equipment to increase engagement based on resident abilities and limitations (Loy et al., 2021). In a nursing home, you can find such adaptations as raised flower beds and weighted garden tools that assist a resident utilizing a wheelchair with limited range of motion to successfully participate in a preferred activity.

Restorative nursing programs help maintain or improve physical functioning, psychosocial issues, and communication skills (De Vries & Lake, 2005) and reduce the resident's risk of falls, injury, and hospitalizations. Regulations state that a licensed nurse must oversee restorative programs; however, RTs may provide specific interventions, making it a collaborative effort between the two disciplines (De Vries & Lake, 2005). RTs can also provide co-treatments with OT/ST/PT in group settings to improve and maintain functional abilities and re-integration into the community.

As described in this and other chapters, the proportion of older adults with cognitive impairment in nursing homes may typically be 50% or higher, and these individuals have been noted to have low participation in recreation activities in nursing homes. Yet evidence has shown the value of such interventions to support quality of life and function in cognitively impaired nursing home residents. For example, Buettner and Ferrairo (1998) examined the impact of TR interventions on nursing home residents diagnosed with dementia. The participants in the experimental group received activities established by a CTRS and nurse manager and showed significant improvements in mental status, level of depression, hand strength, flexibility, and levels of agitation. Recognizing this reality, the ATRA convened an expert panel in 2002 that issued a consensus statement on collaboration between nursing and recreation therapy to promote deeper understanding of dementia-related behaviors coupled with interventions to address unmet needs that may be expressed as disruptive behaviors (Buettner & Kolanowski, 2003).

Overall, research studies completed in nursing homes have demonstrated that older individuals with many diagnoses and comorbidities benefit significantly from therapeutic recreation services (Loy et al., 2021). Therapeutic interventions coupled with an interdisciplinary approach can impact quality indicators including late loss ADLs, range of motion, pressure ulcers, hydration/nutrition, depression, and many others (De Vries & Lake, 2005). When recreation professionals are integrated fully and consistently into the interprofessional care team and care planning process in a nursing home, resident motivation, engagement, and access to What Matters can be more fully enabled.

SOCIAL WORKER

As discussed in the earlier sections, providing person-centered care for patients and residents is the keystone to high-quality care in the nursing home setting, and social workers play an integral part in its delivery. The roles and responsibilities of an LTC social worker are vast and varied and often depend on resident-specific needs. Social workers are skilled at understanding and addressing the needs of residents and families, and their training allows them to recognize the needs from a holistic, whole-person, biopsychosocial, and spiritual perspective. The primary components of social work services in this setting include psychosocial assessment, care planning, care coordination/referrals, advocacy, grievance management, education, cultural competence, discharge planning, supportive counseling, and advance care planning. An LTC social worker is often the conduit for communication between residents, families, community agencies, and the interdisciplinary care team. Social workers play an important role, particularly in supporting nurses, so the team can achieve their shared goal of promoting an optimal level of psychosocial well-being and physical functioning for all persons they care for.

Most social work departments in LTC facilities are staffed by a social work director, who provides leadership and oversight for the department, and unit-based social workers. As put forth by the National Association of Social Workers (2003), a social work director preferably has a master's degree from an accredited school of social work, as well as a minimum of two years postgraduate experience in LTC. Social work staff should, at minimum, have a bachelor's degree from an accredited school of social work, two years of postgraduate experience in LTC, and meet state requirements for social work practice. These professional standards ensure that LTC social workers are equipped with the skills needed to perform their duties.

As mentioned above, social workers in LTC provide myriad services, but there are three we will highlight here: upholding resident rights, discharge planning, and advance care planning.

Resident Rights

The driving force behind every social worker is to enhance and preserve quality of life, and no task emphasizes that more than promoting and protecting resident rights. State and federal regulations require nursing homes to have policies covering the rights of residents, and these rights must be respected by the staff and understood by the resident and family.

Upon admission and annually thereafter, the social worker will review resident rights with the resident and provide ongoing staff education to ensure that nursing home residents are treated with respect and enjoy their continued civil and legal rights. The social worker takes great care in explaining these rights to residents in a way they can understand and with as much explanatory detail as possible. Social workers will also use this time to remind residents that they need to respect the rights of others in the facility as well. The social worker then ensures that the review of resident rights is documented in the resident's record.

Examples of resident rights include the right to (CMS, n.d.):

- Dignity, respect, and a comfortable living environment
- Quality of care and treatment without discrimination
- Be free from abuse, corporal punishment, and involuntary seclusion
- Freedom of choice to make own, independent decisions
- The safeguard of property and money
- Safeguards in admission, transfer, and discharge
- Privacy in communications
- Participate in organizations and activities of choice

- An easy-to-use and responsive complaint procedure
- Exercise all rights without fear of reprisals

A comprehensive list of resident rights is available and posted in every nursing facility. It is important that all professionals and staff providing care and working in nursing homes familiarize themselves with these rights and partner with the social worker to ensure the protection of resident rights for this vulnerable population. Preserving resident rights is the foundation for supporting residents' quality of life.

Discharge Planning

Discharge planning is another important, and often complex, component of social work delivery in LTC. Some might find it surprising that discharge planning is a common element within LTC, but there are many reasons why a patient or resident in the nursing home setting would be discharged from the facility. Most discharges are the result of the patient's conclusion of their short-term rehabilitation course following a hospital stay (this level of care in a nursing home is also referred to as *post-acute*). Other reasons for discharge or transfer might include the following:

- An alternate level of care is more appropriate, especially if the resident's health and functional status has improved and returning to the community is a viable option
- Resident and/or family choose to move to another location
- Discharge or transfer is necessary for the health or safety of the patient or others
- Failure to pay for nursing home services

Whatever the reason prompting the discharge or transfer, it is the responsibility of the nursing home to plan for a safe and orderly discharge, and social workers are the driving force behind making that happen.

Although social workers take the lead in discharge planning, it does not happen in isolation. It is a collaborative process that involves physicians, advanced practice providers (e.g., nurse practitioners and physician assistants), nursing, therapy, dietary, recreation, external agencies, and the patient/resident and family. Social workers will use their knowledge of available resources, coupled with the recommendations of the team, to formulate and implement safe discharge plans.

Residents who transfer to another facility require a thorough referral process to ensure the accepting facility can meet the needs of the person. Nurses are integral in this referral process, as they are most knowledgeable about the medical and care needs of the resident. Patients/residents returning home or to another community-based level of care require extensive care coordination and education for a successful transition. The social worker will arrange various services, such as the following:

- Family training and education
- Transportation
- Durable medical equipment
- Home health services
- Meal delivery
- Other support services

These services are coordinated to meet the requests and needs of the resident and family, as well as the recommendations of the care team. A safe discharge or transfer takes thoughtful collaboration, which can result in a meaningful accomplishment for the team when the resident is able to transition to the next appropriate setting.

Advance Care Planning

It is essential that the care provided in the nursing home is properly aligned with what matters to the resident or surrogate decision-maker who acts as the resident's proxy. What Matters includes preferences for medical treatment and other interventions, which should be aligned to the resident's goals for care. To provide goal-concordant care, the nursing home staff must first know the goals, values, and preferences of those they care for. This knowledge is ascertained through advance care planning and goals of care conversations.

It is the responsibility and privilege of the entire team to engage residents in advance care planning, but it is often the social worker who facilitates and educates around these conversations. Social workers are highly trained when it comes to broaching sensitive topics, respecting cultural backgrounds, navigating complex systems, and empowering others—all key components for effective advance care planning.

Although social workers often initiate and conduct ongoing advance care planning and communicate the resident's care preferences with others, a team approach is essential to high-quality advance care planning.

The advance care planning process is the overall and ongoing discussion about goals, values, and preferences. These preferences then need to be translated into advance care planning documents, which are advance directives and medical orders. Upon admission, social workers provide information about advance directives and assist with preparing, updating, and reviewing them. That initial conversation lays the foundation for the care team to continue these conversations and integrate the resident's values and preferences into plans of care throughout the resident's nursing home stay.

All team members have the responsibility to help the resident or surrogate decision-maker understand their health status and treatment options and help them communicate their goals and treatment preferences. At a minimum, these conversations should take place upon admission or readmission, quarterly thereafter, and with any change in condition.

All members of the interdisciplinary team should be well versed in the essential elements of effective advance care planning/goals-of-care conversations. Social workers support the team in this process by sharing guidance around how to have these conversations and what the individual resident-specific preferences may be. Initiating a goals-of-care conversation is one of the greatest gifts a care team can offer (see the nearby sidebar for helpful information on conducting this conversation). Residents and families often will not be the ones to initiate the discussion, but they are grateful when the nursing home staff do.

Here are a couple additional resources for advance care planning:

- VitalTalk Quick Guides cover tips for having conversations around a variety of topics: https://www.vitaltalk.org/resources/quick-guides/
- The Goals-of-Care Conversation: A Best-Practice, Step-By-Step Approach: https://www.acpdecisions.org/goals-of-care-conversations-a-best-practice-step-by-step-approach/

How to Have a Goals-of-Care Conversation: A Basic Framework

Set the right tone for the conversation by picking a quiet, private place where you can sit down with the resident and take your time. Be sure to leave your own agenda aside and use the time to focus on the resident's thoughts and to be respectful of their cultural background. A good way to start an advance care planning conversation is to say, "I want to make sure I am honoring and respecting your voice, so I want to hear what matters most to you." Also explain the reason for having the conversation and, to minimize alarm when talking about options for medical care, explain that the team wants to proactively understand what their wishes are.

Once the tone is set, proceed with open-ended questions:

- "What is your understanding of your medical condition right now?"
- "What are your goals if your health worsens?"
- "What are your hopes or fears when it comes to your healthcare?"

The responses you get to these types of open-ended questions will help the team understand the person's values and goals, which is the essence of advance care planning. It is then imperative that the treatment preferences discussed in these conversations are properly documented, and any necessary medical orders are obtained.

Social workers not only engage the resident and surrogate decision-makers in the advance care planning process but also serve as a resource for staff who want to hone their skills at this important process. After all, there is no better way to provide person-centered care than to be certain we are honoring and respecting the wishes of those we care for.

PUTTING IT ALL TOGETHER – CASE EXAMPLE

Introduction

To illustrate interprofessional team collaboration in the nursing home setting, let's discuss a brief case story. We hope that this story, based on a real person's nursing home journey, helps the reader envision how interprofessional practice works in everyday practice.

Case Details

Mr. Thomas, an 84-year-old male, resided in LTC for four years after an initial short stay s/p fall with hip fracture and short-stay rehabilitation with return to home for a brief period. The family was unable to support his increasing care needs, so they pursued direct admit to a nursing home from home.

Clinical Picture at Time of Nursing Home Admission

- Occupational/social/leisure:
  - Retired barber
  - Widower x 20 years—misses wife
  - Strong support of daughter who lives locally and is a healthcare professional familiar with nursing home setting
  - Hadn't slept in a regular bed for >15 years (night owl, intermittent sleeper—frequent short naps during day on couch)
  - Pleasant and sociable on basic level; likes his privacy
  - Leisure preferences:
    - Reading newspaper, sitting outdoors, TV (classic movies and action), Philadelphia sports, recreational golf (up until past year due to physical/cognitive decline), going out to breakfast with daughter, visits with family and reminiscing
    - Not a fan of structured activities or groups
- Physical/functional:
  - Unsteady gait short distances with rolling walker in small rancher home
  - Impulsive baseline personality; high fall risk
  - Personal hygiene and basic ADLs barely functioning prior to nursing home admission—accepting of help to keep him safe and clean
- Medical:
  - Type 2 diabetes—fair control with medication and diet
  - Chronic urinary incontinence—atonic bladder

- Progressive dysphagia of unclear etiology
- Eating preferred foods important to him
- Difficulty swallowing pills—on minimal medications at time of admission (h/o declining medications suggested by family doctor due to cost, swallowing difficulties, and complexity of following medication regimen accurately and consistently)
- Cognitive impairment—diagnosed globally with "dementia" at time of nursing home placement; short-term memory severely impaired, other cognitive functions less affected, and does not exhibit agitation or other behavioral dysfunction

Interprofessional Care Plan Based on Admission Presentation

- **Primary goal:** Develop a safe and satisfying routine aligned with what matters most to Mr. Thomas, including mobility opportunities to prevent functional decline and decrease fall risk, preserve ability to go on outings to daughter's home and out for breakfast occasionally (rehabilitative/restorative focus centered on integration of daily routine in new living environment)
- Team member focus:
    - **Physical therapist:** Optimize daily ambulatory mobility through skilled PT for gait and balance training, environmental setup, and nursing staff training in restorative walking program and assist to bathroom at ambulatory level with rolling walker; set up maintenance program to use stationary bike in rehab gym 2-3x/week under distant supervision of nursing restorative staff ; Mr. Thomas enjoyed socializing with rehab and restorative nursing team and amenable to aerobic exercise in this context
    - **Occupational therapist:** Mr. Thomas diagnosed with atonic bladder and urinary catheter was recommended as best approach, so no intervention for urinary incontinence management warranted; he was satisfied with current level of staff support for basic self-care needs—seen for brief course of occupational therapy for patient and nurse caregiver education in establishment of consistent ADL routine aligned with patient's preferences

- **Speech therapist:** Performed comprehensive assessment of swallowing function and recommended least restrictive diet for food and beverages in alignment with what was acceptable to Mr. Thomas, and in communication with patient's daughter (primary advocate) and physician, to ensure preservation of eating enjoyment while optimizing safety
- **Registered dietitian:** Worked with Mr. Thomas to recommend a variety of acceptable food choices that would meet his nutritional needs and preserve his enjoyment of dining experiences
- **Recreation therapist:** Conducted an interview with Mr. Thomas and his family regarding current preferences and available resources and options; advocated for and partnered with nursing and occupational therapy in recommending and implementing a consistent day/night routine aligned with his usual habits and preferences
- **Pharmacist:** Recommended least restrictive medication profile to manage Mr. Thomas's multiple chronic conditions while preserving his wishes to take the fewest medications possible via the safest administration route available (i.e., smaller pills, thickened liquid suspension as available)
- **Social worker:** Provided regular check-ins with Mr. Thomas and his daughter to monitor his satisfaction with transition to nursing home setting; active listener and collaborative problem-solver when challenges arose; communicated expressed needs and concerns to the care team on behalf of patient and family (i.e., consistent team support for patient "napping" tendencies rather than full night sleep; environment that supports ability to get in/out of bed and room as desired throughout the night; decreasing risk of falls and patient dissatisfaction with sleep schedule not aligned with his preferences and usual routine)
- **Nurse:** Instrumental in recommending and implementing effective solution for sleep—use of a larger bed due to Mr. Thomas's size (6'4", 220#), fall risk, h/o claustrophobic tendencies and not sleeping in traditional bed for many years; also, provided day-to-day nursing care and medical interventions aligned with his needs and monitored overall status and function, with early identification and communication of changes to the team

Clinical Progression

- Aging and chronic condition progression over time—gradual decline in function; transitioned from restorative to palliative approach with changing team focus and care management leaders in line with patient needs
- Near end of life transitioned to hospice care aligned with Mr. Thomas's and his family's wishes due to effects of advancing multiple chronic conditions, failure to thrive, and severe dysphagia; social worker led the team in facilitating goals of care/advance care planning conversations throughout the journey from restorative to palliative to hospice to ensure a comprehensive and personalized plan for a successful end of life journey

Discussion

This case illustrates a cohesive team approach focused on supporting optimal safety and function and accessing what mattered most to Mr. Thomas and the people who loved him at every stage of his late life journey.

The patient's daughter, as a trained healthcare professional knowledgeable about care team roles and workflows in nursing home settings and a strong advocate for her father, was an integral part of the team communication and care planning throughout her father's journey, helping to ensure timeliness and completion of assessments, actions, and follow-through by appropriate members of the care team.

Conclusion

The site where Mr. Thomas lived was not formally trained in the 4Ms of Age-Friendly Health Systems (What Matters, Medication, Mentation, and Mobility). If they had been, the focus and consistency of care delivery and interprofessional team collaboration would likely not have relied so heavily on the daughter for guiding the focus and approach, as the focus is aligned, understood, and "baked in" for sites and teams truly applying the Age-Friendly model.

Because of how common it is for individuals residing in nursing home settings to not have someone actively involved and consistently advocating for their needs, evolving to the Age-Friendly (4M) model of interprofessional care delivery as the standard of care in the nursing home setting is critically important.

SUMMARY

As described in previous chapters, LTC settings serve a dual purpose. They are care settings for older adults who need short-term post-acute care (such as rehabilitation following a hip fracture) and also provide care and housing for older adults who are unable to care for themselves independently. Most older adults receiving care or living in LTC have complex, chronic illness and may additionally be cognitively impaired. Because of their complexity, both post-acute patients and long-term residents in an LTC setting benefit from interprofessional team evaluation, assessment, care planning, and intervention that addresses every dimension of their health and wellness. In the highest functioning LTC settings, the interprofessional team is *fully integrated and interdependent*. This means that individual clinicians are not simply practicing side by side (what is often referred to as practicing in "silos"); rather, they are collaborating and consulting with each other, working together to tailor assessments and interventions to help patients and residents recover from illness or injury and achieve and sustain their highest possible quality of life. The LTC setting is unique in its ready access to an array of clinical experts all practicing together in relatively close proximity when compared to hospital care. The RN who practices and leads in an LTC setting has a unique opportunity to work closely with other professionals to fully develop team-based care and bring its benefits to patients and residents.

REFERENCES

Academy of Geriatric Physical Therapy. (2022). *Competencies in the care of older adults at the completion of the entry-level physical therapist professional program of study*. https://aptageriatrics.org/geriatricspt_files/recources/resource_20221101_234151.pdf

Academy Quality Management Committee. (2018, January). Academy of Nutrition and Dietetics: Revised 2017 scope of practice for the registered dietitian nutritionist. *Journal of the Academy of Nutrition and Dietetics, 118*(1), 141–165. https://doi.org/10.1016/j.jand.2017.10.002

Accreditation Council for Education in Nutrition and Dietetics. (2023). *Licensure maps and statutes by state*. https://www.eatrightpro.org/advocacy/licensure/licensure-map-and-statutes-by-state

Administration for Community Living. (2021). *How much care will you need?* https://acl.gov/ltc/basic-needs/how-much-care-will-you-need

American Journal of Occupational Therapy. (n.d.). *What is occupational therapy?* https://www. Aota.org/about/what-is-ot

American Journal of Occupational Therapy. (2020). Occupational therapy practice framework: Domain and process (4th ed.). *American Journal of Occupational Therapy, 74*(2). https://doi.org/10.5014/ajot.2020.74S2001

American Physical Therapy Association. (2023). *APTA guide to physical therapist practice 4.0*. https://guide. Apta.org

American Speech-Language-Hearing Association. (n.d.). *Supervision of clinical fellows*. https://inte.asha.org/practice/supervision/supervision-of-clinical-fellows/

American Speech-Language-Hearing Association. (2016). *ASHA practice policy*. www.Asha.org/policy/

American Therapeutic Recreation Association. (n.d.). *About recreational therapy.* https://www.Atra-online.com/page/AboutRecTherapy Buettner, L., & Ferrario, J. (1998). Therapeutic recreation-nursing team: A therapeutic intervention for nursing home residents with dementia. *Annual in Therapeutic Recreation, 7,* 21–28

Buettner, L., & Ferrario, J. (1998). Therapeutic recreation-nursing team: A therapeutic intervention for nursing home residents with dementia. *Annual in Therapeutic Recreation, 7,* 21–28.

Buettner, L., & Kolanowski, A. (2003). Practice guidelines for recreation therapy in the care of people with dementia. *Geriatric Nursing, 24*(1), 18–25. https://doi.org/10.1067/mgn.2003.19

Cacchione, P. Z. (2020). Age-Friendly Health Systems: The 4Ms framework. *Clinical Nursing Research, 29*(3), 139–140. https://doi.org/10.1177/1054773820906667

Centers for Medicare & Medicaid Services. (n.d.). *Your rights and protections as a nursing home resident.* https://downloads.cms.gov/medicare/Your_Resident_Rights_and_Protections_section.pdf

Centers for Medicare & Medicaid Services. (2017, July 13). *42 CFR 483.45 pharmacy services.* https://www.ecfr.gov/on/2017-07-13/title-42/section-483.45

Centers for Medicare & Medicaid Services. (2023). *State operations manual appendix PP: Guidance for surveyors in long term care facilities.* https://www.cms.gov/medicare/provider-enrollment-and-certification/guidanceforlawsandregulations/downloads/appendix-pp-state-operations-manual.pdf

Cereda, E., Pedrolli, C., Klersy, C., Bonardi, C., Quarleri, L., Cappello, S., Turri, A., Rondanelli, M., & Caccialanza, R. (2016, December). Nutritional status in older persons according to healthcare setting: A systematic review and meta-analysis of prevalence data using MNA((R)). *Clinical Nutrition, 35*(6), 1282–1290. https://doi.org/10.1016/j.clnu.2016.03.008

Commission on Dietetic Registration. (2021). *Definition of terms list.* https://www.cdrnet.org/vault/2459/web/20221215%20Definition%20of%20Terms%20List-December%202022.pdf

Cormi, C., Chrusciel, J., Laplanche, D., Dramé, M., & Sanchez, S. (2020, June). Telemedicine in nursing homes during the COVID-19 outbreak: A star is born (again). *Geriatrics & Gerontology International, 20*(6), 646–647. https://doi.org/10.1111/ggi.13934

Criss, M. G., Wingood, M., Staples, W. H., Southard, V., Miller, K. L., Norris, T. L., Avers, D., Ciolek, C. H., Lewis, C. B., & Strunk, E. R. (2022). APTA Geriatrics' guiding principles for best practices in geriatric physical therapy: An executive summary. *Journal of Geriatric Physical Therapy, 45*(2), 70–75. https://doi.org/10.1519/JPT.0000000000000342

De Vries, D., & Lake, J. (2005). Recreational therapy in long-term care. *Extended Care News, 104,* 18–25.

Dorner, B., & Friedrich, E. (2018). Position of the Academy of Nutrition and Dietetics: Individualized nutrition approaches for older adults: Long-term care, post-acute care, and other settings. *Journal of the Academy of Nutrition and Dietetics, 118*(4), 725–735. doi: org/10.1016/j.jand.2018.01.022

Drulia, T., & Hodge, A. (2021, November). Clinical practice patterns of speech-language pathologists delivering dysphagia services to persons with COPD: Analysis of survey outcomes. *Seminars in Speech and Language, 42*(5), 363–383. https://doi.org/10.1055/s-0041-1735846

Institute for Healthcare Improvement. (2022). *Guide to care of older adults in nursing homes.* https://241684.fs1.hubspotusercontent-na1.net/hubfs/241684/IHI-Age-Friendly-Guide-Nursing-Homes_March28-2022.pdf

Liu, L., Dong, H., Jin, X., & Brooke-Wavell, K. (2022). Tackling dementia: A systematic review of interventions based on physical activity. *Journal of Geriatric Physical Therapy, 45*(4), E169–E180. https://doi.org/10.1519/JPT.0000000000000332

Loy, T., DeVries, D., & Keller, J. (2021). Recreational therapy in nursing homes history, regulations, COVID-19, and beyond. *Therapeutic Recreation Journal, 55*(1). https://doi.org/https://doi.org/10.18666/TRJ-2021-V55-I1-10744

Luppa, M., Luck, T., Weyerer, S., Konig, H. H., Brahler, E., & Riedel-Heller, S. G. (2010, January). Prediction of institutionalization in the elderly: A systematic review. *Age and Ageing, 39*(1), 31–38. https://doi.org/10.1093/ageing/afp202

May, S., Jonas, K., Fehler, G. V., Zahn, T., Heinze, M., & Muehlensiepen, F. (2021). Challenges in current nursing home care in rural Germany and how they can be reduced by telehealth: An exploratory qualitative pre-post study. *BMC Health Services Research, 21*(1), 925. https://doi.org/10.1186/s12913-021-06950-y

Murray, A. M. (2008, April). Cognitive impairment in the aging dialysis and chronic kidney disease populations: An occult burden. *Advances in Kidney Disease and Health, 15*(2), 123–132. https://doi.org/10.1053/j.Ackd.2008.01.010

National Academies of Practice. (2022). *NAP interprofessional practice and education lexicon 2.0.* https://www.napractice.org/assets/docs/NAP%20Lexicon%202.0.pdf

National Association of Social Workers. (2003). *Standards for social work services in long-term care facilities.* https://www.socialworkers.org/LinkClick.aspx?fileticket=cwW7lzBfYxg%3d&portalid=0

National Certification Council for Activity Professionals. (2023). *Certification standards.* https://www.nccap.org/assets/_2023%20NCCAP%20STANDARDS_00262023%20FINAL.pdf

National Council for Therapeutic Recreation Certification. (2018). *Recreational therapy certification requirements by state.* https://www.sru.edu/documents/academics/online-learning/Recreational%20Therapy%20Certification%20Requirements%20by%20State.pdf

National Council for Therapeutic Recreation Certification. (2023). *Certification standards.* https://www.nctrc.org/wp-content/uploads/2023/01/CertificationStandards.pdf

Nursing Explorer. (n.d.). *Nursing schools search.* https://www.nursingexplorer.com/

Pinto, A. R., Silva, R. G., & Pinato, L. (2016). Oropharyngeal swallowing in chronic renal failure. *Codas, 28*(1), 71–76. https://doi.org/10.1590/2317-1782/20162015041

Polinski, J. M., Barker, T., Gagliano, N., Sussman, A., Brennan, T. A., & Shrank, W. H. (2016). Patients' satisfaction with and preference for telehealth visits. *Journal of General Internal Medicine, 31*(3), 269–275. https://doi.org/10.1007/s11606-015-3489-x

Rivelsrud, M. C., Hartelius, L., Bergstrom, L., Lovstad, M., & Speyer, R. (2023, February). Prevalence of oropharyngeal dysphagia in adults in different healthcare settings: A systematic review and meta-analyses. *Dysphagia, 38*(1), 76–121. https://doi.org/10.1007/s00455-022-10465-x

Saedi, E., Gheini, M. R., Faiz, F., & Arami, M. A. (2016, Sept. 15). Diabetes mellitus and cognitive impairments. *World Journal of Diabetes,* 7(17), 412–422. https://doi.org/10.4239/wjd.v7.i17.412

Sheikh, N. (2022, Nov. 15). *The connection between vision and dementia: Understanding the research.* Altoida. https://altoida.com/blog/the-connection-between-vision-and-dementia-understanding-the-research/

Tinetti, M. E., & Kumar, C. (2010, Jan. 20). The patient who falls: "It's always a trade-off." *JAMA, 303*(3), 258–266. https://doi.org/10.1001/jama.2009.2024

US Government. (1987). *42 CFR Part 483: Requirements for states and long-term care facilities, § Omnibus Budget Reconciliation Act.* https://www.govinfo.gov/content/pkg/CFR-2011-title42-vol5/pdf/CFR-2011-title42-vol5-part483.pdf

Yuan, Y., Lapane, K. L., Tjia, J., Baek, J., Liu, S. H., & Ulbricht, C. M. (2021). Physical frailty and cognitive impairment in older adults in United States nursing homes. *Dementia and Geriatric Cognitive Disorders, 50*(1), 60–67. https://doi.org/10.1159/000515140

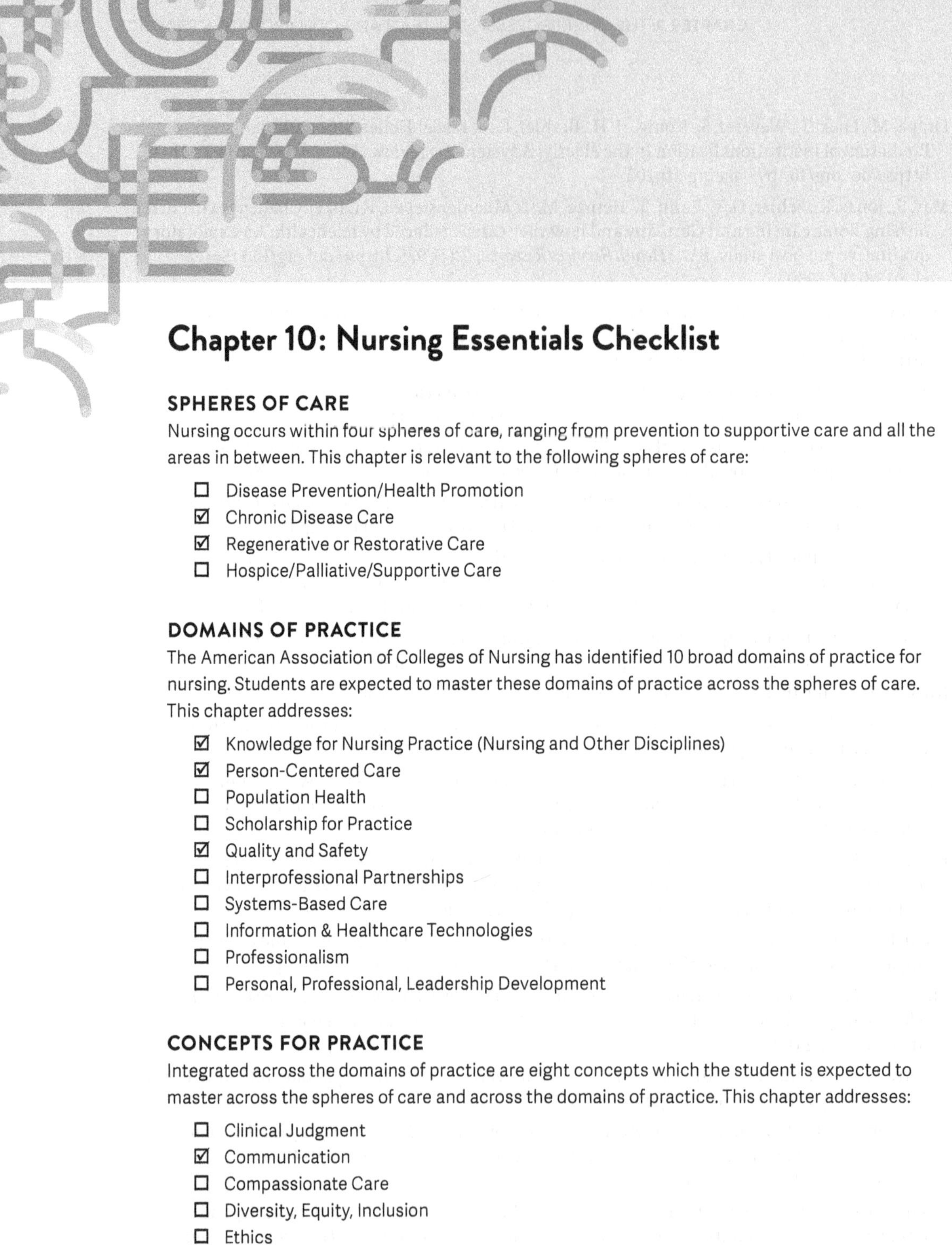

Chapter 10: Nursing Essentials Checklist

SPHERES OF CARE

Nursing occurs within four spheres of care, ranging from prevention to supportive care and all the areas in between. This chapter is relevant to the following spheres of care:

- [ ] Disease Prevention/Health Promotion
- [x] Chronic Disease Care
- [x] Regenerative or Restorative Care
- [ ] Hospice/Palliative/Supportive Care

DOMAINS OF PRACTICE

The American Association of Colleges of Nursing has identified 10 broad domains of practice for nursing. Students are expected to master these domains of practice across the spheres of care. This chapter addresses:

- [x] Knowledge for Nursing Practice (Nursing and Other Disciplines)
- [x] Person-Centered Care
- [ ] Population Health
- [ ] Scholarship for Practice
- [x] Quality and Safety
- [ ] Interprofessional Partnerships
- [ ] Systems-Based Care
- [ ] Information & Healthcare Technologies
- [ ] Professionalism
- [ ] Personal, Professional, Leadership Development

CONCEPTS FOR PRACTICE

Integrated across the domains of practice are eight concepts which the student is expected to master across the spheres of care and across the domains of practice. This chapter addresses:

- [ ] Clinical Judgment
- [x] Communication
- [ ] Compassionate Care
- [ ] Diversity, Equity, Inclusion
- [ ] Ethics
- [ ] Evidence-Based Practice
- [ ] Health Policy
- [ ] Social Determinants of Health

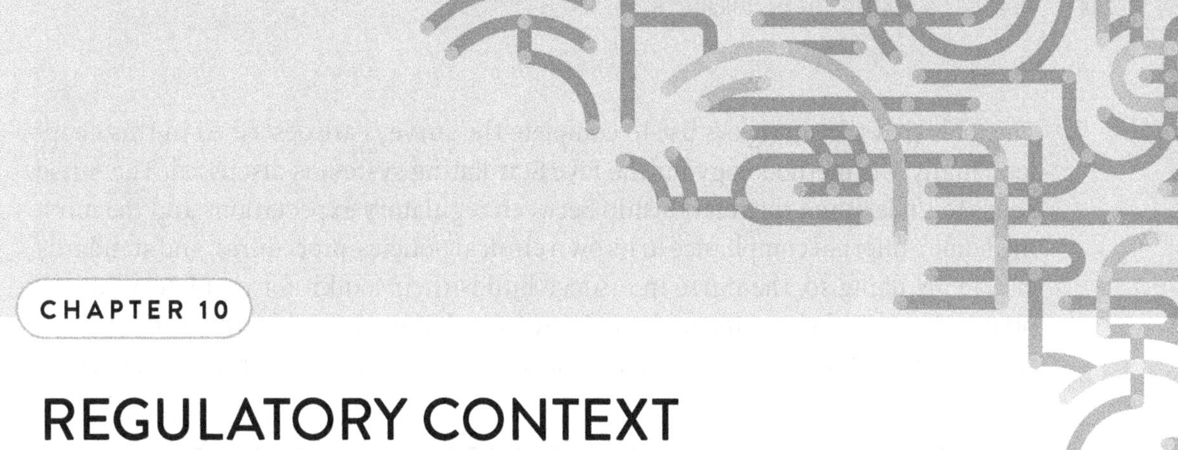

CHAPTER 10

REGULATORY CONTEXT

Julie Britton, DNP, MSN, RN-BC, GCNS-BC, FGNLA
Stefanie Mozgai, RN

OBJECTIVES

1. Discuss how and why the OBRA '89/Nursing Home Reform Act and Final Rule was implemented.
2. Define the purpose, types, and frequency of surveys conducted in long-term/post-acute care facilities.
3. Describe the implications of survey results for a nursing home's Five Star Rating.
4. Appreciate the relationship between regulatory requirements, quality care, and optimal resident outcomes.

INTRODUCTION

This chapter explores how the regulatory/survey process evolved and explains the regulatory framework that is now widely known as the "Final Rule." The Final Rule established several expectations, the most important of which is that providers remain in substantial compliance with Medicare/Medicaid program requirements as well as state law.

We discuss the different types of surveys, what the results for these surveys mean, and the implications of the results. We also explore the concept of being "survey-ready" every day. Preparing for a regulatory survey in a nursing home is an intense, all-hands-on-deck effort that requires expert navigation by the interprofessional team.

The tools that the surveyors use to complete the surveys are described in this chapter. Finally, the methodology for the Five Star Rating system is discussed. The nurse needs to understand the relationship between regulatory expectations and the nursing home's internal compliance to its own clinical policies, procedures, and standards of care. By doing so, the nurse in essence builds their toolkit for regulatory/survey preparedness. By being prepared and knowing what to anticipate, the nurse will be able to connect how providing good clinical care results in good survey outcomes.

NURSING HOME SURVEY AND OBRA BACKGROUND

As a student or practicing nurse in a nursing home, you will hear staff talk frequently about the "state," "CMS," "deficiencies," "quality of care," and "quality of life." These are terms that are most often associated with the survey process. The *survey* is a nuts-and-bolts inspection of everything that occurs in the facility according to federally established rules of participation and regulations. Issues spanning how the care is provided, how clean the center is, or what the temperature of the food is are just a few examples of what surveyors will inspect.

The foundation for the current regulatory requirements is a piece of federal legislation known as OBRA '89, also called the Nursing Home Reform Act. This landmark legislation was designed to improve the quality of life, quality of care, health, and safety for residents in long term/post-acute care (LT/PAC) facilities (Medicare and Medicaid Programs, 2015). The legislation emphasized patient-centered care, providing a homelike environment, and assuring that facilities maintain or improve the quality of the residents' lives.

While a formal survey of nursing home practice and compliance with regulatory requirements takes place annually (or less frequently), the concept of "survey" should be viewed as a routine, daily event. In essence, a facility's performance is being monitored and inspected every day of the year by residents, families, physicians, facility staff, and others. For this reason, you might hear nursing home leaders coach their teams to practice as though it is "survey day, every day."

The History of Nursing Home Regulations

Like other healthcare settings, the LT/PAC industry must conform to rules and regulations to participate in the Medicare program and be licensed as a skilled nursing provider. Due to the extremely high compliance expectations and complexity of regulations in nursing homes, it has been said by many that the LT/PAC industry is one of the most regulated industries in the country, where the pages of regulatory requirements exceed that of even the nuclear power industry (American Medical Directors Association, 2002). To ensure adequate quality of care is provided to residents in LT/PAC facilities, LT/PAC providers must comply with both state and federal regulations (Eliopoulos, 2015).

With the establishment of the Social Security Act in 1935, concerns were raised regarding poor conditions and lack of quality care in nursing homes by the public and political sectors. Licensing/regulations were discouraged due to the need for nursing homes and beds. The thought at the time was that the majority of LT/PAC facilities probably would not meet the basic requirements of the regulatory process and therefore would be forced to close. In the 1950s, a study conducted by the Council of State Governments found that nursing homes were not providing quality services (Institute of Medicine [IOM], 1986), and many were considered substandard. From this study, the US Public Health Service began to consider licensing programs at the state level (IOM, 1986). Through these processes, many nursing homes continued to be labeled as substandard, though the continued fear of enforcement shutting down the operations of nursing homes prohibited pursuit of the issues, as it was thought that it would take time for nursing homes to comply with standards.

By 1961, the US Senate had created the Special Committee on Aging (IOM, 1986). The committee held several hearings on the issues identified in nursing homes, and by 1963, the first federal standards for nursing homes were issued (IOM, 1986). In 1983, Congress asked the IOM to conduct a review of nursing home performance. The 18-month study of nursing home issues by the IOM committee resulted in numerous regulatory recommendations, few of which were supported by evidenced-based research or outcomes (Kapp, 2014). In addition to the IOM committee findings and recommendations, the General Accounting Office published a report detailing its concerns with the lack of Department of Health and Human Services oversight of nursing homes (IOM, 1986).

Congress incorporated the IOM recommendations as part of the Omnibus Budget Reconciliation Act (OBRA) of 1989, also known as the Nursing Home Reform Act. OBRA '89 created a national minimum set of standards of care and rights for people living in certified nursing facilities. These minimum federal health and care requirements for nursing homes were intended to be delivered through a variety of established protocols. OBRA is a baseline that nursing facilities build on to reach not only resident "well-being" but also happiness and fulfillment.

Consolidated Medicare and Medicaid requirements for participation for LTC facilities were first published in the *Federal Register* on February 2, 1989 (Medicare and Medicaid Programs, 2015). These regulations have been selectively revised and updated since that time to incorporate new legislation or to address specific issues. Note that a significant overhaul of LT/PAC regulations didn't occur until 2015.

In 2015, the Centers for Medicare & Medicaid Services [CMS] published the proposed rule "Medicare and Medicaid Programs; Reform of Requirements for Long-Term Care Facilities," outlining substantial changes to the regulations for LTC, the first of its kind since 1991 (Medicare and Medicaid Programs, 2015, p. 42169). The rule is often referred to as the "Final Rule." The long overdue overhaul of nursing home regulatory requirements should stimulate new opportunities to improve care (Unroe et al., 2017).

Resident safety, health outcomes, individual choice, and quality assurance and performance improvement were at the forefront when these regulations were being reviewed for revision. Great strides have been made in these areas in the last two to three decades, in part because of extensive research that has helped enhance quality of care and life for residents who reside in LT/PAC facilities (Medicare and Medicaid Programs, 2015, p. 42169).

Since then, there has been an emergence of significant innovations with focus on patient-centered care and quality assessment practices. An example would be wearable devices that monitor and track a resident's steps, heart rate, and sleep patterns. In addition, the population the LT/PAC facilities serves has changed dramatically, becoming more diverse and more clinically complex. In more recent years, many LT/PAC leaders have likened the care that is provided in the LT/PAC facility to that provided on a medical-surgical or step-down unit of an acute-care hospital.

In constructing the Final Rule, CMS deemed it necessary to evaluate LT/PAC regulations on a comprehensive basis, from both a structural and a content perspective. Regulations were reviewed in an effort to improve the quality of life, care, and services in LT/PAC facilities, optimize resident safety, reflect current professional standards, and improve the consistent flow of the regulations. New requirements were added, and many regulations were revised with intent aimed at aligning requirements to current clinical practice standards to improve resident safety along with the quality and effectiveness of care and services delivered to residents (Medicare and Medicaid Programs, 2015, p. 42169).

As is true with other types of regulatory changes, with the proposed additions and revisions to the regulations, there was a period of time that was open for the public to comment on them. Thousands of public comments were made, which influenced changes in the new requirements and revisions of existing regulations as well as effective date(s) of the proposed regulations. Specifically, many commenters supported the change in focus toward *person-centered care*. This requires facilities to learn more about who the resident is as a person, provide greater support for resident preferences, and give residents increased control and choice.

As has been discussed in previous chapters, the Age-Friendly Health Systems (AFHS) framework and 4Ms, when applied in LT/PAC, place what matters to residents at the center of care. Although not required by regulation, implementing AFHS supports the LT/PAC facility's efforts to comply with the regulatory focus on person-centered care and culture change, ultimately improving both the resident's quality of life and quality of care.

The purpose of the Final Rule was to update regulatory requirements for LT/PAC facilities to meet the needs of both short-stay and LTC residents, as well as the differences in acuity of the population as compared to 25 years ago. In addition to improving quality of care and resident safety, CMS has indicated that the 2015 Final Rule requirements will help reduce procedural burdens on providers (Medicare and Medicaid Programs, 2015, p. 42168).

Purpose/Intent

CMS has stated that the goals for the revision of OBRA '89/Nursing Home Reform Act included aligning clinical practice with the multiple care-delivery models to ensure and allow flexibility to meet the everchanging needs of the diverse populations that LT/PAC facilities are serving (Medicare and Medicaid Programs, 2015, p. 42169). CMS has taken a competency-based approach to ensure as mandated that each resident is provided care to maintain or attain their highest practicable physical, mental, and psychosocial well-being.

To achieve this, CMS requires facilities to assess their facility capabilities/staff competencies and their resident population by completing a facility assessment. This competency-based approach helps the facility to identify gaps in service, is compatible with existing state requirements and business practices, and promotes both efficiency and effectiveness in care delivery. It helps facilities identify the population they are serving and apply the necessary staff education/training/competencies to serve that specific population. The facility assessment also identifies ethnic, cultural, and religious factors needed to meet patient preferences related to activities, food, etc.

Many of the quality of life and quality of care improvement changes in the Final Rule are grounded in the concepts of person-centered care and culture change. Patient-centered care is at the core of nursing in all populations and settings but has a place of unique importance in the LT/PAC setting (Cadmus et al., 2017, p. 12). As the LT/PAC setting continues to undergo necessary culture change, patient-centered care is at the heart of that change.

The recent regulatory changes will result not only in improved quality of life and care for residents but also improvements in the caregiver's quality of work life and in savings to the facility. It is important for the nurse to understand that quality-driven care produces the highest quality experience of care and resident outcomes while at the same time increasing operational efficiencies and reducing operating costs. For example, quality-driven staffing practices can achieve cost savings through reduced turnover and decreased use of contract labor.

Each state has a State Survey Agency (SSA) that is responsible for conducting the majority of surveys in LT/PAC facilities to certify compliance with the federal (CMS) participation requirements. Federal certification requirements under the Medicare program are uniform throughout the United States. However, states and localities may have additional requirements that the LT/PAC facility must meet to continue to operate within those jurisdictions.

Some state licensing requirements may be more stringent or prescriptive than federal requirements. Licensure surveys are conducted to determine a nursing home's compliance with specific state or local laws and regulations. LT/PAC facilities that do not meet state or local requirements for licensure may not be certified for participation in the Medicare/Medicaid programs. In the event of a difference in the stringency of a federal certification requirement and a corresponding state licensing requirement, the LT/PAC facility must comply with the more stringent of the two.

As noted earlier, OBRA '89 established expectations around compliance with regulations. The first is that LT/PAC facilities must remain in "substantial compliance" with Medicare/Medicaid program requirements as well as state law. A survey finding of substantial compliance indicates that the facility complies with the regulations, and there were no deficient practices found. The regulation emphasizes the requirement for ongoing compliance rather than cyclic compliance.

In other words, the enforcement process mandates that policies and procedures be established to remedy deficient practices and to ensure that correction is lasting and the same deficient practice is not detected again on the next survey. LT/PAC facilities need to take the initiative and responsibility for continuously monitoring their own performance to sustain compliance with regulations. Facilities accomplish this through their Quality Assurance and Performance Improvement (QAPI) process. If a deficient practice is noted on survey, the LT/PAC provider must prepare and submit an acceptable plan of correction to achieve and maintain improved quality of care.

Furthermore, the LT/PAC provider must address all deficiencies *promptly*. As noted previously, the standard for federal program participation mandated by the regulation is *substantial compliance*. Because the regulations are in place to protect residents' safety and well-being, the state and CMS will take steps to bring about correction of deficient practices quickly (CMS, 2023c).

TYPES OF SURVEYS

Surveys are conducted by surveyors employed by SSAs who inspect for compliance with federal regulations and any state or local requirements. The State Operations Manual (SOM) is a federal document created by CMS for the purpose of communicating policy regarding survey and certification activities. State surveyors follow the SOM to guide their survey activities. The LT/PAC facility also uses the SOM to guide its practice and compliance.

CMS communicates updates and changes to survey policy to SSAs via Quality, Safety, and Oversight (QSO) memoranda. Nursing facilities also receive the QSO memos so that they are aware of any change in requirements. These memos were previously called Survey and Certification (or S&C) memos.

CMS has outlined the qualifications a surveyor must possess to conduct inspections. These include a background in a health profession such as nursing, social work, pharmacy, or dietary. Surveyors who inspect nursing homes are required to pass the Surveyor Minimum Qualifications Test (SMQT), which tests the surveyors' knowledge, skills, and abilities. Surveyors must pass the SMQT in order to inspect nursing homes independently. Prior to passing the SMQT, a surveyor may function as a team member with at least one other qualified surveyor (CMS, 2019b). CMS outlines these qualifications and the SMQT in Chapter 4 of the SOM.

Standard and Life Safety Code Surveys

There are several different types of surveys, which are defined by CMS in Chapters 2, 5, and 7 of the SOM. It is important to know that to initially certify an LT/PAC facility (e.g., a new facility that is opening), both a standard survey and a Life Safety Code survey must be completed.

Standard Survey

This survey is a periodic, resident-centered inspection that gathers information through interviews and observations about the quality of service provided in a facility to determine compliance with the requirements of participation. The length of a standard survey varies based on number of surveyors, size and layout of the facility, and the number and complexity of concerns that need to be investigated onsite.

The extended survey evaluates additional participation requirements subsequent to finding substandard quality of care during a standard survey. Substandard quality of care means one or more deficiencies related to the particular participation requirements under 42 CFR 483.13 related to resident behavior and facility practices, 42 CFR 483.15, quality of life, or 42 CFR 483.25, quality of care, that constitute either immediate jeopardy to resident health or safety (level J, K, or L); a pattern of or widespread actual harm that is not immediate jeopardy (level H or I); or widespread potential for more than minimal harm but less than immediate jeopardy, with no actual harm (level F). This process is outlined in Chapter 7 of the SOM (CMS, 2023c), which is discussed further later in this chapter. *Immediate jeopardy* means a situation in which the facility's noncompliance with one or more requirements of participation has caused, or is likely to cause, serious injury, harm, impairment, or death to a resident (CMS, 2019a).

Life Safety Code Survey

Life Safety Code (LSC) is a set of fire protection requirements designed to provide a reasonable degree of safety from fire. It covers construction, protection, and operational features designed to provide safety from fire, smoke, and panic.

Revised periodically, the LSC is a publication of the National Fire Protection Association, which was founded in 1896 to promote the science and improve the methods of fire protection (CMS, 2020b). All initial surveys must verify substantial compliance with the regulatory requirements.

Focused Surveys

At times, CMS implements focused surveys that concentrate on specific tasks or care areas. These surveys may be used to inform future activities, assess surveyors' level of knowledge, streamline survey processes, or provide resource tools to facilities. Types of focused surveys include Dementia Care surveys, MDS surveys, and Focused Infection Control (FIC) surveys.

Dementia Care Survey

In 2014, CMS invited SSAs to participate in the pilot of a Focused Dementia Care survey to test new surveyor worksheets and processes focused on dementia care in nursing homes. As described in CMS Survey and Certification memo 16-04 (CMS, 2015), the focused survey examined the process for prescribing antipsychotic medication and assessed compliance with other federal requirements related to dementia care practices in nursing homes.

The pilot was initiated to gain new insights about surveyor knowledge and skills. CMS also looked for ways that the current survey process may be streamlined to identify and cite deficient practice more efficiently and accurately, as well as to recognize successful dementia care programs.

Upon completion of the pilot and a 2015 expansion effort, CMS revised the survey materials and tools based on surveyor feedback and data analysis. In response to feedback from stakeholders and partners of the National Partnership to Improve Dementia Care, CMS shared revised materials with the intent that facilities use these tools to assess their own practices in providing resident care (CMS, 2015).

Minimum Data Set Survey

In 2014, as announced in S&C 14-22-NH, CMS also created a Minimum Data Set (MDS) survey focusing on the regulations related to resident assessments. The MDS is a standardized assessment tool that facilitates care planning and management in nursing homes.

The MDS requirements apply to all residents in Medicare and/or Medicaid certified nursing homes and are the basis for the comprehensive assessment. The MDS regulations relate to assessment accuracy as well as completion and timing of the assessments.

While the primary purpose of the MDS is to serve as the basis for individualized care planning and delivery of person-centered care, CMS recognizes that the MDS also supports Medicare and Medicaid payment rates and quality monitoring (CMS, 2014).

Focused Infection Control Survey

In 2020, in response to COVID-19, CMS issued QSO 20-20-All. The QSO cited here required federal surveyors to perform targeted FIC surveys of facilities in those areas most in need of additional oversight. The FIC survey elements were available to every facility in the country to make them aware of infection control priorities during this time of crisis. Using these elements, facility leaders and teams could perform a voluntary self-assessment of their ability to meet the priorities (CMS, 2020a).

According to the CMS Fiscal Year 2023 Mission & Priorities document, issued in Admin-Info 22-10-All, FIC surveys continue. States must perform annual FIC surveys of 20% of nursing homes based on state discretion or additional data that identify facility and community risk, such as (CMS, 2022a):

- Facilities in counties with high rates of COVID-19 community transmission
- Facilities with multiple weeks of reporting COVID-19
- Special Focus Facilities (SFFs; covered later in this chapter)
- Facilities identified as candidates for the SFF program
- Facilities with allegations or complaints that pose a risk for harm or immediate jeopardy to the health or safety of residents

Abbreviated Standard Survey

The SSA must complete a standard survey of each LT/PAC facility no later than 15 months after the previous standard survey. Facilities with excellent histories of compliance may be surveyed less frequently to determine compliance but no less frequently than every 15 months, and the statewide standard survey average across all facilities in the state must not exceed 12 months. With the COVID-19 pandemic, SSAs were not consistently able to keep up with these time frames. At this writing, some SSAs are almost three years behind in conducting required standard surveys.

Changes in practice may also prompt a standard survey. For example, a change of ownership, management firm, administrator, or director of nursing may prompt the SSA to conduct a standard or abbreviated standard survey within 60 days of the change. In addition, facilities with poor histories of compliance may be surveyed more frequently than 12–15 months to ensure that residents are receiving quality care in a safe environment.

The statewide average interval for each SSA is available through the Certification and Survey Provider Enhanced Reporting system. CMS has an ongoing responsibility to monitor compliance with the survey frequency requirements.

Complaint

As described in detail in Chapter 5 of the SOM, SSAs are required to investigate complaints that allege facility noncompliance with federal and/or state regulatory requirements. The goal of the federal complaint/incident process is to establish a system that will assist in promoting and protecting the health, safety, and welfare of residents receiving healthcare services. If the SSA determines that the allegation(s) fall(s) within the authority of the SSA, the SSA determines the severity and urgency of the allegations, so that appropriate and timely action can be pursued (CMS, 2023b).

Anyone can call the SSA to report a complaint, and facilities are required to post State Ombudsman and SSA phone numbers. For example, complaints could be reported by a patient, family member, physician, or facility staff, to name a few.

All facilities are required to have a grievance process in place. Sometimes, when the SSA comes in on a complaint visit, the facility may already be aware of the issue because a grievance may already have been reported and resolved by the facility's process.

Whenever an issue or concern is raised, the facility should always address it immediately.

Special Focus Facilities

QSO 23-01-NH Sections 1819(f)(8) and 1919(f)(10) of the Social Security Act require CMS to conduct an SFF program that focuses on nursing homes that have a persistent record of noncompliance leading to poor quality of care (CMS, 2022b). The SFF program requires the persistently poorest-performing facilities selected in each state to be inspected no less than once every six months, and increasingly severe (progressive) enforcement actions are taken when warranted. CMS expects that selected facilities will rapidly make and sustain improvements so that they "graduate" from the program.

Once a state selects a facility as an SFF, the SSA, on CMS's behalf, conducts a full, onsite inspection of all Medicare health and safety requirements every six months and recommends progressive enforcement (e.g., fines, denial of Medicare payment) until the nursing home either graduates from the SFF program or is terminated from the Medicare and/or Medicaid program (CMS, 2022b).

CMS SOM Chapter 7

The inspection of LTC facilities is highly prescribed and written in detail in CMS SOM Chapter 7. Due to the need to ensure that an accurate evaluation of the facilities can occur, states have the responsibility for keeping surveys unannounced and their timing unpredictable. This gives the SSA doing the surveying greater ability to obtain valid information because it increases the probability that the surveys will observe conditions and care practices that are typically present (CMS, 2023c).

When the state has cited deficiencies during the course of a survey, the SSA may, as necessary, conduct a post-survey revisit to determine if the facility now meets the requirements for participation. The deficiencies that are cited indicate what regulations a facility is out of compliance with (Acello, 2005, p. 31).

Upon completion of any type of survey, the surveyors may informally provide on their exit their preliminary findings indicating noncompliance with any requirements/regulations. The surveyors may describe the specific findings of the deficient practice but will not always disclose the scope and severity. The SSA will provide the facility with a Form 2567, which is also known as "Statement of Deficiencies and Plan of Correction." The 2567 contains the deficiency (deficiencies), a regulatory reference, as well as the evidence that supports the deficiency. The SSA has 10 working days to provide the 2567 to the facility. The facility then has 10 calendar days to respond with a "Plan of Correction" (POC), which outlines the following:

- How the facility will correct the deficiency
- The ongoing monitoring of the corrective action
- Who is responsible for the corrective action
- The date the correction will be completed

The SSA reviews the POC for completeness. The SSA may ask the facility to submit additional information, if needed. Once the POC is deemed acceptable, the SSA may conduct a revisit to determine if the facility is in compliance.

A center has an option to dispute a deficiency that they believe is not warranted through the Informal Dispute Resolution (IDR) process. If the facility wishes to pursue an IDR, the formal request needs to be submitted within 10 days of receipt of the 2567.

Noncompliance with regulations may occur for a variety of reasons and can result in harm to residents or put residents at risk for harm. When facilities fail to maintain substantial compliance, CMS uses various enforcement remedies to address a facility's responsibility to promptly achieve, sustain, and maintain compliance with all federal requirements (CMS, 2023c).

Chapter 7 of the SOM also implements the nursing home enforcement regulations. The resulting enforcement action depends on the severity of the deficiencies identified. The remedies can range from civil monetary penalties (fines) to the termination of the Medicare Provider Agreement. The remedy is selected to best achieve the purpose of attaining and sustaining compliance based on the circumstances of each case and recommendations from the SSA. The choices of enforcement remedies include the following:

- Civil monetary penalties
- Directed inservice training
- Directed POC

- Appointment of temporary management
- Denial of payment for all new Medicare and Medicaid admissions
- Denial of all payment for all Medicare and Medicaid residents
- State monitoring
- Termination of the Medicare Provider Agreement

Termination of a facility's provider agreement must be imposed when the facility is not in substantial compliance six months after the last day of the survey identifying deficiencies or within no more than 23 days if immediate jeopardy is identified and not removed (CMS, 2023c).

THE SURVEY PROCESS

As discussed previously, facilities should be survey-ready every day. To help nursing home staff prepare for surveys, tools are available that can provide guidance on what will be surveyed. Surveyors also prepare for a survey, and knowing that process can help nurses better understand the process overall.

Ways LT/PAC Facilities Prepare for Survey

Facilities use a variety of practices, audits, and reports to be survey-ready. An example of a tool that facilities may use is the set of Critical Element Pathways (CEPs). CEPs provide detailed investigative guidance for specific regulatory requirements and are used by surveyors to determine compliance for specific care areas. Because the SSA uses the CEPs for resident/staff interviews and observations, it is a best practice for nursing facilities to use the same tools that surveyors will use to assess their compliance. CEPs serve as a guide to quality care and can help identify areas for improvement. Nurses should become familiar with the CEPs and use them in everyday practice.

The following mandated CEPs are completed by surveyors at each annual/standard survey:

- Dining observation
- Infection control
- Kitchen
- Medication administration

- Medication storage
- QAA/QAPI
- Resident council meeting
- Sufficient and competent nurse staffing
- Beneficiary notice
- Immunizations

Many facilities conduct a "Quality Review/Mock Survey" in preparation for survey. These typically simulate the same survey process the SSA conducts, using the same practices and tools. Survey drills are also a great way to be prepared as well. This ongoing preparation drives resident quality of care.

Other ways to be survey-ready:

- Continuous training with all staff
- Monthly staff communication meetings
- An effective QA/QAPI program
- Active resident council
- An effective customer service program
- An effective grievance program
- Frequent rounding
- Completion of mandated CEPs
- Complete CEPs for any other high-risk areas
- Keep survey book up to date at all times
- Make sure all staff knows their job functions before surveyors enter the facility
- Have a plan for weekend, holiday, and after-hour surveys
- Train staff on what to expect during the survey
- Train staff on how to respond to surveyors when questions are asked
- Review the list of questions surveyors could ask

How Surveyors Prepare for Survey

The following outlines what the surveyors review to prep for a survey:

- MDS data of current residents are used to identify problems to investigate during survey, observe resident progress, and determine effectiveness of interventions
- Review of deficiencies from last standard survey
- Review of complaints and facility reported incident
- Review of any active enforcement against the facility
- Review of any waivers
- 32 residents are included in the initial pool of residents to review
- Vulnerable residents (dependent on staff such as a resident who has Alzheimer's, dependent on staff for care, or is quadriplegic) are added
- New admissions in the last 30 days are included
- At least one resident who smokes, one resident who is receiving dialysis, one resident on hospice, one resident on a ventilator, and two residents who are on transmission-based precautions are added
- Three closed records of discharged residents are added
- Based on the census, the sample of residents will range from 8–35 (for census 175 and greater)

What to Expect on Survey

You are the night nurse/nursing supervisor working at an LT/PAC facility. At 6 a.m., a state surveyor arrives to conduct a complaint investigation that alleges short staffing on the night shift. The administrator and director of nursing won't arrive for another hour. Are you prepared to respond to the surveyor's questions, and do you know what to expect during the course of an investigation?

If the nurse does not know the answer to the surveyor's questions, it is very appropriate to let the surveyor know they are not sure but will get back to them with an answer. Facilities typically have a "survey readiness binder" accessible at all times in the event that surveyors enter the facility when the administrator and/or director of nursing are not present. The point person, usually a nurse, should know where the binder is so they can provide necessary information to the surveyors.

CMS requires that at least 10% of each SSA standard health survey must begin either on the weekend or in the early morning/evening hours before 8 a.m. or after 6 p.m. All CMS inspections are unannounced. The state has the responsibility for keeping surveys unannounced and their timing unpredictable. This gives the state agency doing the surveying greater ability to obtain valid information because it increases the probability that the surveys will observe conditions and care practices that are typically present (CMS, 2023c).

Upon arrival at the center, the survey team will meet with the administrator and/or director of nursing. They will do the following:

- Conduct an entrance conference (surveyors will ask for the Entrance Conference Checklist worksheet, which is a standard form and includes information that surveyors will use to guide the survey. Examples of information include medication administration times, staffing sheets for certain time periods, menus, etc.)
- Tour the facility (tour will include all aspects of the facility)
- Complete medication administration observations
- Attend resident council and/or meet with the resident council president
- Complete resident and staff interviews
- Complete resident and staff observations
- Review policies and procedures noted on Entrance Conference Checklist
- Review medical records

Surveyors use CEPs for conducting resident/staff interviews and observations.

How Survey Results Are Measured/ The 2567 Statement of Deficiencies

As inspection is being conducted, surveyors will evaluate whether noncompliance with any regulation exists. The survey team must use its professional judgment and evidence gathered from observations, interviews, and record reviews to carefully consider the scope and severity of any deficiencies. Upon exit, the surveyors will issue a form 2567, which outlines the scope and severity of any deficient practices that the surveyors identified. Deficient practices are identified using "F-tags," which correspond to a specific regulation (see CMS, 2021 for a list of F-tags).

The severity level reflects the impact of the deficiency and is categorized by four levels of harm:

- No actual harm with potential for minimal harm
- No actual harm with potential for more than minimal harm that is not immediate jeopardy
- Actual harm that is not immediate jeopardy
- Immediate jeopardy to resident health or safety

Immediate jeopardy means a situation in which the facility's noncompliance with one or more requirements of participation has caused, or is likely to cause, serious injury, harm, impairment, or death to a resident.

The scope level of a deficiency reflects how many residents were affected by the deficiency. There are three scope levels assigned to a deficiency:

- Isolated
- Pattern
- Widespread

The SSA determines the scope and severity levels for each deficiency cited at a survey (CMS, n.d.). See Table 10.1.

TABLE 10.1 Assessment Factors Used to Determine the Seriousness of Deficiencies Matrix

	ISOLATED	PATTERN	WIDESPREAD
Immediate jeopardy to resident health or safety	**J** PoC Required	**K** PoC Required	**L** PoC Required
Actual harm that is not immediate	**G** PoC Required	**H** PoC Required	**I** PoC Required
No actual harm with potential for more than minimal harm that is not immediate jeopardy	**D** PoC Required	**E** PoC Required	**F** PoC Required
No actual harm with potential for minimal harm	**A** **No** PoC Required No remedies Commitment to Correct Not on CMS-2567	**B** PoC Required	**C** PoC Required

Substandard quality of care means one or more deficiencies related to participation requirements under §483.10 "Resident rights", paragraphs (a)(1) through (a)(2), (b)(1) through (b)(2), (e) (except for (e)(2), (e)(7), and (e)(8)), (f)(1) through (f)(3), (f)(5) through (f)(8), and (i) of this chapter; §483.12 of this chapter "Freedom from abuse, neglect, and exploitation"; §483.24 of this chapter "Quality of life"; §483.25 of this chapter "Quality of care"; §483.40 "Behavioral health services", paragraphs (b) and (d) of this chapter; §483.45 "Pharmacy services", paragraphs (d), (e), and (f) of this chapter; §483.70 "Administration", paragraph (p) of this chapter, and §483.80 "Infection control", paragraph (d) of this chapter, which constitute either immediate jeopardy to resident health or safety; a pattern of or widespread actual harm that is not immediate jeopardy; or a widespread potential for more than minimal harm, but less than immediate jeopardy, with no actual harm.

Substantial compliance

IMPLICATIONS OF SURVEY RESULTS

As is true for hospitals, CMS uses a Five Star Quality Rating system to measure, benchmark, and report quality. CMS created the system for nursing homes to help consumers, their families, and caregivers compare nursing homes more easily and to call attention to areas about which consumers may want to ask questions, such as staffing practices and wounds and falls rates.

A facility's survey results are considered the cornerstone of the federal Five Star Rating system (Davidson, 2023, p. 14). Many consumers are now shopping on Care Compare (https://www.medicare.gov/care-compare/?redirect=true&providerType=Nursing-Home), a publicly available website that compares nursing homes using the Five Star data on survey, quality, and staffing information, to find an LT/PAC facility.

The methodology to determine a facility's star rating is very complex. The facility's surveys from the prior 36 months are factored into its star rating for the survey domain. The types of surveys included are the three most recent annual surveys, any complaint surveys, and FIC surveys. The number, scope, and severity of deficiencies on each of these surveys are weighted according to CMS algorithms to determine the facility's survey rating (CMS, 2023a).

Five Star Rating Scoring Rules for Survey/Health Inspection Results

Nurses need to be aware how survey results impact a facility's Five Star Rating. Health inspection reports (surveys) receive their own star rating, and these are weighted most heavily in the facility's combined star rating. Points are assigned to deficiencies according to their scope and severity, and the points are then used to generate the star rating. More serious, widespread deficiencies receive more points, with additional points assigned for substandard quality of care. Deficiencies from Life Safety Code or Federal Comparative surveys are not included. However, results of a state survey during a Federal Oversight survey are included. There are also scoring rules for repeat surveyor visits to determine compliance. These are beyond the scope of this chapter.

Survey Scoring Rules Summary

More recent standard surveys are weighted more heavily than earlier surveys, with the most recent period (rating cycle 1) being assigned a weighting factor of 1/2, the previous period (rating cycle 2) having a weighting factor of 1/3, and the second prior period (rating cycle 3) having a weighting factor of 1/6. Differential weighting is also applied to complaint surveys and FIC surveys. The weighting of surveys by cycle is important to know because a facility's overall star rating is impacted.

The rating for survey/health inspections is based on the relative performance of *all facilities* within a state. CMS determines the ratings using these criteria for the performance of facilities within a state:

- Top 10% of facilities receive 5 stars
- Middle 70% receive a rating of 2, 3, or 4 stars with an equal number in each rating category
- Bottom 20% of facilities receive 1 star

The rating is updated monthly on Care Compare. The health inspection cut point tables are updated monthly and posted on CMS.gov.

A facility's survey star rating could change due to the following:

- A new health inspection survey
- A complaint investigation for an FIC survey that results in one or more deficiency citations
- A second, third, or fourth revisit
- Resolution of an Informal Dispute Resolution resulting in changes, and "aging" of complaint and/or FIC survey deficiencies

Rating Methodology for Facilities With Abuse Deficiencies

Care Compare includes an abuse icon that identifies facilities that meet either of the following criteria:

1. Harm level abuse citation in the most recent survey cycle: Cited for abuse where residents were found to be harmed (scope/severity of G or higher) on the most recent survey or on a complaint or FIC survey within the past 12 months
2. Repeat abuse citations: Cited for abuse where residents were found to be potentially harmed (scope/severity of D or higher) on the most recent standard survey or on a complaint or FIC survey within the past 12 months and on the previous (i.e., second most recent) standard survey or on a complaint survey in the prior 12 months (i.e., from 13 to 24 months ago)

Nursing homes that receive the abuse icon can achieve a maximum of 2 stars in their survey/health inspection rating and a maximum of 4 stars in their overall rating. The abuse icon (and the cap on the survey/health inspection rating) will be removed as of the first monthly website refresh following the point at which a nursing home no longer meets the abuse icon criteria.

SCENARIO A Nurse Preparing a Resident's Medications

Nurses spend a good bit of their time administering medications and performing treatments. As part of the annual/standard survey, the surveyor will conduct medication administration observations. The surveyor will choose the nurse they will observe.

A surveyor observes a nurse prepare a resident's medications. The nurse walks into the resident's room without knocking and does not check the resident's identification band. The nurse calls the resident by name and informs them they have their medications. The nurse observes the resident swallow their medication and leaves the room and documents on the resident's medication administration record (MAR). The nurse then proceeds to start reviewing the next resident's MAR. The surveyor stops the nurse and informs them they did not verify the resident's identity prior to administering medication. The nurse responds that they verified the resident by the photo that is part of the resident's MAR. Although the nurse verified the resident's identity, there are other areas of concern with this scenario.

Can you identify the areas of concern?

- For failing to knock on the resident's door prior to entering the resident's room, the facility will receive a deficiency under F 557 Resident Rights-Respect/Dignity/Right to Have Personal Property. The nurse needs to know that a resident's room is their home and that it must be treated as such.
- The nurse also failed to perform hand hygiene after leaving the resident's room and prior to reviewing the next resident's MAR. Not performing hand hygiene will result in F 880 Infection Control deficiency. Hand hygiene must be practiced vigilantly at all times.

SCENARIO Mealtime in the Dining Room

The surveyors are observing the dinner meal in the dining room. There are two certified nursing assistants, one RN, one speech therapist, and one recreation aide (RA). There are 20 residents, and of those 20, 14 are totally dependent for meals. The meals are being delivered to three of the residents at one of the tables while one resident does not receive their meal until the others have almost completed their meal. The RA, who is standing, is assisting a resident with their meal, and this resident was assessed as dependent for meals. Several residents are at tables where the table height is too low, and their wheelchair does not fit under the table. The residents are then sitting alongside the table.

Can you identify what the issues are in this scenario?

- Insufficient staff to provide the meal assistance, which is needed for the 14 residents who are dependent on staff for their meals. The facility will receive a deficiency for F 725 Nursing Services–Sufficient Staff. The nurse needs to know there must be a sufficient number of staff to serve the residents in the dining room.
- The RA is practicing out of their scope, as they have not been deemed competent to feed a dependent resident, resulting in a deficiency for Training Requirements. Staff who are assigned to dining room duties and will be assisting residents with their meals need to be deemed competent to do so.
- The facility will also receive Resident Rights–Respect/Dignity deficiency for the RA standing and not sitting while feeding the resident, and for the residents at the one table not being served at the same time. The nurse needs to know the resident's dining room is their "restaurant," and everyone at the table should be served at the same time.
- The facility will also receive F 558 Resident Rights–Reasonable Accommodations of Needs/Preferences for the tables not being at proper height for wheelchairs. The proper table height is required so residents can sit comfortably at their seat, regardless if they are in a regular dining room chair or wheelchair.

SUMMARY

CMS enforces LT/PAC facility compliance with regulations designed to ensure the health, safety, and well-being of residents who live and/or receive care there. CMS meets this obligation in part by contracting with SSAs to conduct surveys. Federal regulations describe the minimum standards that a facility must meet. The SSA also assures compliance with state or local regulations. An example of a state regulation could be staffing. Some states have specific staffing requirements, which are more stringent than federal requirements. Because of this discrepancy, the facility may receive a state deficiency for staffing but not a federal deficiency. In short, facilities that focus on quality and have control mechanisms in place to ensure systems and processes are sustained fare better with their survey outcomes.

What will be evaluated during a survey is not a mystery. The regulations clearly state the standards that must be met, and the survey will determine if the facility is in compliance (Eliopoulos, 2015, p. 229). To assure compliance with regulations, nurses should be familiar with regulations and adhere to practices that support them. CMS indicates the minimum standards that an LT/PAC facility must meet. Nursing leaders must strive for high standards that incorporate evidence-based and best practices to support optimal care and operations.

Being survey-ready every day will ensure quality of care, patient and employee satisfaction, and exceptional clinical, financial, and survey outcomes. When the right actions are taken every day to support quality and safety, excellent outcomes will follow.

REFERENCES

Acello, B. (2005). *The long-term care nursing desk reference.* HCPRO, Inc.

American Medical Directors Association. (2002). *White paper on the survey process.* https://paltc.org/amda-white-papers-and-resolution-position-statements/white-paper-survey-process

Cadmus, E., Salmond, S., Hassler, L., Bohnarczyk, N., & Black, K. (2017). *Developing a residency in post-acute care.* Sigma Theta Tau International.

Centers for Medicare & Medicaid Services. (n.d.). *Nursing home enforcement.* https://www.cms.gov/Medicare/Provider-Enrollment-and-Certification/SurveyCertificationEnforcement/Nursing-Home-Enforcement

Centers for Medicare & Medicaid Services. (2014, April 18). *S&C: 14-22-NH.* https://www.cms.gov/Medicare/Provider-Enrollment-and-Certification/SurveyCertificationGenInfo/Downloads/Survey-and-Cert-Letter-14-22.pdf

Centers for Medicare & Medicaid Services. (2015, Nov. 27). *S&C: 16-04-NH.* https://www.cms.gov/Medicare/Provider-Enrollment-and-Certification/SurveyCertificationGenInfo/Downloads/Survey-and-Cert-Letter-16-04.pdf

Centers for Medicare & Medicaid Services. (2019a). *State operations manual appendix Q.* https://www.cms.gov/Regulations-and-guidance/Guidance/Manuals/downloads/som107ap_q_immedjeopardy.pdf

Centers for Medicare & Medicaid Services. (2019b). *State operations manual chapter 4.* https://www.hhs.gov/guidance/sites/default/files/hhs-guidance-documents/11936_som107c04.pdf

Centers for Medicare & Medicaid Services. (2020a). *QSO 20-20-All.* https://www.cms.gov/files/document/qso-20-20-all.pdf

Centers for Medicare & Medicaid Services. (2020b). *State operations manual chapter 2.* https://www.hhs.gov/guidance/sites/default/files/hhs-guidance-documents/som107c02.pdf

Centers for Medicare & Medicaid Services. (2021). *List of revised F-tags.* https://www.cms.gov/Medicare/Provider-Enrollment-and-Certification/GuidanceforLawsAndRegulations/Downloads/List-of-Revised-FTags.pdf

Centers for Medicare & Medicaid Services. (2022a). *Admin Info: 22-10-All.* https://www.cms.gov/files/document/admin-22-10-all.pdf

Centers for Medicare & Medicaid Services. (2022b). *QSO-23-01-NH.* https://www.cms.gov/files/document/qso-23-01-nh.pdf

Centers for Medicare & Medicaid Services. (2023a). *Design for Care Compare nursing home Five-Star Quality Rating system: Technical users' guide.* https://www.cms.gov/medicare/provider-enrollment-and-certification/certificationandcomplianc/downloads/usersguide.pdf

Centers for Medicare & Medicaid Services. (2023b). *State operations manual chapter 5.* https://www.cms.gov/Regulations-and-Guidance/Guidance/Manuals/Downloads/som107c05pdf.pdf

Centers for Medicare & Medicaid Services. (2023c). *State operations manual chapter 7.* https://www.hhs.gov/guidance/sites/default/files/hhs-guidance-documents/som107c07.pdf

Davidson, M. S. (2023, March 24). A growing threat to nursing home safety. *Newsweek.*

Eliopoulos, C. (2015). *Fast facts for the long-term care nurse: What nursing home and assisted living nurses need to know in a nutshell.* Springer Publishing.

Institute of Medicine. (1986). *Improving the quality of care in nursing homes*. National Academies Press. https://www.ncbi.nlm.nih.gov/books/NBK217556/

Kapp, M. B. (2014). Are nursing home regulations like cobwebs? *The Gerontologist, 54*(5), 886–890.

Medicare and Medicaid Programs. (2015, July 16). *Reform of requirements for long-term care facilities, 80 Fed. Reg. 42167, to be codified at 42 CFR. pts. 405, 431, 447, 482, 483, 485, & 488*. Centers for Medicare & Medicaid Services. https://www.federalregister.gov/documents/2015/07/16/2015-17207/medicare-and-medicaid-programs-reform-of-requirements-for-long-term-care-facilities

Unroe, K. T., Ouslander, J. G., & Saliba, D. (2017). Nursing home regulations redefined: Implications for providers. *Journal of the American Geriatric Society, 66*(1), 191–194. https://doi.org/10.1111/jgs.15128

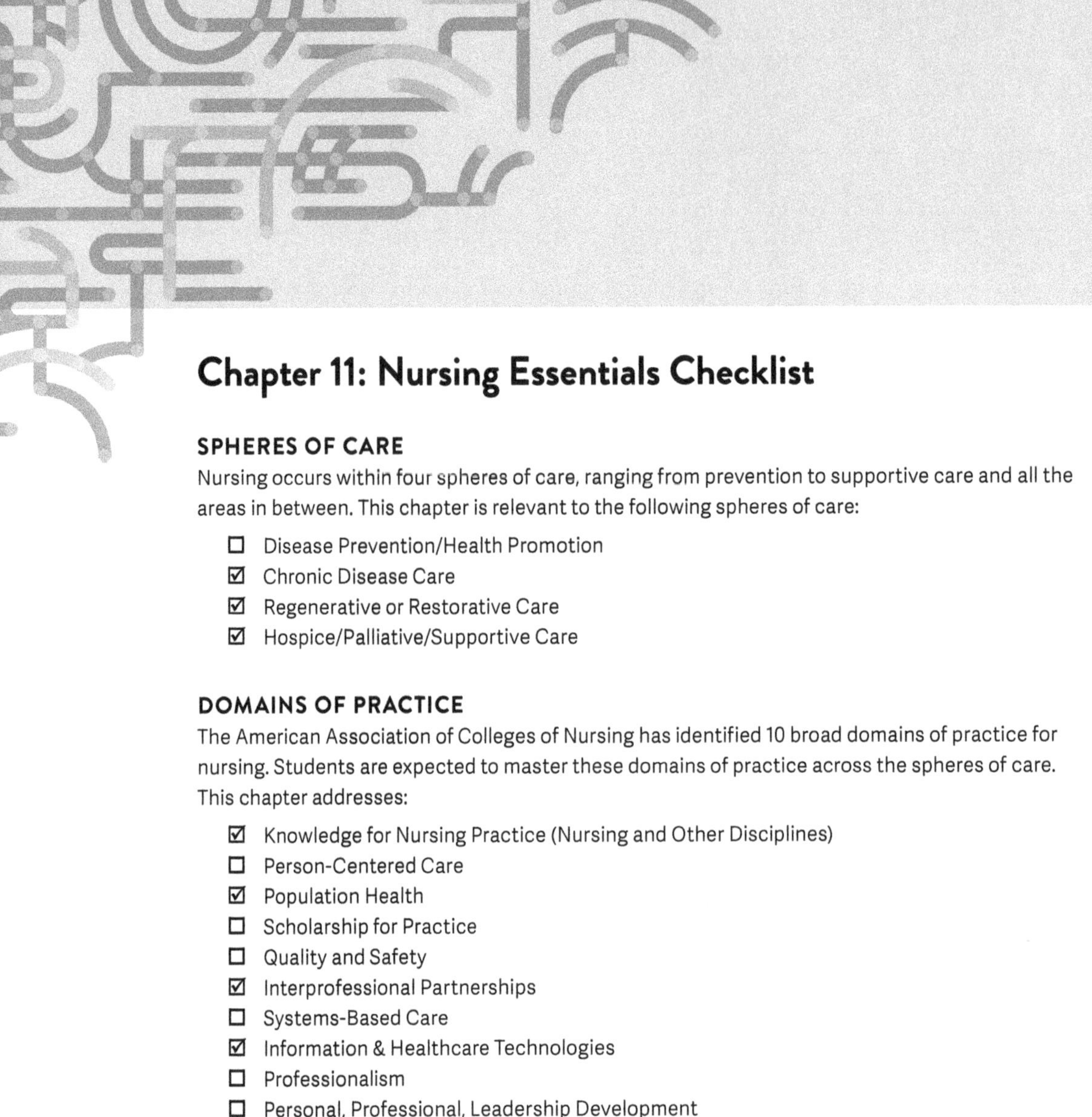

Chapter 11: Nursing Essentials Checklist

SPHERES OF CARE

Nursing occurs within four spheres of care, ranging from prevention to supportive care and all the areas in between. This chapter is relevant to the following spheres of care:

- ☐ Disease Prevention/Health Promotion
- ☑ Chronic Disease Care
- ☑ Regenerative or Restorative Care
- ☑ Hospice/Palliative/Supportive Care

DOMAINS OF PRACTICE

The American Association of Colleges of Nursing has identified 10 broad domains of practice for nursing. Students are expected to master these domains of practice across the spheres of care. This chapter addresses:

- ☑ Knowledge for Nursing Practice (Nursing and Other Disciplines)
- ☐ Person-Centered Care
- ☑ Population Health
- ☐ Scholarship for Practice
- ☐ Quality and Safety
- ☑ Interprofessional Partnerships
- ☐ Systems-Based Care
- ☑ Information & Healthcare Technologies
- ☐ Professionalism
- ☐ Personal, Professional, Leadership Development

CONCEPTS FOR PRACTICE

Integrated across the domains of practice are eight concepts which the student is expected to master across the spheres of care and across the domains of practice. This chapter addresses:

- ☐ Clinical Judgment
- ☑ Communication
- ☐ Compassionate Care
- ☐ Diversity, Equity, Inclusion
- ☐ Ethics
- ☐ Evidence-Based Practice
- ☑ Health Policy
- ☐ Social Determinants of Health

CHAPTER 11

FINANCING LONG-TERM CARE

Nancy D. Zionts, MBA
Sophie A. Campbell, MSN, RN, CRRN, RAC-CT, CNDLTC
Brian Stever, BSN, RN, RAC-CT

OBJECTIVES

1. Differentiate between qualifications and payment for short-term post-acute care versus long-term care in nursing homes.
2. Appreciate the nurse's role in timely and accurate documentation in the health record to support nursing home reimbursement.
3. Describe the structure and contribution of the Minimum Data Set in payment to nursing homes for care delivered.
4. Delineate the differences between nonprofit and for-profit nursing homes.

INTRODUCTION

At this point in your education, as you are perhaps considering working as a licensed RN caring for residents in long-term care (LTC), you have been exposed to a whole range of courses—many focused on clinical conditions you will face on the front line, and others on principles of nursing, teamwork, communications, and so forth. And now, you turn the page in this book and the chapter title is "Financing Long-Term Care." You might be tempted to ask, "Why would I need this information? I will be a member of the nursing staff, not administration or finance." The challenge we face as authors in just these few pages is to explain to you why financing of LTC is relevant and even a core part of your role. We describe how LTC services are billed and paid for, how that affects the role of nurses, and why the accurate documentation of services delivered to residents is so important.

HOW NURSES ARE PAID

Before we talk about how an LTC organization gets paid and how reimbursement is made to LTC, do you know how nurses are paid?

For the most part, that is a simple answer: You will be paid a wage based on your job title and role, experience, specialties, and working status (whether you are full time or part time or hourly). Some LTC providers pay a salary to all management staff positions, which is most often the role of the RN in LTC. However, LTC providers separate wages by specific positions:

- **Salaried positions:** "Exempt" from overtime, salaried employees receive the same pay each pay period regardless of the hours they work.
- **Hourly positions:** "Non-exempt" from overtime, hourly employees are paid at a specific rate for each hour worked, and they are eligible for overtime pay for logging more than full-time hours in a work week.

Which type of position you have will be determined between you and your manager when you accept a role in LTC. That is the good news. On a shift-by-shift basis, you do not have the pressure of worrying about the number of residents in your facility, how long they are there, and what their diagnoses are.

WHY LEARN ABOUT NURSING HOME FINANCING?

So, if your salary is secured, why learn about nursing home financing?

Your job is to use your best clinical judgment to focus on what matters to each resident and their care needs, and how best you can deliver care to address those needs. But that does not mean you don't have to know how your organization is financed, and how what you do every shift influences the payments your organization receives.

First, while you may be starting off on the front line, given the nature of the LTC environment, you may find yourself moving up the career ladder very quickly. Contrary to other environments like acute care, the distance between the entry-level positions in a nursing home and administrative or managerial positions is very short. That is to say, you will be responsible for administrative functions at the point of care (knowing what your resident needs and addressing those needs while executing critical thinking skills to plan care and manage changes of condition), and you may grow into an administrative position (clinical manager, unit manager, shift supervisor, assistant director of nursing, or director of nursing) fairly quickly.

Second, just as what you do as a clinician can be directly correlated with how well your residents progress through their disease processes and course of treatment, what you do can also be correlated to how much your organization will be paid for the delivered care. While that seems like a lot of pressure, our message to you is simple:

- Focus on using your clinical judgment to deliver what the resident needs.
- Make sure that you very carefully and accurately document the care need, your responses, the time spent, and the resources consumed in their care.

If you do those things, the financing will take care of itself. Quality of resident care is first, and the reimbursement follows the care.

As you read this chapter, keep the above points in mind, and remember your clear role in financing

HOW FINANCING AND YOUR ROLE AS PART OF THE NURSING STAFF INTERSECT

The rest of this chapter outlines the many different types of reimbursements and payors, services that are or are not covered by those payors, and the detailed documentation required to justify those payments.

The Financing System in Long-Term Care Is Complex

Far from being simple, financing the care in nursing homes demands that managers balance many often competing and equally important elements in an environment known for complex funding. Nursing homes, like other healthcare settings, face onerous and conflicting regulations and a range of arrangements with different payment sources, care limits (hours per day, per week, etc.), matching reimbursement requirements and consumer copays, levels of family engagement (or not), requirements to show progress to continue services and payment, and reporting requirements and quality targets/incentives.

The financing landscape in LTC is ever-evolving. Although the primary payors are federal (Medicare, the Veterans Administration, PACE [Program for All Inclusive Care for the Elderly]), even they have different programmatic guidelines and requirements. In addition, each state has Medicaid programs (medical assistance for persons with disabilities or income below a certain threshold) for their residents who qualify, and those also come with their own regulations and payment guidelines that require compliance to ensure accurate reimbursement.

Even within Medicare, there are Medicare Advantage plans that offer different payments that come with different "strings attached" or rules and regulations for providers. And many states have implemented Mandatory Medicaid Managed Care Programs for Long Term Services and Supports, meaning there are insurers contracted by the state reviewing the care delivered and determining and making payments to the LTC facility.

You may on any given day be caring for 10 residents—all with different payment programs covering the care you provide—from fee-for-service to global payments to daily rates to incentive programs. To be sure, it is a challenging reimbursement environment, with providers experiencing financial pressures. That fact is not new, but the specific pressures and demands to receive reimbursement on providers are ever-changing.

The Varied Payors for Nursing Homes: Who Pays for What?

In this section, we cover how the nursing home is paid. The staff payments have to come from somewhere, and those staff salaries come from the payments that the nursing home receives, generally lumped under the umbrella term *reimbursement.* Many factors go into determining how nursing homes are reimbursed, including the level of care the resident is receiving (short-term post-acute versus long-term care), the payment sources for the care, the length of their stay, and whether they are admitted after an acute-care stay or direct from the community.

Private Pay

One of the payment types for LTC in a nursing home is personal payment or "out-of-pocket" payments. This is not strictly a reimbursement but rather a direct payment. In this case, the nursing home sends a bill or invoice to the resident, their family, financial power of attorney, or someone who is managing and responsible for the finances each month to pay for the care and services delivered at the nursing home. Residents or their families can use personal savings, retirement funds, interest on investments or bank accounts, or money from the sale of the resident's home and personal property.

Short-Stay Residents and Medicare/Insurance Plans

Medicare as a reimbursement is provided by a federal program, funded by deductions that we each pay from our salaries when we have a job. It is available to people age 65 or older and younger people with specific disabilities and medical health conditions who have qualified. Medicare provides payment for the skilled nursing portion of the nursing home stay (short stay/post-acute care) and for specific care and services for the LTC resident in the nursing home. For example, a resident who has been in the nursing home for several years but needs services from rehabilitation therapy would have those services paid for by Medicare under the Medicare Part B portion (Medicare Part A pays for the skilled nursing care in the nursing home). To learn more about Medicare, go to Medicare.gov.

When a patient is admitted to the nursing home for a short-term admission, referred to as short-term stay, short-term rehabilitation, post-acute stay, or skilled nursing, there are more options for reimbursement than when the patient stays at the nursing home as a long-stay resident and lives there. The short-term stay is a transition for a patient between hospital care/surgery and being able to manage in the community. Typically, this care is more intensive and is at a higher cost to the nursing home, which would translate to a higher bill to the patient's insurance plan. This level of care is usually reimbursed to the nursing home by either a federal government payment (the most common being Medicare) or by a commercial insurance payor.

If the resident has switched from Medicare provided by the federal government to a Medicare Advantage Plan/Managed Care Plan—such as Highmark, Humana, Aetna, or many other choices—then the Minimum Data Set (MDS) tool will be submitted to this payor for reimbursement to the nursing home for resident care, and that is also based on the care delivered and diagnoses (see the "Minimum Data Set 3.0" section later in this chapter for a definition of and coding information for MDS). This is the same with a commercial insurance payor. Commercial plans are not required to pay the same as Medicare, but they are usually very similar to what the federal Medicare program reimburses. These payors also require pre-authorization (prior approval) for the patient who is their beneficiary to be admitted to the nursing home. They also require *re-authorization*, which is a review of the current status of the skilled nursing patient to determine if they will authorize additional days of short-term care reimbursement to the nursing home. This is often done using medical record documentation.

Long-Stay Residents and Medicaid

Residents who remain in the nursing home for LTC, which means they are making the nursing home their home, have their care and services reimbursed to the nursing home through other payor sources. Usually, this payor source is Medicaid. This reimbursement is managed at the state level but is a combined state and federal program. Medicaid covers the cost of room and board at the nursing home (or the cost of living there and the medical needs for the residents).

Who Is Eligible for Medicaid?

Medicaid eligibility by the resident in the nursing home depends on their assets and income levels. Each state determines the eligibility requirements of the residents and the asset qualification levels. Most residents need to "spend down" their assets before they are eligible for Medicaid. This type of reimbursement is usually the same amount for each LTC resident who is a Medicaid beneficiary. To learn more about Medicaid as a reimbursement source, visit Medicaid.gov.

What Services Can Be Billed for in Nursing Homes

There are many clinical conditions and services that *can* be provided in a nursing home for which the nursing home will be reimbursed or paid for. It is a matter of ensuring the patient/resident care is represented in the medical record documentation and knowing which entity will be paying the nursing home for the care. It would seem, at first blush, that a nursing home would not be the place for many highly skilled care services, but looking at all levels of care, the following are included in the consolidated reimbursement to the nursing home:

- Room and board
- Meals
- Medical supplies

- Medications
- Activities
- Social services
- Dietitian services
- Nursing services
- Pastoral care/worship services
- Rehabilitation therapy treatment services
- Restorative nursing services
- Physician assessment visits

In addition to these basic services provided and paid for in the nursing home, residents can also receive services from a podiatrist, optometrist, dentist, psychologist, or psychiatrist, either in the nursing home or through an outside appointment. Nursing home residents can also be transferred to a hospital or clinic for services that are excluded from the consolidated billing such as radiation therapy, dialysis, blood transfusions, and emergency services. Some of the clinical care areas that are included in nursing home care and reimbursed to the nursing home include:

- Intravenous (IV) therapy
- Wound care services (pressure ulcers, arterial ulcers, venous ulcers, surgical wounds, or burn care)
- Chemotherapy treatment
- Tracheostomy care
- Ventilator care for either weaning or dependency
- Isolation for infectious diseases
- Oxygen administration
- Respiratory therapy
- Enteral feedings—nasogastric or through gastrostomy
- Behavioral management and interventions

- Specific diagnosis care related to diabetes, COPD, hemiplegia/hemiparesis, quadriplegia, septicemia, pneumonia, coma, respiratory failure, multiple sclerosis, Parkinson's disease, and cerebral palsy

Respite Care

Another level of care that can be found in a nursing home is *respite care*. This is a service that some but not all nursing homes provide as temporary relief to primary caregivers who are caring for persons living in the community. For example, adult children caring for a parent in their home who will be taking a vacation can place their parent in the nursing home for a short, temporary stay called *respite*. Each nursing home maintains their own guidelines or criteria on the acceptable length of stay for respite care.

Medicare does not typically reimburse the nursing home for respite stays except for persons enrolled in a hospice program. There is the potential for some combinations of care levels that can result in a respite stay in a nursing home being reimbursed by Medicare for a very limited number of days. Most insurance plans do not pay nursing homes for respite stays. Medicaid may provide some level of reimbursement to the nursing home, but that varies per state and the level of care the resident is receiving. Respite stays in the nursing home are usually paid for as private pay or reimbursed to the nursing home by the family, resident, or the assets of the resident.

Hospice and Palliative Care

Nursing homes also provide hospice care services and palliative care services. These service levels are very similar yet different. *Hospice* is provided to residents who meet certain criteria in the last six months of their lives. *Palliative care* is intended to focus on the resident's quality of life and matches the medical care for the symptoms of serious illnesses such as COPD, cancer, heart failure, dementia, and others to the residents' *goals for care*.

Palliative is a level of care only recognized within the plan of care for the resident in the nursing home and does not result in a differentiation for payment sources. Palliative care is usually provided directly to LTC nursing home residents by LTC staff or by outside medical consultants (physicians and advanced practice providers), and the resident care is reimbursed to the facility by the same methods as LTC.

Hospice care is also provided in a nursing home and is end-of-life care. Hospice care focuses on comfort and quality of life, with care decisions directed by the advanced directive of the resident. Residents may elect not to receive certain treatments or care, such as readmission to the hospital for a change in condition. Hospice care is provided for residents with six months or less to live if the disease follows its expected course who have opted to receive palliation for their qualifying diagnosis.

A resident of the nursing home receiving hospice care will receive the majority of care from the nursing home caregivers, with the hospice team assisting as a cohesive part of the care management team. Hospice services can include treatment orders, plans of care, social services, pastoral care, and activities of daily living assistance on a specific number of days per week. Reimbursement to the nursing home for this level of care is sometimes made by Medicare under the hospice benefit, sometimes made by the hospice directly to the nursing home, and sometimes reimbursed by Medicaid. Some private insurance plans do have hospice coverage.

Consolidated Billing Under Medicare: What Is Excluded

As previously stated, the majority of skilled nursing stays are reimbursed to the nursing home by the federal Medicare program/Medicare Advantage Plans or other commercial insurance payors. Medicare and the Medicare Advantage Plans utilize something called *consolidated billing*, which was part of the Balanced Budget Act of 1997 and became law effective for nursing homes on or after July 1, 1998. This required the nursing home to submit one "consolidated" bill for all care and services for skilled residents. This creates a situation where duplicate bills cannot be sent for the same services. If a nursing home accepts a resident for care, all care is included in the consolidated bill except for the documented exclusions in a coordination of care system. The consolidated billing resembles the bundled payments that hospitals use.

The excluded services from consolidated billing are those that are not expected to be provided in a nursing home setting. These services will be reimbursed by the federal government to the provider of the services, but they do not have to be included under consolidated billing for the nursing home. For example, a nursing home resident has bloodwork completed during the skilled nursing stay and is transferred to the hospital for a CT scan. The bloodwork is considered part of consolidated billing and will be reimbursed to the nursing home, along with all other skilled resident care. However, the CT scan is an exclusion to consolidated billing and will not be included in the consolidated billing reimbursement bill from the nursing home to the federal government for Medicare. The CT scan will be paid to the hospital or outpatient center that completed it, but that site will have to independently bill Medicare for payment because CT scans are an exclusion.

Excluded services to consolidated billing for the nursing home skilled residents include:

- Physician services—these include the physician visits to the nursing home to assess the residents as well as the physician component of reading an X-ray, reviewing a swallow study, and many others
- Physician assistants working under the supervision of a physician
- Qualified psychologists
- Certified registered anesthetists
- Hospice care related to a terminal condition
- Cardiac catheterizations
- CT scans
- Magnetic resonance imaging (MRI)
- Radiation therapy services
- Angiography
- Ambulatory surgery that includes the use of an operating room
- Emergency services
- Dialysis services
- Epoetin/darbepoetin alfa when administered during dialysis
- Medically necessary ambulance services for dialysis transports
- Certain lymphatic and venous procedures
- Chemotherapy *
- Radioisotope services *

- Custom prosthetic devices *
- Ambulance transportation to the nursing home for an admission or from the nursing home for a discharge

**These exclusions are not broad categories. There are only certain and specific items in these categories that are excluded from consolidated billing.*

Note that a new list of consolidated billing exclusions is provided each calendar year by the federal government. Exclusions are both added to and eliminated from the list following review by the federal government.

The Reimbursement Bottom Line for Nursing Staff

It is important for nursing staff to collect information about payment source(s) at the time of admission, which will provide the foundation for accurate billing and timely reimbursement for the care and services the facility has provided.

But the bottom line is the same: The role of the nurse in the nursing home is to provide the highest level of quality resident care that is safe, based on standards of practice, and compliant with regulatory requirements, and facility policies and the reimbursement will follow.

NURSING STAFF AND DOCUMENTATION: WHERE FINANCING AND THE CARE YOU PROVIDE INTERSECT

Regardless of how the facility you work for is paid, what you as a staff member need to focus on in any senior living services or LTC location is the care of the person and documenting what you have done and what resources have been expended in care of your residents.

As discussed above, reimbursement for the skilled nursing stay is based on the patient/resident conditions and level of care required and provided. These items must be documented in the medical record as support for the care delivered and require that interdisciplinary team members, especially nursing, "show your work." Documentation is the only validation that the care provided matches assessed needs. Assessment data are collected using the MDS tool.

The Payment Structures for Nursing Homes

Over the years, the methodology for nursing facility payment has changed. The Centers for Medicare & Medicaid Services (CMS) originally paid nursing facilities based on a "fee-for-service" model, where a facility would submit claim information for each resident and receive payment based on each individual service provided. For example, a resident's physical, occupational, speech therapy, and any other skilled services items were billed separately based on the allowable payment rate for that service, adjusted for location in the country. This model was difficult to monitor and control, so the federal government enacted the Balanced Budget Act of 1997. This new act mandated the implementation of a per diem Prospective Payment System, or PPS (CMS, 2022b, 2023b). This allowed for a more streamlined way of payment. Over the years, that payment structure has changed and improved.

The Current System: Patient-Driven Payment Model or PDPM

The current reimbursement system for nursing homes for skilled residents is the Patient-Driven Payment Model (PDPM). This went into effect October 1, 2019. Under PDPM, consolidated billing remains in effect for paying nursing homes for care of skilled nursing or short-term residents, but in this system, the various cost drivers of resident care are recognized and accounted for. PDPM includes a component for medical diagnoses and clinical conditions, recognizing that medical conditions require different care levels. It also includes two components for rehabilitation therapy. One component is a combination of physical and occupational therapies and the second is for speech language pathology. These rehabilitation therapy components focus on the diagnoses and clinical conditions that resulted in the need for the rehabilitation therapy, which are clinical care factors.

There is also a nursing care component to levels of reimbursement by amount of nursing time required (intensity) or skill levels. And finally, there is the resident functional mobility level. This factor adjusts payment for skilled care that requires more staff time, energy, and equipment to assist residents who are less functionally mobile than for those who are more functionally mobile. The PDPM reimbursement system relies on coding in the MDS assessment tool, and that tool relies on medical record documentation completed by nursing home team members related to the care and services provided for the residents.

The PDPM model is much more complex than previous models because it utilizes a six-category classification system to place a resident into a variety of case mix groupers (a *grouper* refers to a classification scheme that places "like" patients together based on projected resource consumption). The categories are:

1. Physical Therapy
2. Occupational Therapy
3. Speech Language Pathology
4. Nursing Services
5. Non-Therapy Ancillary Services
6. Non-Case Mix

Because there are so many categories, it means there are approximately 28,000 variations available in which to classify a single person! Some details (CMS, 2022a):

- Each category is created based on specific issues/services the resident is experiencing or utilizing, such as their primary diagnosis and other diagnoses associated with their care, their functional ability, special treatments, procedures, or programs they may have during their stay.
- The codes are a set of letters of the alphabet in each category. Physical Therapy and Occupational Therapy classify in the same letter of the alphabet, Speech Language Pathology is another letter, Nursing Services is another, and Non-Therapy Ancillary Services is classified separately.
- These groupers combine into the Health Insurance Prospective Payment System (HIPPS) codes. HIPPS rate codes, representing specific sets of patient characteristics (or case mix groups), are used by health insurers to make payment determinations under several prospective payment systems.
- Case mix groups are developed based on research into utilization patterns among various provider types. For the payment systems that use HIPPS codes, clinical assessment data are the basic input.

Minimum Data Set 3.0

How does a patient/resident classify into these case mix groupers? Skilled nursing facilities (SNFs) use the MDS, a mandatory standardized assessment. In 2010, CMS implemented MDS version 3.0. This version of the MDS was created in a way that would allow a more agile platform to be used. Previously, if questions were to be added, they had to be added to the end of a section or a new section had to be created. There was no way the document could expand and allow the questions to be folded into the area where they were most relevant. Now, each time an appropriate change is needed, the form can absorb those questions.

The MDS 3.0 is the most comprehensive documentation tool for LTC. Organized into sections, each section reviews a specific area of a resident's situation. The Resident Assessment Instrument Manual version 1.17.1 provides guidance on how to code the information for the resident. Table 11.1 displays the intent for each section of the MDS (CMS, 2023a).

TABLE 11.1 Coding Resident Information With the MDS

MDS SECTION	TITLE	INTENT
A	Identification Information	Obtain key information to uniquely identify each resident, nursing home, type of record, and reasons for assessment.
B	Hearing, Speech, and Vision	Document the resident's ability to hear, understand, and communicate with others and whether the resident experiences visual, hearing, or speech limitations and/or difficulties.
C	Cognitive Patterns	Determine the resident's attention, orientation, and ability to register and recall information.
D	Mood	Identify signs and symptoms of mood distress.
E	Behavior	Identify behavioral symptoms that may cause distress or are potentially harmful to the resident, or may be distressing or disruptive to facility residents, staff members, or the environment.
F	Preferences for Customary Routine and Activities	Obtain information regarding the resident's preferences for his or her daily routine and activities.
G	Functional Status	Assess the need for assistance with activities of daily living (ADLs), altered gait and balance, and decreased range of motion.
GG	Functional Abilities and Goals	Assess the need for assistance with self-care and mobility activities.

MDS SECTION	TITLE	INTENT
H	Bladder and Bowel	Gather information on the use of bowel and bladder appliances, the use of and response to urinary toileting programs, urinary and bowel continence, bowel training programs, and bowel patterns.
I	Active Diagnoses	Code diseases that have a relationship to the resident's current functional, cognitive, mood or behavior status, medical treatments, nursing monitoring, or risk of death.
J	Health Conditions	Document health conditions that impact the resident's functional status and quality of life.
K	Swallowing/ Nutritional Status	Assess conditions that could affect the resident's ability to maintain adequate nutrition and hydration.
L	Oral/Dental Status	Record any oral or dental problems present.
M	Skin Conditions	Document the risk, presence, appearance, and change of pressure ulcers as well as other skin ulcers, wounds, or lesions. Also includes treatment categories related to skin injury or avoiding injury.
N	Medications	Record the number of days that any type of injection, insulin, and/or select medications was received by the resident.
O	Special Treatments, Procedures, and Programs	Identify any special treatments, procedures, and programs that the resident received during the specified time periods.
P	Restraints and Alarms	Record the frequency that the resident was restrained by any of the listed devices at any time during the day or night; record the frequency that any of the listed alarms were used.
Q	Participation in Assessment and Goal Setting	Record the participation of the resident, family, and/or significant others in the assessment, and to understand the resident's overall goals.
V	Care Area Assessment (CAA) Summary	Document triggered care areas, whether or not a care plan has been developed for each triggered area, and the location of care area assessment documentation.
X	Correction Request	Request to modify or inactivate a record already present in the QIES ASAP database.
Z	Assessment Administration	Provide billing information and signatures of persons completing the assessment.

From CMS, 2023a

Why Your Documentation Matters

Documentation does matter. The way in which nurses and other team members document the services they provide will ensure that the organization is reimbursed accurately for those services. And although the RN might not complete every section, an RN must certify the MDS as complete and accurate.

Documentation Supports Eligibility

Residents admitted into an SNF under Medicare Part A must meet certain criteria for continuation of that stay. Medicare Part A covers skilled nursing care if the following conditions are met (Medicare.gov, n.d.):

- The resident has Part A and has days left in their benefit period to use.
- The resident has had a qualifying hospital stay (three midnights as an inpatient in a hospital).
- The resident's doctor has decided that the resident needs daily skilled care, AND it must be given by, or under the supervision of, skilled nursing or therapy staff.
- The resident receives these skilled services in an SNF that is certified by Medicare.
- The skilled services are provided on a daily basis (five days per week for therapy and seven days per week for nursing).
- The resident needs these skilled services for a medical condition that is either:
    - A hospital-related medical condition treated during their qualifying three-day inpatient hospital stay, even if it was not the reason they were admitted to the hospital
    - A condition that started while they were getting care in the SNF for a hospital-related medical condition (e.g., if they develop an infection that requires IV antibiotics while they are getting SNF care)

Types of skilled services include but are not limited to:

- **Stroke recovery:** rehabilitation therapy, helping patients regain motor skills and speech functions

- **Parkinson's care:** specific care required to attend advanced Parkinson's cases (does not apply for all facilities)
- **General wound care:** wound cleaning and antibiotics administration for infection
- **Acute medical conditions:** services offered to help cases where an illness, infection, or injury threatens the patient's health
- **General rehabilitation:** speech, physical, and occupational therapy, and other services to help patients recover after an extended illness or invasive operation

What Good Documentation Looks Like

Most electronic health records used in SNFs have some type of daily skilled documentation included in their programming. A good daily skilled note as well as weekly summary/review of progress toward goals should be included in the process. The documentation should support that SNF care was reasonable and necessary by illustrating these points:

- Reasons for skilled stay—for example, medically complex condition (surgical wound care, pressure injury care, etc.)
- Intensity of therapy provided with tolerance
- Less than 24 hour/day care would impose safety risks and/or adverse impact on resident's medical condition

Conditions/observations that do not support continued skilled care:

- Custodial care or maintaining
- Poor or fair rehab potential
- Inability to follow directions
- Refusal to participate in treatment (investigate why this occurs and document that in the note as well)
- "Resting comfortably, no complaints of pain"
- Chronic condition
- Lack of motivation

- Little change or status quo
- Plateau
- Ambulating "ad lib"

Here is an example of a good skilled note:

> Mr. Collins is a 69-year-old male retired stunt driver admitted to the community s/p bladder cancer with surgical removal of a malignant tumor. He has received intermittent catheterization due to bladder retention caused by the surgical procedure. He is also on a scheduled toileting program to improve his continence. He is receiving radiation outpatient twice weekly and is monitored for radiation dermatitis at the site. He is moderately depressed from his loss of independence due to cancer as noted from his PHQ-9 score of 11. He had a CVA two years ago with associated dysphagia with occasional coughing while eating but has no other limitations. He also has a history of smoking two packs of cigarettes daily for 35 years and has COPD based on this history, with oxygen use. He stated that he cannot lie flat due to shortness of breath; therefore, the staff have placed the head of the bed elevated each night, which is documented in the plan of care. While in the hospital, he acquired a stage 3 pressure injury on his sacrum due to lack of movement in bed. He is receiving wound care daily. There is a potential for his wound to take a while to heal due to a diagnosis of DM type 2.

In this note, you see all areas that are important to the resident and his daily care. A weekly summary of this same information could be written as:

> Resident continues to require intermittent catheterization due to bladder retention. The last catheterization was two days ago. His toileting program has improved his continence, and currently, he is incontinent less than once daily. The skin at the radiation site continues to be clean and dry with no signs of breakdown. His last radiation treatment is scheduled for a week from today. His depression has improved since he is less incontinent, and his cancer is responding. His swallowing is improving since he has been treated by speech therapy, but he does continue to have occasional coughing with liquids. The stage 3 pressure injury is resolving with dietary changes and daily wound treatments. The wound edges are clean, and the overall size has decreased by 25% in the last week.

Though these daily skilled notes are for residents under Medicare A/Managed Care Insurance payors, *any resident* that is in LTC can have the same type of note written. Many states still use some type of case mix index to reimburse a facility for their services provided. So, how does what you document equate to how you are reimbursed?

Each resident MDS is coded based on the information provided during the allowed time frame of that MDS. Most areas are coded for either a seven- or 14-day window. If we were to take the information just from the note written about Mr. Collins and place it on his MDS for reimbursement, we would see a HIPPS code of KEFC1. This HIPPS code places him at a very complex level of care; therefore, the SNF facility reimbursement will be higher than the average daily rate and will appropriately reimburse the nursing facility for the intensity of Mr. Collins' care.

Nonprofit Nursing Homes Versus For-Profit Nursing Homes

Quite simply, a for-profit nursing home, although subject to the same regulatory requirements, is operated as a business, intended to create a financial return for its owners or shareholders. In comparison, nonprofit nursing homes are accountable to a community board that is responsible for a mission and that operates to reinvest any excess revenues over expenses into the community and services that will benefit the people who live there. And when revenues are insufficient to meet the expenses demands, nonprofit boards often engage in community fundraising to cover the difference and maintain their operations.

SUMMARY

As you consider what you have read in this chapter, remember your role in financing is clear:

- Focus on using your clinical judgment to deliver the highest level of quality resident care that is safe, based on standards of practice, and compliant with regulatory requirements and facility policies.
- Make sure that you have very carefully and accurately documented the care need, your actions, the time spent, and the resources consumed in care to best represent the status of the resident and their care needs.

If you do those things, the financing will take care of itself.

REFERENCES

Centers for Medicare & Medicaid Services. (2022a). *Definition and uses of Health Insurance Prospective Payment System codes (HIPPS codes).* https://www.cms.gov/Medicare/Medicare-Fee-for-Service-Payment/ProspMedicareFeeSvcPmtGen/Downloads/hippsuses.pdf

Centers for Medicare & Medicaid Services. (2022b). *Prospective Payment Systems – General information.* https://www.cms.gov/Medicare/Medicare-Fee-for-Service-Payment/ProspMedicareFeeSvcPmtGen

Centers for Medicare & Medicaid Services. (2023a). *Minimum Data Set (MDS) 3.0 Resident Assessment Instrument (RAI) manual.* https://www.cms.gov/Medicare/Quality-Initiatives-Patient-Assessment-Instruments/NursingHomeQualityInits/MDS30RAIManual

Centers for Medicare & Medicaid Services. (2023b). *Skilled nursing facility PPS.* https://www.cms.gov/medicare/payment/prospective-payment-systems/skilled-nursing-facility-snf

Medicare.gov. (n.d.). *Skilled nursing facility (SNF) care.* https://www.medicare.gov/coverage/skilled-nursing-facility-snf-care

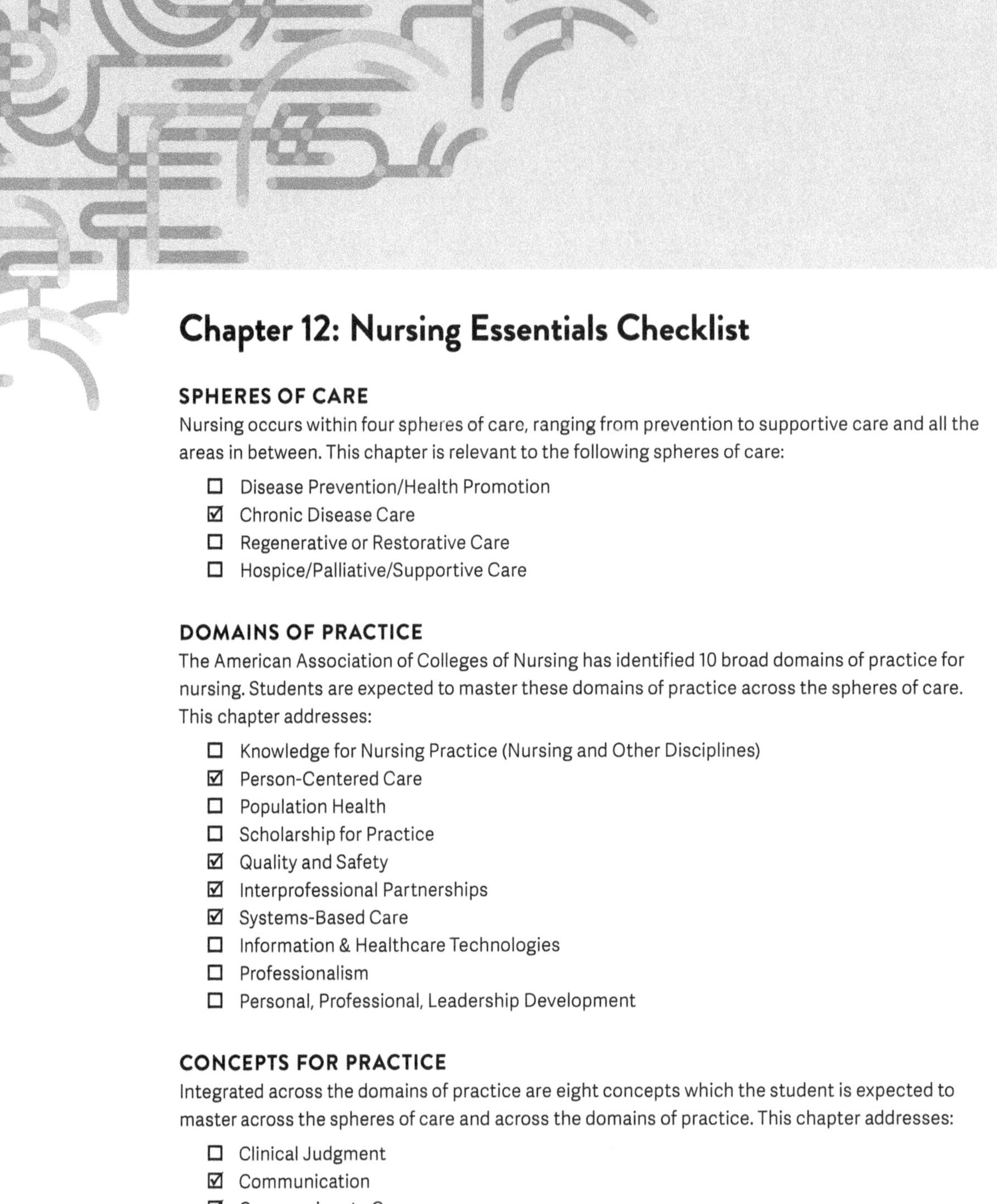

Chapter 12: Nursing Essentials Checklist

SPHERES OF CARE

Nursing occurs within four spheres of care, ranging from prevention to supportive care and all the areas in between. This chapter is relevant to the following spheres of care:

- ☐ Disease Prevention/Health Promotion
- ☑ Chronic Disease Care
- ☐ Regenerative or Restorative Care
- ☐ Hospice/Palliative/Supportive Care

DOMAINS OF PRACTICE

The American Association of Colleges of Nursing has identified 10 broad domains of practice for nursing. Students are expected to master these domains of practice across the spheres of care. This chapter addresses:

- ☐ Knowledge for Nursing Practice (Nursing and Other Disciplines)
- ☑ Person-Centered Care
- ☐ Population Health
- ☐ Scholarship for Practice
- ☑ Quality and Safety
- ☑ Interprofessional Partnerships
- ☑ Systems-Based Care
- ☐ Information & Healthcare Technologies
- ☐ Professionalism
- ☐ Personal, Professional, Leadership Development

CONCEPTS FOR PRACTICE

Integrated across the domains of practice are eight concepts which the student is expected to master across the spheres of care and across the domains of practice. This chapter addresses:

- ☐ Clinical Judgment
- ☑ Communication
- ☑ Compassionate Care
- ☑ Diversity, Equity, Inclusion
- ☐ Ethics
- ☑ Evidence-Based Practice
- ☐ Health Policy
- ☑ Social Determinants of Health

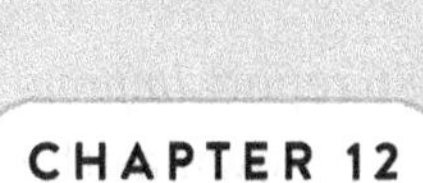

CHAPTER 12

IMPROVING QUALITY IN NURSING HOMES

Melissa Batchelor, PhD, RN, FNP, FGSA, FAAN
Liza L. Behrens, PhD, RN
Karen Eshraghi, MSW
Howard B. Degenholtz, PhD, FGSA
Marilyn Rantz, PhD, RN, FAAN

OBJECTIVES

1. Explain the purpose of quality measures for nursing home care.
2. Define the measures used to assess a facility's culture of safety.
3. Describe the process for implementing quality improvement programs in nursing homes.
4. Explain the NASEM conceptual model of quality of care in nursing homes.

INTRODUCTION

In the United States, nursing homes play a unique role within the long-term care continuum, serving as both a healthcare delivery and home setting. Older adults who live in nursing homes (residents) are often living with multiple chronic health conditions with complex care needs that can no longer be met in their home with the support of family, friends, and/or community resources. There is a pervasive stigma around nursing homes deeply rooted in historically poor care delivery and ageism. The negative myths and stereotypes associated with nursing home care are so deeply ingrained in American society that it is common for people to express that they do not ever want to become a resident in one. There is a significant need to address this stigma. Improving the quality and safety of care delivered and received in nursing homes is one way to do this.

Federal regulation of nursing homes began after the release of the 1986 report *Improving the Quality of Nursing Home Care* by the Institute of Medicine (now known as the National Academies of Science, Engineering, and Medicine [NASEM]), leading to passage of the Omnibus Reconciliation Act of 1987. These regulations are now developed and monitored at the federal level by the Centers for Medicare & Medicaid Services (CMS), and compliance oversight is provided by individual state government agencies (e.g., state department of health). However, even with 35+ years of regulation, providing high-quality nursing home care remains elusive to many of our nation's 15,000 nursing home communities.

The global COVID-19 pandemic in 2020 thrust nursing homes into the media spotlight for egregious quality and safety deficiencies that directly led to the death of thousands of residents and staff. The pandemic exposed many of the nursing home industry's long-existing challenges, including poor infection control practices, failures in regulation and oversight, and inadequate staffing (to name a few). The most recent evidence-based report, *The National Imperative to Improve Nursing Home Quality*, by NASEM, set forth a vision for high-quality nursing home care. Their primary goal was that residents of nursing homes should "receive care in a safe environment that honors their values and preferences, addresses goals of care, promotes equity and assesses benefits and risks of care and treatments" (NASEM, 2022, p. 6). This chapter provides a basic description of the quality and safety measures used in nursing homes and how these data can be used by the individual facility and the public to assess the quality of care being provided.

QUALITY MEASURES

CMS has placed a national priority to assure that skilled nursing home providers across the nation provide care in accordance with aims and goals for quality improvement. According to CMS, the purpose of quality measurement is to provide Medicare beneficiaries with accountability and transparency through public reporting. Although there may be varying perspectives of what is "quality care" based on important priorities and preferences, skilled nurse providers are gauged on a national level by certain quality clinical indicators that are deemed critical to the performance of nursing home teams to provide good quality care.

The vision of the national quality measurement system is to provide high standards for safe, equitable, and accessible quality care within a framework designed to improve systems of care in the nursing home setting. Individual measures provide meaningful insights about standards associated with goals for quality of care and life. When all the individual quality measures are aggregated together, it provides a picture of the nursing home's level of clinical performance in comparison to state and national averages (CMS, 2016, 2022).

The drawback, however, is that this quality measure system does not capture resident and family perspectives on important quality of living considerations that are equally important to overall quality of care, such as home-like environment, quality of food, social environment, cleanliness, and so on (Mukamel et al., 2021).

Quality measure reporting is a public service through CMS that helps consumers with selecting and evaluating the quality of skilled nursing home providers. The available tools and resources help educate the public about why these quality metrics are germane to a safe and healthy environment. Care Compare is an example of a web-based tool available on Medicare.gov that helps consumers select providers in a specific geographic region (CMS, n.d.-a). For example, selecting a nursing home that provides the best quality of care for a loved one can be a daunting task for family members. This decision is often made in a time of duress given the advancing healthcare needs of the senior requiring skilled level care. Care Compare provides a starting point in the process of finding the right home for a loved one.

The Resident Assessment Instrument/Minimum Data Set

Knowing about the quality measures empowers interdisciplinary teams to identify opportunities to make a difference in impacting the goals of care in the nursing home setting. Quality measures are derived from a comprehensive standardized tool called the Resident Assessment Instrument/Minimum Data Set (RAI/MDS). This standardized clinical assessment tool is implemented in the electronic medical record for nursing home teams to evaluate resident-level indicators, such as clinical conditions and functional and emotional well-being. See Chapter 11 for information about specific sections within the RAI/MDS.

The interdisciplinary team participates in the MDS clinical assessment process in conjunction with resident and family, but it is ultimately the MDS coordinator who ensures that the MDS assessment is submitted accurately and in a timely fashion. Nursing home providers are required to complete and submit this resident assessment at specific time intervals: upon admission, quarterly, annually, or if there has been a significant change (CMS, 2023).

Quality measures are measurement tools that help nursing home providers indicate the extent to which proper care is provided to residents. This performance data reports on key process and outcome measures associated with good clinical care. Each quality measure has clearly defined specifications and uses a calculated methodology to determine fluctuations in the submitted MDS clinical assessments. Quality measures are risk-adjusted and sensitive to demographic and clinical characteristics not related to the outcomes.

Long-Stay Versus Short-Stay Quality Measures

Quality measures are grouped into short- and long-stay measures dependent on the resident's length of stay in the skilled nursing home (See Table 12.1). Short-stay measures are for episodes of 100 or fewer days, whereas long-stay measures are for episodes greater than 100 days. Short-stay measures provide data-driven insights about the nursing home's performance in key clinical areas associated with a successful post-acute stay, such as making functional gains, preventing hospitalization, avoidance of antipsychotic medication, and so on.

Long-stay measures demonstrate the nursing home's performance in key clinical areas related to quality of life and care in the nursing home when vital supports are needed for residents who have limitations in their ability to live independently and safely (CMS, 2022).

TABLE 12.1 Quality Measures

LONG-STAY QUALITY MEASURES*	SHORT-STAY QUALITY MEASURES*
Number of Hospitalizations per 1,000 Long-Stay Resident Days	Percent of Short-Stay Residents Who Were Re-Hospitalized After a Nursing Home Admission
Number of Outpatient Emergency Department Visits per 1,000 Long-Stay Resident Days	Percent of Short-Stay Residents Who Have Had an Outpatient Emergency Department Visit
Percent of Residents Who Received an Antipsychotic Medication	Percent of Residents Who Newly Received an Antipsychotic Medication
Percent of Residents Experiencing One or More Falls With Major Injury	Changes in Skin Integrity Post-Acute Care: Pressure Ulcer/Injury
Percent of High-Risk Residents With Pressure Ulcers	Percent of Residents Who Made Improvements in Function
Percent of Residents With a Urinary Tract Infection	Percent of Residents Who Were Assessed and Appropriately Given the Seasonal Influenza Vaccine
Percent of Residents Who Have or Had a Catheter Inserted and Left in Their Bladder	Percent of Residents Who Were Offered and Declined the Seasonal Influenza Vaccine*
Percent of Residents Whose Ability to Move Independently Worsened	Percent of Residents Who Did Not Receive, Due to Medical Contraindication, the Seasonal Influenza Vaccine*
Percent of Residents Whose Need for Help With Activities of Daily Living Has Increased	Percent of Residents Who Were Assessed and Appropriately Given the Pneumococcal Vaccine
Percent of Residents Assessed and Appropriately Given the Seasonal Influenza Vaccine	Percent of Residents Who Received the Pneumococcal Vaccine*
Percent of Residents Who Were Offered and Declined the Seasonal Influenza Vaccine*	Percent of Residents Who Were Offered and Declined the Pneumococcal Vaccine*
Percent of Residents Who Did Not Receive, Due to Medical Contraindication, the Seasonal Influenza Vaccine*	Percent of Residents Who Did Not Receive, Due to Medical Contraindication, the Pneumococcal Vaccine*
Percent of Residents Who Were Assessed and Appropriately Given the Pneumococcal Vaccine	
Percent of Residents Who Received the Pneumococcal Vaccine*	

(continues)

TABLE 12.1 *(continued)*

LONG-STAY QUALITY MEASURES*	SHORT-STAY QUALITY MEASURES*
Percent of Residents Who Were Offered and Declined the Pneumococcal Vaccine*	
Percent of Residents Who Did Not Receive, Due to Medical Contraindication, the Pneumococcal Vaccine*	
Percent of Residents Who Were Physically Restrained	
Percent of Low-Risk Residents Who Lose Control of Their Bowels or Bladder	
Percent of Residents Who Lose Too Much Weight	
Percent of Residents Who Have Symptoms of Depression	
Percent of Residents Who Used Antianxiety or Hypnotic Medication	

** These measures are not publicly reported but available for provider preview. CMS, 2022*

Shared Decision-Making to Increase Quality of Care

Shared decision-making approaches in the nursing home setting are beneficial throughout the care-delivery journey from a senior moving into a new home to ongoing care planning review, as it involves the resident, family, and care team in making healthcare decisions together. It is a quality process that provides benefits such as improved health outcomes or increased resident and family satisfaction as it promotes meaningful engagement and resident autonomy (Cranley et al., 2020).

The SHARE model is a promising, five-step shared decision-making model that can be used by clinical teams to determine what matters to residents. SHARE (1) *S*eeks the resident's participation to (2) *H*elp explore and compare treatment options, (3) *A*ssesses the resident's values and preferences to (4) *R*each a decision based on the benefits, risks, and harms of each option, and (5) *E*valuate the resident's decision. Using this model of communication based the resident's priorities and preferences co-creates a plan of care based on evidenced-based best practices, and the relevant interventions are tailored for each resident-level goal of care (Agency for Healthcare Research and Quality [AHRQ], 2023). Despite the many advantages to shared decision-making, there has been little uptake to widespread implementation in nursing homes (Cranley et al., 2020).

SAFETY MEASURES

According to the US Government, safety for nursing home residents is equated to the elimination of adverse events—that is, any undesirable or unanticipated event that could potentially or actually result in serious injury or death for the resident due to medical care (CMS, 2016). According to the Department of Health and Human Services, Office of Inspector General (OIG), one out of every five residents who receive skilled nursing home care experience a preventable adverse event during their stay (Levinson, 2014). Although not all adverse events are preventable in nursing care, some are.

Examples of preventable adverse events in nursing care may include (CNA, 2023; Levinson, 2014):

- **Substandard treatment:** For example, provision of care that does not align with evidence-based nursing practice for pressure injury prevention
- **Inadequate resident monitoring:** This includes falls due to lack of adequate monitoring by nursing staff
- **Failure or delay in the provision of care:** Such as a failure to recommend to move the resident to a higher level of care

Adverse events are reported by nursing home administrators or directors of nursing through state level reporting systems. The Institute for Healthcare Improvement (IHI), with support of OIG, has developed the IHI Global Trigger Tool for Measuring Adverse Events to help nursing homes identify, track, and address adverse events related to the active delivery of care (Griffin & Resar, 2009).

Cultivating a Culture of Safety

Another way safety is measured in nursing homes is through the *culture of safety*. The culture of safety in a nursing home represents the commitment of frontline staff through leadership to minimize adverse events despite the complex and hazardous work environment (Gaur et al., 2022). AHRQ has developed and tested the Nursing Home Survey on Patient Safety Culture, now known as the AHRQ Survey on Patient Safety Culture (SOPS) for nursing homes (AHRQ, 2023; Gartshore et al., 2017).

This publicly available survey has been found to be a valid and reliable way to measure staff perceptions of a nursing home's safety culture in 12 core domains of teamwork, staffing, compliance with procedures, training and skills, nonpunitive response to mistakes, handoffs, communication about incidents, communication openness, supervisor expectations and actions promoting safety, overall perceptions of resident safety, management support for resident safety, and organizational learning (AHRQ, 2023). Research evidence links a strong culture of safety to a higher health and quality rating in nursing home communities (Yount et al., 2022).

Complying With Safety Protocols

Additionally, nursing homes that are certified to receive Medicare and/or Medicaid undergo an unannounced Life Safety Code (LSC) survey and a Standard Health Care Facilities Code (HCFC) survey annually. The LSC survey evaluates the degree to which the nursing home is designed to protect and provide resident safety from fire, smoke, and panic responses. Similarly, the HCFC survey evaluates the organizational safety practices around facilities, materials, equipment, and appliances.

Surveys are conducted by individual states to verify a nursing home community's compliance with federal standards for care. Nursing homes may receive a deficiency citation for noncompliance of varying event scopes (e.g., isolated, pattern, widespread) and severities (e.g., Level 1, no actual harm with potential for minimal harm, to Level 4, immediate jeopardy). Dependent upon event scope and severity, nursing homes are often given three to six months to develop and implement a plan of corrective action to address the safety issues (CMS, 2023).

By virtue of life experience, scope of practice, healthcare training, and close proximity to direct patient care, nurses are uniquely positioned to leverage existing safety measures and balance resident safety with the preferences, values, and wishes of nursing home residents using person-centered risk management strategies (Behrens et al., 2020, 2022, 2023).

QUALITY IMPROVEMENT PROGRAMS AND PROCESSES IN NURSING HOMES

Quality improvement programs and processes in nursing homes are a means to evaluate and correct care provided to residents and include Quality Assurance and Performance Improvement (QAPI) and Continuous Quality Improvement (CQI) activities (Dyck et al., 2014). As mentioned earlier, these processes are mandated by law, with the goal of making care more efficient, effective, safe, clean, and so on (Dyck et al., 2014; Langley et al., 2009).

CQI and QAPI are often used interchangeably in the nursing home setting. *CQI* is the underlying change theory and method guiding improvements in healthcare delivery (Kyrkjebø & Hanestad, 2003). *Quality assurance* (QA) is the ongoing process of nursing homes to ensure that acceptable levels of care are met per standards of care (CMS, n.d.-b). *Performance improvement* (PI) is the study of and improvement of nursing home care processes with the goal of delivering better services or outcomes, identifying and fixing problems and barriers related to care delivery, and, most importantly, improving resident quality of life (CMS, n.d.-b).

As a nurse working in a nursing home community, you may be asked to participate in part or all of your nursing home's QAPI program. There are five elements to a QAPI program in a nursing home (CMS, n.d.-b):

1. Design and scope of the program
2. Governance and leadership
3. Feedback, data systems, and monitoring
4. Performance improvement projects (PIPs)
5. Systematic analysis and systemic action

QAPI should be systematic, continuously evaluate care against evidence-based standards, and continuously correct care delivery (Dyck et al., 2014). *Quality indicators* are quantitative measures that serve as surrogates for quality care measures to assess the structural factors affecting performance of care (i.e., care environment), the process of care delivery that staff perform, and the impact on patient outcomes (Nakrem et al., 2009).

Evidence-based guidelines for person-centered nursing care suggest monitoring indicators for resident well-being, satisfaction with care, and a therapeutic care setting. These outcomes are nurse-sensitive quality indicators that are appropriate for QAPI programs in nursing homes (Sillner et al., 2021).

CASE STUDY A QAPI Team Works to Improve Performance

TK is the nursing home administrator of a large nursing home. Each month, the QAPI team meets to review both the long- and short-stay quality measures. The quality measure data provide meaningful information to help the team know where to prioritize staff resources and time for making improvements. Given negative trending in one of the short-stay measures, the functional gains measure, TK assigned a PIP team of key team members from the rehabilitation unit of the nursing home to formulate a performance improvement plan.

Following a thorough assessment using root-cause analysis, the PIP team charted an interdisciplinary plan of action with the goal of improving the percentage of short-stay residents that made improvements in function. Using a PDSA (plan-do-study-act) approach, opportunities for improvement were identified, such as increasing daily rounding to communicate on patient functional status, providing caregiver education on MDS coding, and devising new workflows between nursing and rehabilitation disciplines.

The PIP team reported regularly at the QAPI meetings on the successes and challenges in the project and regularly trended performance improvements in the quality measure.

MODELS OF QUALITY CARE IN NURSING HOMES

Quality of care in nursing homes has had much scrutiny and many attempts to describe what it really means. As illustrated in the beginning of this chapter, people know what they want and can articulate what that is. However, a clear conceptual model of quality of care in nursing homes was developed from the research evidence on the topic (Donabedian, 1988; Fulmer, 2018; Institute of Medicine, 2001; National Quality Forum, 2021; Rantz et al., 2008; Rantz et al., 1998; Rantz et al., 1999; Rauch et al., 2019).

Following is the illustration of the NASEM report *Conceptual Model of Quality Nursing Home Care* (NASEM, 2022, p. 39).

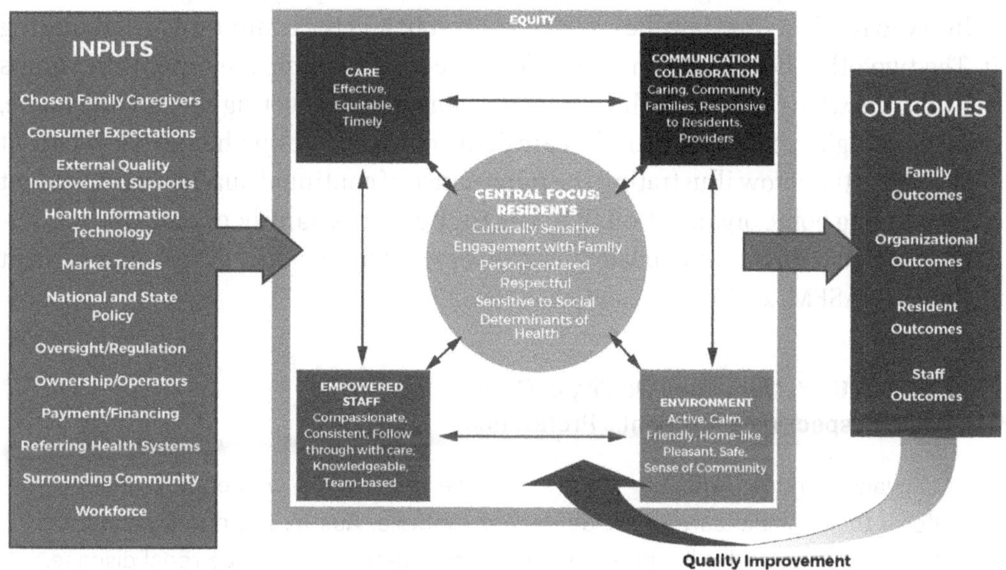

FIGURE 12.1 Conceptual model of the quality of care in nursing homes.

In the center of the model is a key central focus on the residents of the nursing home. This should be apparent when visiting or living in the facility. There should be people who are observed interacting with residents and family members in a respectful way, with messages that are heard and can be interpreted as culturally sensitive and person-centered. In the model's center box are four other key categories (NASEM, 2022):

1. Care that is effective, timely, and equitable
2. Communication that is caring and responsive to residents, families, providers, and community

3. Empowered staff who are knowledgeable, consistent, compassionate, and team-based and who follow through with care
4. An environment that is calm yet active, friendly, and pleasant; that has community involvement; and is home-like

The box around the center of the model also illustrates the nursing home in which quality care is happening; the nursing home promotes equity throughout their care delivery to residents and families, as well as for staff and the community surrounding it. The two other boxes, one on each side of the nursing home, represent the inputs and outcomes. On the left are illustrated the many inputs affecting the nursing home, and on the right are outcomes of the care delivery of the nursing home. A key part of the model is the arrow illustrating the importance of continual quality improvement of the nursing home organization that uses the outcomes (family, organizational, resident, staff) to improve and update care-delivery systems using quality improvement methods (NASEM, 2022).

CASE STUDY Upholding Quality of Care While Respecting a Resident's Preferences

Clinicians working in nursing homes can use the NASEM conceptual model to inform their clinical care to residents. For example, Austin, the nurse caring for MJ, who has opted for hospice care as she experiences end-stage renal disease, reflected on the various aspects of the conceptual model and decided to apply it to his practice. He called the care team together for a brief brainstorming and care-planning session to help develop ways to provide care that best met MJ's personal preferences for being engaged as much as possible with her family and with some staff who had become, for her, "like family."

The team came up with several approaches to help MJ "be her best" and "look her best" to use her limited energy to visit when she could with family. This required shifting some care routines and assignments to maximize her best energy times to be with the people she enjoyed, while still getting the personal care and hygiene she needed. Both MJ and her family were appreciative of the efforts. When she died, both family and some key staff were there for her, as she wanted.

This scenario reflects the conceptual model as well as the conclusion of the report *The National Imperative to Improve Nursing Home Quality* by NASEM (2022, p. 498):

> Nursing homes should deliver comprehensive, person-centered, interdisciplinary team-based care that meets or exceeds established quality standards and supports strong connections to health care and social service systems and resources, family, friends, and the community more broadly . . . promotes quality of life; aligns with residents' medical, behavioral, and social care needs; reflects residents' values and preferences; promotes autonomy; and manages risks to ensure residents' safety.

The 4Ms Framework

The Age-Friendly Health System's 4Ms (What Matters, Medication, Mentation, and Mobility), introduced in Chapter 2, were initially developed to improve quality of care in acute-care settings but are applicable to the nursing home setting. In 2021, the Institute for Healthcare Improvement (IHI) published *Age-Friendly Health Systems: Guide to Care of Older Adults in Nursing Homes,* along with a companion document, *Age-Friendly Health Systems: A Workbook for Nursing Home Teams* (IHI, 2022a, 2022b). These two documents, also introduced in Chapter 2, provide guidance for nursing home administration (the guide) and staff (the workbook) for improving the quality of care delivered using the 4Ms framework. Table 12.2 highlights the 4Ms with basic descriptions of additional measures that the interdisciplinary team can use to assess residents and interventions that can be used to improve the quality of life for residents.

TABLE 12.2 The 4Ms in Nursing Homes

4MS	WHO	WHAT	INTERVENTION(S)
What Matters	Nurse Social worker MD/NP/PA Care manager Chaplain Activities director Therapy department (PT/OT/ST)	Ask questions about the residents' priorities and goals while in the nursing home. Align the priorities and goals with the medical and nursing care provided.	Review What Matters to the resident with the quarterly MDS and care plan meetings. Develop methods to monitor if care delivery matches what is in the care plan.

(continues)

TABLE 12.2 *(continued)*

<table>
<tr><th>4MS</th><th>WHO</th><th>WHAT</th><th>INTERVENTION(S)</th></tr>
<tr><td>Medication</td><td>Licensed nurses
MD/NP/PA
Pharmacist</td><td>Review all over-the-counter sedatives and sleep medications with particular attention to medications on the BEERS Criteria such as:
• Anticholinergics (e.g., diphenhydramine)
• Antipsychotics, neuroleptics
• Benzodiazepines or other anxiolytics
• Mood stabilizers
• Muscle relaxants
• Opioids
• Tricyclic or other antidepressants</td><td>Medication reconciliation
Deprescribing
Pharmacy consult
Train staff to report any change in condition that could be related to medications.</td></tr>
<tr><td>Mentation: Dementia</td><td>Nurse
Social worker
MD/NP/PA
Behavioral/mental health consultant</td><td>Screening tools include:
• Mini-Cog
• SLUMS
• MOCA
• MMSE
• MDS BIMS Score</td><td rowspan="2">Staff training to deliver nonpharmacological interventions to prevent and mitigate unsafe behavior(s)
Behavioral health referral
Physical assessment and medication review by primary care provider</td></tr>
<tr><td>Mentation: Depression</td><td>Nurse
Social worker
MD/NP/PA
Behavioral/mental health consultant</td><td>Screening tools include:
• GDS
• PHQ-2
• PHO-9</td></tr>
</table>

4MS	WHO	WHAT	INTERVENTION(S)
Mentation: Delirium	Nurse Social worker MD/NP/PA Behavioral/mental health consultant	Screening tools include: • UB-2 • UB-CAM • CAM	Train staff to recognize hyper- and hypoactive delirium as a medical emergency. Investigate for potential underlying, reversible cause(s) (e.g., medication changes, infection, constipation). Ensure residents have and use adaptive equipment (e.g., glasses, hearing aids, dentures). Prevent sleep disturbances.
Mobility	Nurse Social worker MD/NP/PA Care manager Therapy department (PT)	Timed Get Up and Go (TUG) JH-HLM POMA	Encourage frequent, daily ambulation in a safe environment. Physical therapy Remove catheters and/or other tethering devices. Avoid high-risk medications, chemical and/or physical restraints.

Balancing Quality and Safety With What Matters to the Resident

Every family member or care partner would agree: "I want my loved one to have the best possible care and to be kept safe! I don't want to worry about someone not helping them when they need to go to the bathroom or with meals or changing their clothes—and when they ask for help, that someone shows up so that they don't fall and get hurt!" These basic care sentiments are the real concerns of many families and friends, and all these concerns are directly related to the quality of care (or lack thereof) provided in nursing homes.

Honoring each resident's values and preferences is key to their perspective of getting "quality care" while also receiving care that meets their physical, health, and emotional needs. Sometimes there are conflicts that occur, particularly when resident values and preferences do not clearly align with the goals and treatments typically used to manage health conditions. Essentially, the clinician working with the resident needs to carefully balance "treatment" that the resident may view as unnecessary or "not what I want to do!"

These situations require communication and explanation of the risks and benefits of treatment options with the resident and their designated family members or representatives who help with healthcare decisions (Ersek et al., 2022; Rantz et al., 2023). All discussions are done with respect and empathy, being clear to recognize the resident's right to make decisions as best they are able for themselves and with the support of their designated family. Often, the most successful discussions take place with the resident and family present, as well as other members of the interdisciplinary team, especially the social worker.

CASE STUDY Resident Takes an Active Role in Decision-Making About Her Own Care

Here's an example in which the resident MJ took an active part in the decision-making regarding her own care. MJ is 91 years old and moved into the nursing home two years ago with congestive heart failure and early kidney disease. When she arrived, she could get up from a chair independently, walk over 100 feet with a walker, and use the bathroom independently. Over the past year, her labs have indicated increasing severity of her kidney disease such that her primary care provider is now recommending beginning hemodialysis. This will require transportation three times a week to the dialysis center. Although the provider explained the importance of the treatment and MJ initially agreed, today is her first transport and she is refusing to leave for the treatment. MJ tells her nurse that she has changed her mind; she does not want to be "tied to that machine" for the rest of her life and that no one can make her go today.

Austin, MJ's nurse, talked with MJ to be sure she understood the implications of not getting treatment, that her health condition would worsen, and that she was facing end-of-life decisions. She said she understood. He then scheduled a care conference with other staff of the nursing home including the social worker, nursing supervisor, direct-care worker (who is most involved with MJ's care), primary care provider, MJ's key family members, and MJ herself. Most could be there in person; others connected by videoconference. During the discussion, MJ explained her desire to accept her condition as an end-of-life condition; she wanted to be comfortable in her own room in the place she felt was home. Hospice services were ordered by the provider to be extra support for MJ, but Austin assured her that the nursing home staff would be there with her as she wanted and needed them.

Situations such as the following arise often in nursing homes: the desire for some people to smoke, have private consensual sexual relationships, go for an outdoor walk without supervision, or watch TV late at night. These situations require assessing the safety of the actions of the resident and the safety of other residents living in the environment, as well as other factors. See the nearby case study for an example of how NH staff navigated a similar situation.

Consider these questions when confronted with such situations:

- What is the resident requesting?
- What is the decision-making capacity of the resident around this preference?
- Do family or healthcare providers need to be involved in the decisions to provide additional information about the impact of health status on what the resident wants to do?
- Will the actions of one person violate the safety, comfort, or environment of others?
- Are there cognitive status issues that could interfere with decision-making?

The environment of the nursing home is critical to balancing safety, quality of care, and quality of life (Anderiesen et al., 2014; Anderson et al., 2020). There are obvious things in the environment that contribute to quality of care. One of the most requested features is, "I want my own room. I have lived in my own home, and I want my own space here, too." Fulfilling this desire will require that many nursing homes remodel spaces to provide for private rooms. Additional remodeling will require private baths be added to each room, an essential element for infection management as well as resident privacy preferences.

The physical environment of the nursing home should feel and look homelike, have easy access to the outdoors, have good and natural lighting, be well-maintained, and have pleasant smells. Many visitors, pets, and residents should be freely moving about while engaged in activities of interest. In general, nursing homes are encouraged to be rebuilt as smaller facilities that represent more homelike environments (Rijnaard et al., 2016; Waters, 2021). These smaller environments tend to enhance mobility and engagement with staff, other residents, and visitors.

SUMMARY

Safety in nursing homes sometimes appears to override other priorities; however, it should be of equal importance to personal choice and goals of care. Clinicians who work in nursing homes must learn to balance resident personal choices, the goals of care, and the rights of other residents, as well as health and physical care needs. Learning to carefully review the many aspects of all care priorities and balance safety with personal choice and goals of care is essential to providing high-quality care. Exploring with the resident, family, and staff the shared risk and decisions that recognize personal preferences and choices is critical. Using that approach will help balance the rights of other residents and staff with the priorities of quality and safety while assuring personal preferences and choices.

REFERENCES

Agency for Healthcare Research and Quality. (2023). *Nursing home survey on patient safety culture.* https://www.ahrq.gov/sops/surveys/nursing-home/index.html

Anderiesen, H., Scherder, E. J., Goossens, R. H., & Sonneveld, M. H. (2014, November). A systematic review—Physical activity in dementia: The influence of the nursing home environment. *Applied Ergonomics, 45*(6), 1678–1686. https://doi.org/10.1016/j.apergo.2014.05.011

Anderson, D. C., Grey, T., Kennelly, S., & O'Neill, D. (2020, November). Nursing home design and COVID-19: Balancing infection control, quality of life, and resilience. *Journal of the American Medical Directors Association, 21*(11), 1519–1524. https://doi.org/10.1016/j.jamda.2020.09.005

Behrens, L. L., Boltz, M., Kolanowski, A., Sciegaj, M., Madrigal, C., Abbott, K., & Van Haitsma, K. (2020, Nov. 23). Pervasive risk avoidance: Nursing staff perceptions of risk in person-centered care delivery. *The Gerontologist, 60*(8), 1424–1435. https://doi.org/10.1093/geront/gnaa099

Behrens, L. L., Boltz, M., Sciegaj, M., Kolanowski, A., Jones, J. R., Paudel, A., & Van Haitsma, K. (2022). Nursing staff perceptions of outcomes related to honoring residents' "risky" preferences. *Research in Gerontological Nursing, 15*(6), 271–281. https://doi.org/10.3928/19404921-20220930-01

Behrens, L. L., Madrigal, C., & Dellefield, M. E. (2023, February). Assessment of nursing staff learning needs around person-centered risk management in nursing homes. *Journal of Gerontological Nursing, 49*(2), 7–12. https://doi.org/10.3928/00989134-20230106-02

Centers for Medicare & Medicaid Services. (n.d.-a). *Find & compare providers near you.* https://www.medicare.gov/care-compare/

Centers for Medicare & Medicaid Services. (n.d.-b). *QAPI description and background.* https://shorturl.at/gpqY5

Centers for Medicare & Medicaid Services. (2016). *Medicare and Medicaid programs; reform of requirements for long-term care facilities.* https://www.federalregister.gov/documents/2016/10/04/2016-23503/medicare-and-medicaid-programs-reform-of-requirements-for-long-term-care-facilities

Centers for Medicare & Medicaid Services. (2022). *Quality measures.* https://www.cms.gov/medicare/quality-initiatives-patient-assessment-instruments/nursinghomequalityinits/nhqiqualitymeasures

Centers for Medicare & Medicaid Services. (2023). *State operations manual chapter 7 – Survey and enforcement process for skilled nursing facilities and nursing facilities.* https://www.cms.gov/Regulations-and-Guidance/Guidance/Manuals/Downloads/som107c07pdf.pdf

CNA. (2023). *Aging services 2018 claim report: Valuing employees, minimizing risk.* https://go.cna.com/2018.10.29_KD_AgingServices-ClaimReport_200GatedLP.html

Cranley, L. A., Slaughter, S. E., Caspar, S., Heisey, M., Huang, M., Killackey, T., & McGilton, K. S. (2020, September). Strategies to facilitate shared decision-making in long-term care. *International Journal of Older People Nursing, 15*(3), e12314. https://doi.org/10.1111/opn.12314

Donabedian, A. (1988). The quality of care. How can it be assessed? *Journal of the American Medical Assocation, 260*(12), 1743–1748. https://doi.org/10.1001/jama.260.12.1743

Dyck, M. J., Schwindenhammer, T., & Butcher, H. K. (2014, July). Quality improvement in nursing homes. *Journal of Gerontological Nursing, 40*(7), 21–31. https://doi.org/10.3928/00989134-20140414-99

Ersek, M., Unroe, K. T., Carpenter, J. G., Cagle, J. G., Stephens, C. E., & Stevenson, D. G. (2022, February). High-quality nursing home and palliative care—One and the same. *Journal of the American Medical Directors Association, 23*(2), 247–252. https://doi.org/10.1016/j.jamda.2021.11.027

Fulmer, T. (2018, Aug. 7). *Discovering the 4Ms: A framework for creating Age-Friendly Health Systems.* John A. Hartford Foundation. https://www.johnahartford.org/blog/view/discovering-the-4ms-a-framework-for-creating-age-friendly-health-systems/

Gartshore, E., Waring, J., & Timmons, S. (2017, Nov. 21). Patient safety culture in care homes for older people: A scoping review. *BMC Health Services Research, 17*(1), 752. https://doi.org/10.1186/s12913-017-2713-2

Gaur, S., Kumar, R., Gillespie, S. M., & Jump, R. L. P. (2022, February). Integrating principles of safety culture and Just Culture into nursing homes: Lessons from the pandemic. *Journal of the American Medical Directors Association, 23*(2), 241–246. https://doi.org/10.1016/j.jamda.2021.12.017

Griffin, F., & Resar, R. (2009). *IHI Global Trigger Tool for measuring adverse events.* Institute for Healthcare Improvement. https://www.ihi.org/resources/Pages/Tools/IHIGlobalTriggerToolforMeasuringAEs.aspx

Institute for Healthcare Improvement. (2022a). *Age-Friendly Health Systems: Guide to care of older adults in nursing homes.* https://241684.fs1.hubspotusercontent-na1.net/hubfs/241684/IHI-Age-Friendly-Guide-Nursing-Homes_March28-2022.pdf

Institute for Healthcare Improvement. (2022b). *Age-Friendly Health Systems: A workbook for nursing home teams.* https://241684.fs1.hubspotusercontent-na1.net/hubfs/241684/IHI-Age-Friendly-Workbook-Nursing-Homes_March28-2022%20%28002%29.pdf

Institute of Medicine. (1986). *Improving the quality of care in nursing homes.* National Academies Press.

Institute of Medicine. (2001). *Crossing the quality chasm: A new health system for the 21st century.* National Academies Press. https://doi.org/10.17226/10027

Kyrkjebø, J. M., & Hanestad, B. R. (2003, January). Personal improvement project in nursing education: Learning methods and tools for continuous quality improvement in nursing practice. *Journal of Advanced Nursing, 41*(1), 88–98. https://doi.org/10.1046/j.1365-2648.2003.02510.x

Langley, G., Moen, R., Nolan, K., Norman, C., & Provost, L. (2009). *The improvement guide: A practical approach to enhancing organizational performance* (2nd ed.). Jossey-Bass.

Levinson, D. R. (2014, March 19). *Adverse events in skilled nursing facilities: National incidence among medicare beneficiaries.* US Department of Health and Human Services, Office of the Inspector General. https://oig.hhs.gov/oei/reports/oei-06-11-00370.pdf

Mukamel, D. B., Saliba, D., Weimer, D. L., & Ladd, H. (2021, August). Families' and residents' perspectives of the quality of nursing home care: Implications for composite quality measures. *Journal of the American Medical Directors Association, 22*(8), 1609–1614.e1601. https://doi.org/10.1016/j.jamda.2020.10.004

Nakrem, S., Vinsnes, A. G., Harkless, G. E., Paulsen, B., & Seim, A. (2009, June). Nursing sensitive quality indicators for nursing home care: International review of literature, policy and practice. *International Journal of Nursing Studies, 46*(6), 848–857. https://doi.org/10.1016/j.ijnurstu.2008.11.005

National Academies of Sciences, Engineering, & Medicine. (2022). *The national imperative to improve nursing home quality: Honoring our commitment to residents, families, and staff.* National Academies Press. https://doi.org/doi:10.17226/26526

National Quality Forum. (2021). *National Quality Forum home page.* https://www.qualityforum.org/Home.aspx

Rantz, M., Ersek, M., & Kaskie, B. (2023). Care delivery, quality measurement, and quality improvement in nursing homes: Issues and recommendations from the National Academies' report on the quality of care in nursing homes. *Public Policy & Aging Report, 33*(Suppl. 1), S11–S15. https://doi.org/10.1093/ppar/prac027

Rantz, M. J., Aud, M. A., Zwygart-Stauffacher, M., Mehr, D. R., Petroski, G. F., Owen, S. V., Madsen, R. W., Flesner, M., Conn, V., & Maas, M. (2008). Field testing, refinement, and psychometric evaluation of a new measure of quality of care for assisted living. *Journal of Nursing Measurement, 16*(1), 16–30. https://doi.org/10.1891/1061-3749.16.1.16

Rantz, M. J., Mehr, D. R., Popejoy, L., Zwygart-Stauffacher, M., Hicks, L. L., Grando, V., Conn, V. S., Porter, R., Scott, J., & Maas, M. (1998, February). Nursing home care quality: A multidimensional theoretical model. *Journal of Nursing Care Quality, 12*(3), 30–46. https://doi.org/10.1097/00001786-199802000-00007

Rantz, M. J., Zwygart-Stauffacher, M., Popejoy, L., Grando, V. T., Mehr, D. R., Hicks, L. L., Conn, V. S., Wipke-Tevis, D., Porter, R., Bostick, J., Maas, M., & Scott, J. (1999, October). Nursing home care quality: A multidimensional theoretical model integrating the views of consumers and providers. *Journal of Nursing Care Quality, 14*(1), 16–37. https://doi.org/10.1097/00001786-199910000-00004

Rauch, J., Baxter, M., Quave, D., Yount, N., & Shaller, D. (2019). *2019 chartbook: What consumers say about their experiences with their health plans and medical care.* Agency for Healthcare Research and Quality. https://cahpsdatabase.ahrq.gov/files/2019CAHPSHealthPlanChartbook.pdf

Rijnaard, M. D., van Hoof, J., Janssen, B. M., Verbeek, H., Pocornie, W., Eijkelenboom, A., Beerens, H. C., Molony, S. L., & Wouters, E. J. (2016). The factors influencing the sense of home in nursing homes: A systematic review from the perspective of residents. *Journal of Aging Research, 2016*, 6143645. https://doi.org/10.1155/2016/6143645

Sillner, A. Y., Madrigal, C., & Behrens, L. (2021, Feb. 1). Person-centered gerontological nursing: An overview across care settings. *Journal of Gerontological Nursing, 47*(2), 7–12. https://doi.org/10.3928/00989134-20210107-02

Waters, R. (2021, March). The big idea behind a new model of small nursing homes. *HealthAffairs, 40*(3), 378–383. https://doi.org/10.1377/hlthaff.2021.00081

Yount, N., Zebrak, K. A., Famolaro, T., Sorra, J., & Birch, R. (2022, January). Linking patient safety culture to quality ratings in the nursing home setting. *Journal of Applied Gerontology, 41*(1), 73–81. https://doi.org/10.1177/0733464820969283

Chapter 13: Nursing Essentials Checklist

SPHERES OF CARE

Nursing occurs within four spheres of care, ranging from prevention to supportive care and all the areas in between. This chapter is relevant to the following spheres of care:

- ☑ Disease Prevention/Health Promotion
- ☑ Chronic Disease Care
- ☑ Regenerative or Restorative Care
- ☑ Hospice/Palliative/Supportive Care

DOMAINS OF PRACTICE

The American Association of Colleges of Nursing has identified 10 broad domains of practice for nursing. Students are expected to master these domains of practice across the spheres of care. This chapter addresses:

- ☐ Knowledge for Nursing Practice (Nursing and Other Disciplines)
- ☑ Person-Centered Care
- ☐ Population Health
- ☐ Scholarship for Practice
- ☑ Quality and Safety
- ☐ Interprofessional Partnerships
- ☑ Systems-Based Care
- ☑ Information & Healthcare Technologies
- ☐ Professionalism
- ☑ Personal, Professional, Leadership Development

CONCEPTS FOR PRACTICE

Integrated across the domains of practice are eight concepts which the student is expected to master across the spheres of care and across the domains of practice. This chapter addresses:

- ☐ Clinical Judgment
- ☑ Communication
- ☐ Compassionate Care
- ☐ Diversity, Equity, Inclusion
- ☐ Ethics
- ☑ Evidence-Based Practice
- ☑ Health Policy
- ☐ Social Determinants of Health

CHAPTER 13

NURSING HOME HEALTH INFORMATION TECHNOLOGY

Gregory L. Alexander, PhD, RN, FAAN, FACMI, FIAHSI

OBJECTIVES

1. Introduce the nursing student and staff to nursing home health information technology.
2. Describe the policies affecting the design and utilization of health information technology in nursing homes.
3. Discuss the advantages of health information technology for quality of care and efficiencies in the nursing home.

INTRODUCTION

Health information technology (IT) is an important part of the landscape in nursing home work. Professional nurses, students, and the entire clinical workforce in these settings must be aware of how health IT is developing and the functions that the technology provides in these care delivery systems. Furthermore, nursing home leaders and staff should be aware of the ever-changing federal policy that influences the adoption, sustainability, and scalability of health information technology over time. This chapter provides an introduction for nursing home staff and students to health information systems used in nursing homes, current policies that are impacting the adoption of these systems into clinical care, and some of the functions, advantages, and efficiencies that can be recognized by using nursing home technology.

FEDERAL POLICY DRIVING TECHNOLOGY ADOPTION IN U.S. NURSING HOMES

Health information technology (IT) is a solution for better quality of care in nursing homes. However, scalable sustained IT adoption is constrained by inadequate investment, infrastructure, and a trained IT workforce.

Inputs to Nursing Home Quality: The Case for Health Information Technology

In the United States, over 3 million Americans rely on nursing home services in any given year within more than 15,500 facilities (Centers for Medicare & Medicaid Services [CMS], 2017). The mission of CMS is to provide effective healthcare and promote quality of care for nursing home residents (CMS, 2017). However, the Office of the Inspector General reported that one in three Medicare beneficiaries are harmed by adverse events within 35 days of nursing home admission (Levinson, 2014). Nearly 60% of harmful events are preventable episodes associated with substandard treatment, inadequate monitoring, and delayed or failure to give necessary care (Levinson, 2014), due, in part, to missing or inadequate information communicated at nursing home admission and discharge (King et al., 2013; Popejoy et al., 2014; Vogelsmeier, 2014).

Authors of the JASON report suggested health IT (e.g., electronic health records [EHRs]) and health information exchange as a solution for reducing harmful errors and facilitating communication among providers (JASON, 2014). This report aligns with others—for example, the recent National Academies of Sciences, Engineering, and Medicine (NASEM) panel addressing nursing home quality, which recommended IT for all nursing homes to improve safety and quality of care (NASEM, 2022a).

Key Points of Failure for IT Adoption in Nursing Homes

Substantial constraints in the current system impact the ability to adopt health IT in all US nursing homes. Alexander and McMullen identified four points of failure that will require actionable steps to build quality using health IT in nursing homes (Alexander & McMullen, 2023).

Policies That Promote Differences in Capabilities and Infrastructures and Disparities in Resident Outcomes

The first point of failure includes policies that promote differences in capabilities and infrastructures and disparities in resident outcomes. Key policies and reforms that do not benefit all sectors of healthcare will likely lead to these differences. For instance, meaningful use legislation that was part of the American Reinvestment and Recovery Act financed adoption of IT in acute and ambulatory care but not nursing home settings (US Department of Health and Human Services, 2022). While this legislation led to substantial increases in IT adoption (e.g., EHRs) and certainly improved quality and safety of care in the settings the policy influenced, nursing homes were left behind.

Downstream from this legislation, there are still wide differences in health *IT maturity*, defined as the capabilities, use, and level of integration of IT in nursing home care delivery systems. For example, in a national nursing home study assessing IT maturity, approximately 10% of the facilities in the study ($N = 719$) reported an IT maturity stage of 1 or lower, meaning that those facilities had, at the most, disparate or fragmented IT systems that typically have distinct functionalities that are not well integrated into care delivery (Alexander, Liu, et al., 2022). Differences in IT maturity have been shown to increase disparities in nursing home resident outcomes (e.g., antibiotic use and urinary tract infections; Cohen, Powell, Deroche, et al., 2022; Cohen, Powell, Dick, et al., 2022).

Infrastructure Requirements

The second point of failure regards the infrastructure requirements to implement and sustain nursing home IT. Recent studies have highlighted the inadequate investment in infrastructure required to implement nursing home IT (Ko et al., 2018). In particular, nursing home staff in some studies have reported that too little resources were available, such as availability of computers, the absence or slowness of internet, insufficient connectivity, and lack of system integration (Alexander et al., 2007; Bezboruah et al., 2014; Rantz et al., 2006; Vogelsmeier et al., 2008).

Lag Time in Implementation and Sustained Use of Interoperable Systems

Poor infrastructure also contributes to the third point of failure, which includes a growing concern for lag time in implementation and sustained use of interoperable systems to improve health information exchange and data-sharing among organizations. One study identified that the six nonemergent use cases for health information exchange most communicated by nursing home staff were (Alexander et al., 2015):

1. Scheduling appointments
2. Laboratory specimen drawing
3. Pharmacy orders and reconciliation
4. Social work discharge planning
5. Admissions and pre-admissions
6. Pharmacy-medication reconciliation

Insufficient resources that prevent health information exchange and data-sharing for these clinical workflows have negative impacts on continuity of care and care coordination as nursing home residents move between care-delivery settings. An NH's inability to exchange data in a timely manner affects the ability of staff to make critical decisions to prevent negative outcomes (e.g., avoidable hospitalizations; Vogelsmeier et al., 2021). Evidence-based studies have identified major themes that contribute to nursing home technology implementation, including benefits of using EHR technology (i.e., increased efficiencies and improved and open communication; Alexander, Liu, et al., 2022; Schoville, 2017).

The Lack of Workforce Readiness to Adopt IT in Nursing Homes

The fourth point of failure is workforce readiness to adopt nursing home IT. The NASEM report titled *The National Imperative to Improve Nursing Home Quality: Honoring Our Commitment to Residents, Families, and Staff* (NASEM, 2022b) specifically called out education and training of workforce as a critical factor to improve quality of care in nursing homes (NASEM, 2022c). Authors of the report specified that IT training is a key factor in the ability of IT to contribute to nursing home quality, safe care delivery, and staff productivity (NASEM, 2022a). In addition, there are significant opportunities for interdisciplinary team collaborations supported by IT that facilitate health data-sharing capabilities that enable everyone to access shared documentation. Recommendations were made for CMS and the Health Resources and Services Administration to provide financial support for development and implementation of workforce training to include core health IT competencies in important areas such as telehealth, clinical decision support, and interoperability (NASEM, 2022a).

NURSING HOMES AND THE TECHNOLOGY ENVIRONMENT

Frameworks that help us understand existing states of nursing home IT maturity are necessary to identify structural disparities impacting nursing home quality and resident outcomes. IT deployment in the face of a public health emergency (e.g., the COVID-19 pandemic) was an important factor in gaining access to care.

Framework and Attributes for Nursing Home IT Maturity

An opportunity to overcome these points of failure toward IT adoption is to create frameworks and attributes of IT maturity that can help monitor trends in adoption and associated disparities that occur when failures arise. *IT maturity* is a measure of change among three dimensions explaining IT capabilities, use, and integration among three healthcare domains, including resident care, clinical support (i.e., IT systems supporting laboratory, pharmacy, and radiology), and administrative activities (Alexander, Deroche, et al., 2022; see Figure 13.1).

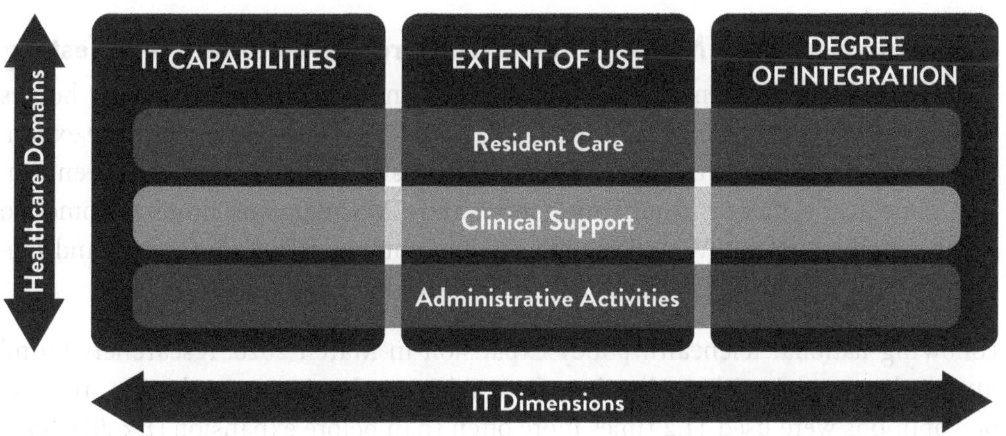

FIGURE 13.1 HIT maturity measurement matrix.

IT maturity is further categorized into stages, from stage 0, where EHRs are nonexistent, to stage 6 in facilities where residents and caregivers may have access to integrated datasets for higher levels of accountable care (Alexander & Wakefield, 2009). This definition of IT maturity is consistent with the concepts from Nolan's stage theory used to characterize trends in IT over time (Nolan, 1973). As mentioned, widespread nursing home IT adoption has not been achieved due to unbalanced national policies that do not promote meaningful use with financial incentives in nursing homes, as in hospital and ambulatory care settings (Kruse et al., 2015; Office of the National Coordinator for Health Information Technology, 2015).

The lack of incentives can create wider structural differences, leading to process variation that impacts resident outcomes. Longitudinal assessments are critical to truly understand nursing home IT maturity. In fact, researchers found alternating patterns of total IT maturity over three years among 815 nursing homes; that is, 71% of nursing homes exhibited a net positive increase, 19% had a net negative decrease, and 10% had consistently negative patterns of IT maturity over time (Alexander et al., 2019; Alexander et al., 2017). The reason for this variation may be the lack of financial meaningful use incentives, infrastructure, resource availability, or competence of workforce about IT systems, mentioned previously (Walker et al., 2016).

Opportunities for IT Maturity Infrastructure Development and Testing

As a result of the pandemic, there have been changes in IT use in nursing homes (Alexander et al., 2020; Powell & Alexander, 2021). These changes include the expansion of Medicare payments for telehealth, increasing collaborations between academic medical centers and nursing homes, and CMS requiring nursing homes to electronically report COVID-19 metrics to the Centers for Disease Control and Prevention (CDC; Archbald-Pannone et al., 2020; CDC, 2021; CMS, 2020).

Following national telehealth policy expansion in March 2020, researchers found nursing home telehealth applications for resident evaluation, consultation, and second opinions were used 11.2 times more often than before expansion ($p < .01$); however, 16% of nursing homes did not have telehealth, and this was more likely to occur in rural nursing homes (Alexander et al., 2020). Similar findings have been confirmed by other researchers exploring the explosive growth of telehealth since the pandemic started (Mehrotra, 2021).

Technology adoption, especially in the face of emergent conditions, yields positive and negative outcomes that must be recognized, identified, and addressed. For instance, in prior work, 21 nursing home administrators and clinicians from 16 nursing homes that rapidly expanded telehealth during the pandemic identified desirable (i.e., avoiding nursing home resident and staff travel, efficient resource utilization, improved access to care, and enhanced communication) and undesirable (i.e., worsening social isolation, difficulty for residents with cognitive impairment, workflow-technical-usability challenges, and increased burden on nursing home staff and infrastructure) consequences of swift IT adoption (Powell & Alexander, 2021).

While there is pending legislation to make permanent the expansion of telehealth (H.R. 341), nursing home IT best practices in this changing environment are not clear. Opportunities to create evidence-based models of care incorporating telehealth in nursing home care-delivery systems are much needed.

Recognizing IT Structural Disparities That Impact Quality of Nursing Home Care

Currently, despite IT's promise for improving nursing home care, few studies have linked change in nursing home IT maturity to health disparities and resident outcomes. Further, nursing home IT maturity is not consistently reported in public reporting systems about the care quality in nursing homes. Emerging differences in nursing home IT use in performance-based systems of care are not clear.

There have been substantial changes in IT use in nursing homes in recent years (Alexander et al., 2020; Powell & Alexander, 2021). For instance, federal policies launched in 2018 established performance-based accountability measures for hospital readmission rates in nursing homes, which has resulted in more facilities adopting EHRs and other electronic tools (e.g., clinical decision support) for frontline staff to use (Shetty et al., 2020). At the same time, researchers have found wide variation in IT maturity in US nursing homes. Nearly 68% of nursing homes reported the ability to connect staff electronically with other staff internal to the organization (IT maturity stage 3 or less), while 32% had more advanced capabilities (IT maturity stage 4 or higher) to connect staff in the nursing home with people external to the facility, including resident care systems that provided an electronic connection with clinics and staff outside their facilities (Alexander & Powell, 2021).

Crucial differences in IT maturity were reported, such as that IT maturity is greater in larger nursing homes (> 120 beds) versus smaller (< 60 beds; $p = .0008$), and nursing homes in metropolitan areas have significantly greater IT maturity than those in rural areas ($p < .0001$); type of nursing home ownership (i.e., for-profit versus nonprofit) did not differ (Alexander & Powell, 2021).

A few researchers have analyzed associations between nursing home IT maturity trends (2013–2017) and antibiotic use nationally, controlling for nursing home and resident characteristics, including infection. Researchers have linked IT maturity survey data with resident level Minimum Data Set assessments yielding 219,461 regular assessments within 90 days of IT maturity survey completion on 80,237 unique, older adult long-stay residents in 816 nursing homes. Researchers determined through multivariate models that IT maturity was associated with antibiotic use (AOR: 1.072, 95% CI: 1.025, 1.122; Cohen, Powell, Deroche, et al., 2022). For every 10-point increase in the maturity score, the expected odds of antibiotic use increased by 7%. Additionally, researchers used these data to test associations between IT maturity and urinary tract infections. Controlling for nursing home and resident characteristics, IT maturity was associated with less urinary tract infections (AOR: 0.906, 95% CI: 0.843, 0.973; Cohen, Powell, Deroche, et al., 2022).

The investigators concluded that using IT to relieve administrative burden, such as data documentation tasks, was thought to lead to decreased urinary tract infections. Their findings suggest that nursing homes with better documentation systems may have potential for measurement bias as they are more likely to record urinary tract infections (Cohen, Powell, Dick, et al., 2022).

Specialized Technologies for Nursing Home Systems

Technology, whether a fully integrated EHR or a point of care (POC) system supporting clinical activities, is crucial for documenting and tracking the patient's plan of care. System integration of these IT systems and their processes into the staff's workflow is vital if we are to provide the highest quality of nursing home care.

Point of Care Systems

Point of care (POC) systems include nursing home information systems that allow staff to enter or access clinical data at a location where their residents receive care. POC systems can be more efficient for nursing home staff to use because the information system is readily available at a location where they should be spending their time, at the bedside. POC systems may replace older systems of documentation such as paper charts, which have historically been located at central nursing stations or on carts that may be pushed around by staff to and from the central nursing station.

Technology vendors have made available nursing home POC systems, especially for clinical support areas in the nursing home such as laboratory, pharmacy, and radiology departments. These POC systems are critical, as most nursing homes, unless they are affiliated with a hospital, do not have an onsite clinical support department. Implementation of POC systems is crucial, as they need to be designed to support existing clinical workflows or dangerous workarounds can creep into clinical processes, creating patient safety issues (Vogelsmeier et al., 2008).

Clinical Charting With a Patient Scheduling Use Case

Documentation of clinical problems and activities by nursing home staff is vital for care planning and continuity of care, as nursing home patients frequently experience changes in conditions that require immediate care, treatment, ongoing communication, and follow-up. The documentation of clinical events has been reported to have a high degree of ambiguous information, leaving both the patient and staff in vulnerable positions (Tate et al., 2023). Consider the use case (see Figure 13.2), adapted from Alexander et al., 2015, which illustrates the flow of clinical information about a nursing home patient who has a personal medical appointment outside of a facility and requires transportation assistance to the appointment.

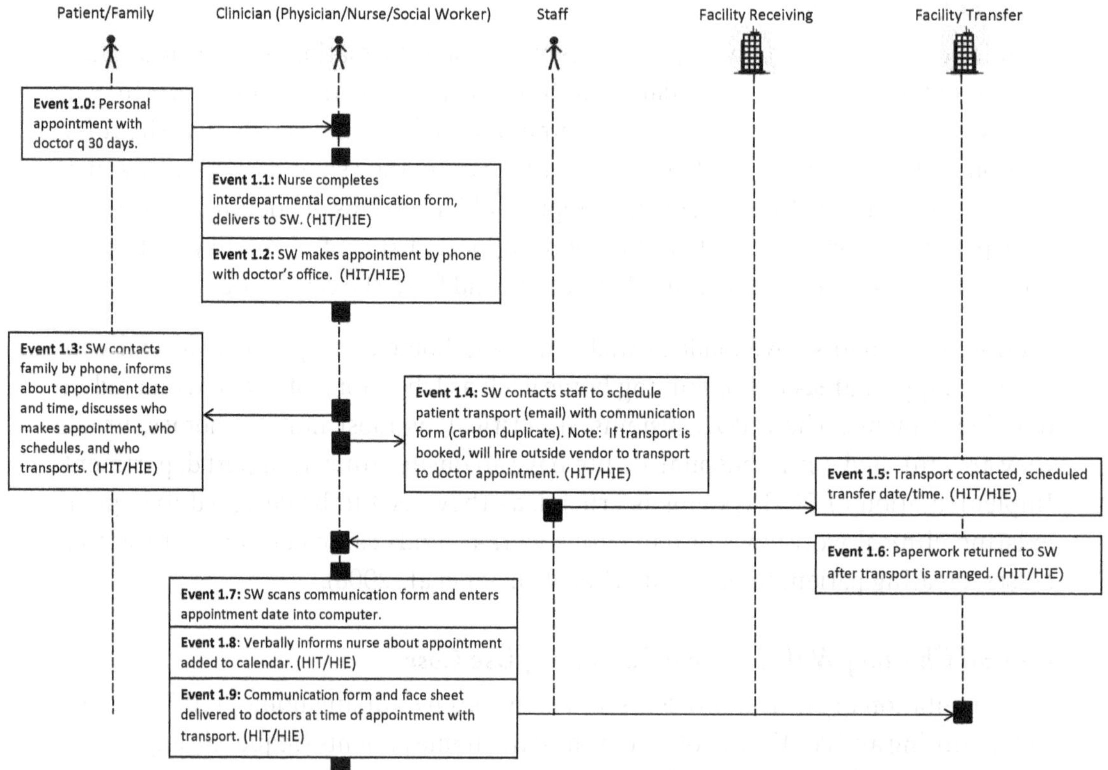

FIGURE 13.2 Use case, nonemergent appointment.

This nonemergent use case starts with a scheduled appointment that occurs every 30 days and includes clinical communication that travels between the nurse, social worker, transport personnel, caregivers, and physician who are caring for the patient. The communication generated about this appointment in a facility with little IT capability (low IT maturity) requires the use of carbon copies, paper-based sources of information being transferred or faxed from one person to another. Disparate, less integrated IT systems may support some of these operations.

Conversely, in a facility with robust IT capabilities (high IT maturity) in resident care that includes health information exchange (i.e., a system to allow secure, real-time clinical data-sharing between end users; Abramson et al., 2014), many of these steps in this lengthy process could be eliminated or made to be more efficient to share data about the patient's appointment schedule and what occurred during the appointment.

Medications Management and Pharmacy Order Communication Use Case

Medications management processes in nursing homes enable nursing staff to manage important drugs used to treat patient conditions. IT capabilities supporting medication management include many of the processes shown in Table 13.1. These include important clinical decision support tools that provide patient-specific information that is intelligently filtered at appropriate times to provide critical information while clinical decisions are being made.

TABLE 13.1 Computerized Processes in Nursing Home Pharmacy Systems

COMPUTERIZED PROCESS	CONTEXT FOR USE OF COMPUTERIZED PROCESS
eMAR (electronic Medication Administration Record)	Automatically documents the administration of medication into certified EHR technology
Duplication order checking	Checks for duplicate orders for tests and medications referring to the same patient stored in an EHR
Medication ordering and purchasing	Medication order renewal or review constitutes prescribing when documented in the system with the date and time the action occurred
Patient drug profile lookup	Tool to review and prioritize patients' drug profiles through integration into the daily pharmacist workflow in the EHR
Refill reports	Allows a clinician to review and confirm a history of electronic and printed prescriptions and refills
Intravenous admixtures management	IV workflow management system featuring barcode scanning of IV mixtures, lot/expiration information, compounding record documentation, and IV administration reporting capabilities
Drug interaction checking	Pinpoints contradictions between medications and other drugs prescribed to a patient
Do not crush alerts	Embedded directions or instructions for contradictions for crushing medications before administration
Pharmacy consulting services	Electronic consultations for pharmacy staff services and type of consultations needed
Allergy alerts	Provides clinicians with an alert or reminder if the patient has a documented allergy to the prescribed drug
Crossmatch with Beers criteria	Tracks for the appropriateness of prescribing medications against evidence-based Beers criteria
Look-alike–sound-alike medication alerts	A clinical decision support tool in the EHR to prevent medication errors caused by confusion between drug products that look and/or sound alike

An example of a clinical workflow for a non-stat pharmacy order communication use case by an external stakeholder (outside the NH) is illustrated in Figure 13.3 (adapted from Alexander et al., 2015). In this use case, the flow of information about a new pharmacy order received from a doctor is traced from patient/family to clinician and to the external pharmacy where the drugs will be retrieved after the order is received. In a facility with few IT capabilities, this process begins with handwritten medication administration orders that are passed along to an external pharmacy via a fax and followed up with a phone call to assure that the new drug order was received. Once confirmed, the clinician notifies other staff by recording the new order on a 24-hour report and paper MAR, which is then circulated to appropriate staff to make them aware of a new order and to expect new drugs to be delivered for administration.

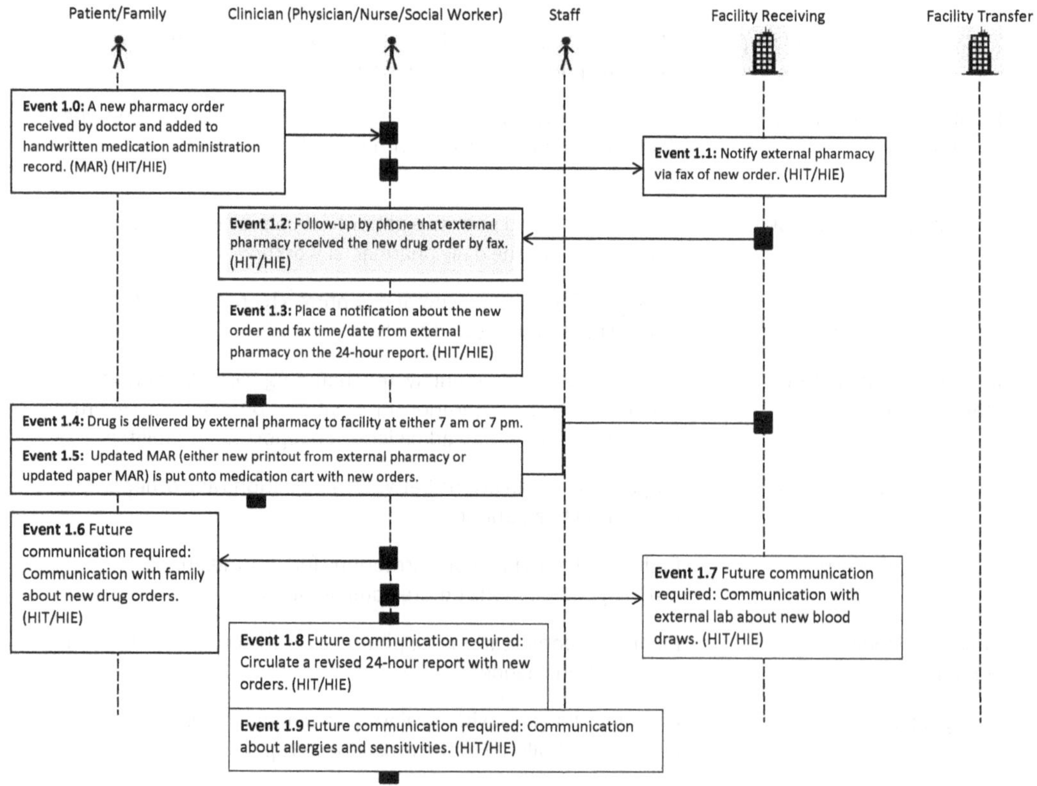

FIGURE 13.3 Non-stat pharmacy order communication (external stakeholder).

Depending on the types of drugs being ordered and administered, there could be future required communications to other external stakeholders, including laboratory personnel for blood sampling to monitor drug effects. In a nursing home with a high level of IT maturity, where pharmacy processes are well integrated into resident care, including many of the processes shown in Table 13.1, many of the workflows for pharmacy orders and communication could become more efficient and safer for clinicians to perform when undertaking medication management activities.

Interoperability and a Use Case for Evaluating Nursing Home Admissions

Interoperability is the ability of clinical information systems and software systems to exchange electronic clinical data accurately, effectively, and consistently in real time to support clinical decisions made by staff (US Department of Health and Human Services, 2020). Nursing home IT systems that support the robust exchange of clinical data continue to be in their early stages of development and implementation in nursing homes (Adler-Milstein et al., 2021; Alexander, Galambos, et al., 2022). Interoperable clinical IT systems have the potential to improve clinical workflows, such as resident transitions of care between hospitals and nursing homes (Henry et al., 2018). Gaps in clinical information that occur during transitions can lead to harmful events and adverse outcomes for nursing home residents.

The Improving Medicare Post-Acute Care Transformation Act of 2014 was created to build interoperable systems by supporting the use of standardized data that is needed to perform exchange of clinical data among different providers (Alexander & McMullen, 2023). The Office of the National Coordinator for Health Information Technology reported in 2017 that 66% of nursing homes had EHRs, which are necessary for optimal data exchange. However, only 18% of nursing homes had patient health information integrated from external stakeholders, indicating that little data-sharing had occurred in facilities surveyed (Henry et al., 2018). Another use case to show the importance of interoperable systems and how data exchange could be useful is illustrated in the nonemergent use case for nursing home admissions in Figure 13.4.

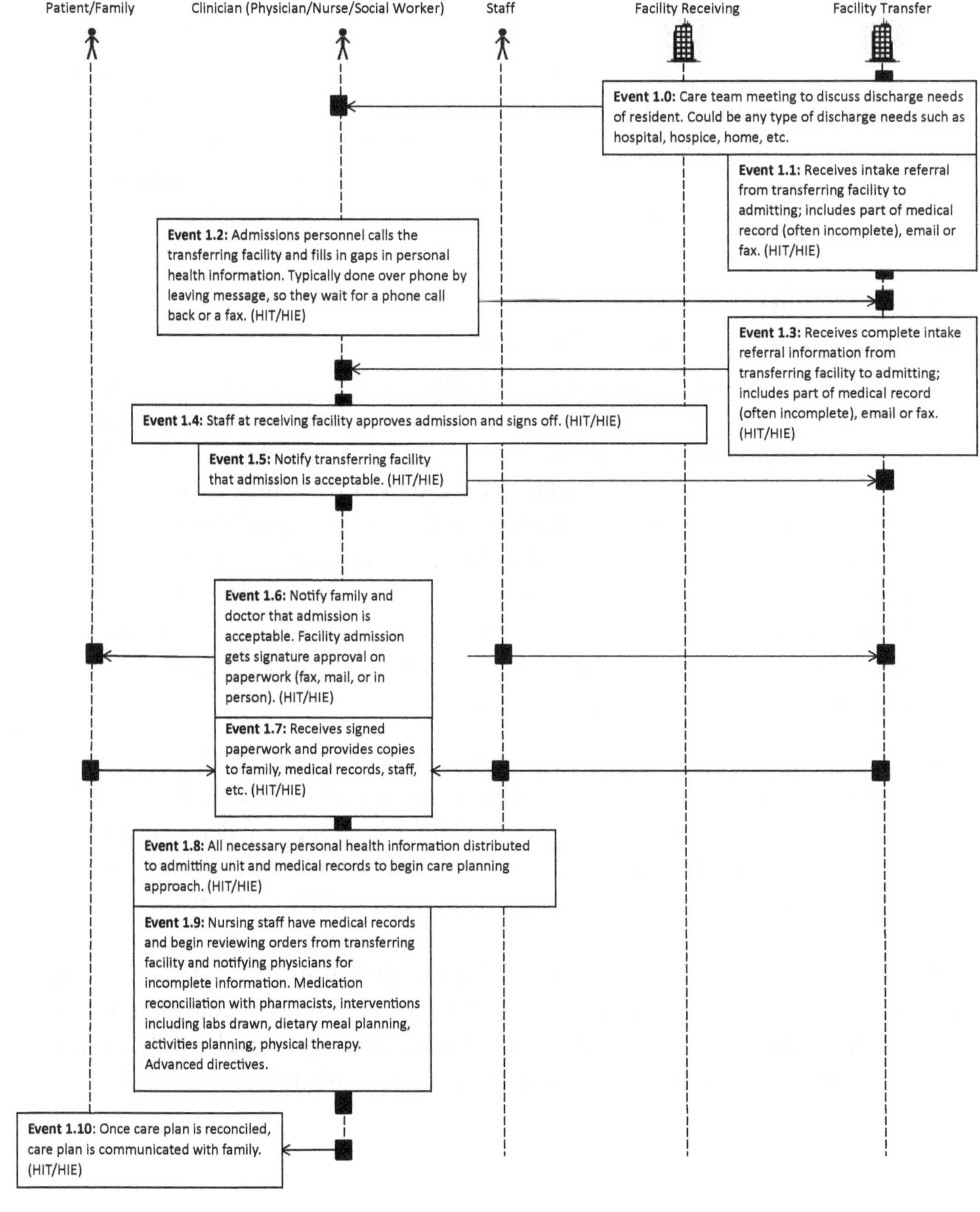

FIGURE 13.4 Use case, nonemergent, admissions and pre-admissions.

This use case illustrates a nursing home with low IT capabilities and a clinical workflow that begins with a care team from an external facility (e.g., hospital, hospice, etc.), which is transferring a patient to an NH. The care team generates a referral from the transferring facility to a receiving facility, which often includes different parts of the medical record that are often incomplete on transfer.

The incompleteness of the medical record makes it difficult for the nursing home (the receiving facility) to make decisions about admittance based on the care requirements of the patient. For example, if the patient is obese and special lifting equipment is needed to transfer the patient, that would be important for the nursing home to know before admitting the patient. Often these gaps in the clinical information must be filled, requiring several calls or perhaps even an in-person visit by a nursing home administrator to the transferring facility before the admission decision is made.

In nursing homes that have high levels of IT maturity with interoperable systems that provide health information exchange, the administrator who is involved in making admission decisions can look at the clinical record from the transferring facility online and determine if the nursing home has the right resources to care for the patient being transferred.

Interoperable systems that enable health data-sharing save time and resources for the nursing home staff during decisions about nursing home admissions. Furthermore, these systems may protect patients from being transferred to a nursing home where inadequate or insufficient resources are available to meet the patient's needs.

CURRENT STATE AND EVOLUTION OF NURSING HOME TECHNOLOGY

Use of nursing home technology (e.g., EHRs and telehealth) is rapidly changing the context of how care is delivered. Whether you're a professional staff member or a student working or studying in this environment, it is important to be aware of these changes and how they are impacting work.

Nursing Home Electronic Health Records

Compared to 2017, when estimates from the Office of the National Coordinator for Health Information Technology reported that 34% of nursing homes had no EHR (Henry et al., 2018), more recent evidence (2019) indicates that only 10% of nursing homes report nonexistent EHRs or isolated discrete IT systems that lack clinical data integration (Alexander, Liu, et al., 2022). This same study also illustrates that there is still room for improvement, as 55% of facilities ($n = 719$) reported limited interoperability and ability to share data with external facilities. More positively, 32% reported having robust clinical IT systems that were enabling more sophisticated IT capabilities like health data-sharing and clinical decision support systems to help predict patient risk.

Telehealth

The COVID-19 pandemic has created an urgent need for nursing home systems to integrate technology that supports patient care while protecting patients who, during the pandemic, were isolated from people who care about them. Following the start of the pandemic, regulatory agencies lifted rules regulating the use of telehealth in clinical activities to protect patients from the spread of the virus and also to help support physical and emotional conditions experienced by isolated nursing home residents.

Immediately following the pandemic, many more nursing homes were using telehealth in their clinical environments compared to before the start of the pandemic (Powell et al., 2022). Unfortunately, there was little evidence about how to implement and use telehealth in nursing homes prior to the pandemic and after policies were implemented to support its use. This rapid deployment led to studies documenting the promises and pitfalls of its use to treat clinical patients in nursing homes (Powell & Alexander, 2021). Promises included benefits of avoiding travel, saved resources, improved access to care, and enhanced communication (Powell & Alexander, 2021).

Conversely, some of the realized pitfalls included patients preferring in-person visits versus virtual, worsening social isolation, difficulties for patients with cognitive decline, workflow challenges, staff burden, and poor infrastructure to support telehealth (Powell & Alexander, 2021). These outcomes need further research to help inform clinical leaders in practice how to use telehealth effectively and efficiently.

SUMMARY

National initiatives that have raised awareness of the poor quality of care in nursing homes in the US have led to actions by important coalitions of people who want to improve the quality of nursing home care for the millions of older adults who live in these facilities. An important recommendation that these groups are addressing is IT implementation in all US nursing homes. There is still much to be learned about why nursing home leaders choose to implement clinical IT systems, which systems they choose to implement, and how IT systems impact clinical staff and the patients who use them.

Professional nurses who are considering placement in a nursing home, or nursing students who are completing a nursing home rotation as part of their educational activities, should be aware that not all nursing homes are alike. There is much variation in the processes of care across nursing homes that are supported by IT systems. Professional nurses seeking employment and nursing students completing rotations in nursing homes need to be fully aware of these differences as they participate in interviews or complete internship rotations.

For professional nurses, the use of IT and nursing home IT capabilities could be an important point to discuss during the interview process to clarify expectations prior to assuming clinical roles. For student nurses, variations in IT capabilities and IT use might be an important highlight of a student rotation as students move through different clinical settings. Important aspects of care delivery might be how data are shared by the multidisciplinary team and how patient data are shared as important clinical decisions about patient care are being determined.

REFERENCES

Abramson, E. L., McGinnis, S., Moore, J., Kaushal, R., & HITEC investigators. (2014). A statewide assessment of electronic health record adoption and health information exchange among nursing homes. *Health Services Research, 49*(1 Pt 2), 361–372.

Adler-Milstein, J., Raphael, K., O'Malley, T., & Cross, D. A. (2021). Information sharing practices between U.S. hospitals and skilled nursing facilities to support care transitions. *JAMA Network Open, 4*(1), e2033980. https://doi.org/doi:10.1001/jamanetworkopen.2020.33980

Alexander, G. L., Deroche, C. B., Powell, K. R., Mosa, A. S. M., Popejoy, L., Koopman, R., & Liu, J. (2022). Development and pilot analysis of the nursing home HIT maturity survey and staging model. *Research in Gerontological Nursing, 15*(2), 93–99.

Alexander, G. L., Galambos, C., Rantz, M., Shumate, S., Vogelsmeier, A., Popejoy, L., & Crecelius, C. (2022). Value propositions for health information exchange toward improving nursing home hospital readmission rates. *Journal of Gerontological Nursing, 48*(1), 15–20.

Alexander, G. L., Liu, J., & Powell, K. (2022). Examining structural disparities of health information technology use in U.S. nursing homes. *JMIR Aging, 5*(3), e37482. https://doi.org/10.2196/37482

Alexander, G. L., Madsen, R., Deroche, C. B., Alexander, R., & Miller, E. (2019). Ternary trends in nursing home information technology and quality measures in the U.S. *Journal of Applied Gerontology, 39*(10), 1134–1143. https://doi.org/https://doi.org/10.1177/0733464819862928

Alexander, G. L., Madsen, R., & Newton, M. (2017). Analyzing change in nursing home information technology sophistication. *Journal of Gerontological Nursing, 43*(1), 17–21.

Alexander, G. L., & McMullen, T. L. (2023). Probing into federal policies and national academies' recommendations to adopt health information technology in all nursing homes. *Public Policy & Aging Report, 33*(S1), S28–S34.

Alexander, G. L., & Powell, K. (2021). *Digital maturity in U.S. nursing homes.* HIMSS Global Health Conference and Exhibition, Las Vegas, Nevada.

Alexander, G. L., Powell, K., & Deroche, C. B. (2020). An evaluation of telehealth expansion in U.S. nursing homes. *Journal of the American Medical Informatics Association, 28*(2), 342–348. https://doi.org/10.1093/jamia/ocaa253

Alexander, G. L., Rantz, M., Flesner, M., Diekemper, M., & Siem, C. (2007). Clinical information systems in nursing homes: An evaluation of initial implementation strategies. *Computers Informatics Nursing, 25*(4), 189–197.

Alexander, G. L., Rantz, M., Galambos, C., Vogelsmeier, A., Flesner, M., Popejoy, L., Mueller, J., Shumate, S., & Elvin, M. (2015). Preparing nursing homes for the future of health information exchange. *Applied Clinical Informatics, 6*(2), 248–266.

Alexander, G. L., & Wakefield, D. S. (2009). Information technology sophistication in nursing homes. *Journal of the American Medical Directors Association, 10*(6), 398–407.

Archbald-Pannone, L. R., Harris, D. A., Albero, K., Steele, R. L., Pannone, A. F., & Mutter, J. B. (2020). Covid-19 collaborative model for an academic hospital and long-term care facilities. *Journal of the American Medical Directors Association, 21*(7), 939–942. https://doi.org/10.1016/j.jamda.2020.05.044

Bezboruah, K. C., Paulson, D., & Smith, J. (2014). Management attitudes and technology adoption in long-term care facilities. *Journal of Health Organization & Management, 28*(3), 344–365.

Centers for Disease Control and Prevention. (2021, Jan. 19). *Nursing home COVID-19 data dashboard.* https://www.cdc.gov/nhsn/covid19/ltc-report-overview.html

Centers for Medicare & Medicaid Services. (2017). *Nursing homes.* https://www.cms.gov/medicare/provider-enrollment-and-certification/certificationandcomplianc/nhs.html

Centers for Medicare & Medicaid Services. (2020). *General provider telehealth and telemedicine tool kit.* https://www.cms.gov/files/document/general-telemedicine-toolkit.pdf

Cohen, C. C., Powell, K., Deroche, C. B., Agarwal, M., Stone, P., & Alexander, G. L. (2022). Examining nursing home information technology maturity and antibiotic use among long-term care residents. *Journal of the American Medical Directors Association, 23*, 1019–1024.e1012.

Cohen, C. C., Powell, K. R., Dick, A. W., Stone, P., & Alexander, G. L. (2022). The association between nursing home IT sophistication and UTI among long-term residents. *The Journal of Applied Gerontology, 41*(7), 1695–1701. https://doi.org/10.1177/07334648221082024

Henry, J., Plypchuck, Y., & Patel, V. (2018, November). Electronic health record adoption and interoperability among U.S. skilled nursing facilities in 2017. *ONC Data Brief, 41.* Office of the National Coordinator for Health Information Technology.

JASON. (2014). *A robust health data infrastructure.* Agency for Healthcare Research and Quality. https://www.healthit.gov/sites/default/files/facas/hitpc_jasonreport_2014-06-10.pdf

King, B. J., Gilmore-Bykovskyi, A. L., Roiland, R. A., Polnaszek, B. E., Bowers, B. J., & Kind, A. J. H. (2013). The consequences of poor communication during hospital to skilled nursing facility transitions: A qualitative study. *Journal of the American Geriatrics Society, 61*(7). https://doi.org/10.1111/jgs.12328

Ko, M., Wagner, L., & Spetz, J. (2018). Nursing home implementation of health information technology: Review of the literature finds inadequate investment in preparation, infrastructure, and training. *The Journal of Health Care Organization, Provision, and Financing, 55*, 1–10.

Kruse, C. S., Mileski, M., Alaytsev, V., Carol, E., & Williams, A. (2015). Adoption factors associated with electronic health record among long-term care facilities: A systematic review. *BMJ Open, 5*(1), e006615.

Levinson, D. R. (2014). *Adverse events in skilled nursing facilities: National incidence among Medicare beneficiaries.* Office of the Inspector General. https://oig.hhs.gov/oei/reports/oei-06-11-00370.pdf

Mehrotra, A. (2021, April 28). *Looking ahead: What should the telemedicine regulatory and payment landscape look like after the pandemic?* US House of Representatives. http://waysandmeans.house.gov/wp-content/uploads/2021/04/Ateev-Mehrotra-Testimony.pdf

National Academies of Sciences, Engineering, and Medicine. (2022a). Health information technology. In *The national imperative to improve nursing home quality: Honoring our commitment to residents, families, and staff* (pp. 453–494). The National Academies Press. https://doi.org/https://doi.org/10.17226/26526

National Academies of Sciences, Engineering, and Medicine. (2022b). *The national imperative to improve nursing home quality: Honoring our commitment to residents, families, and staff.* The National Academies Press. https://doi.org/https://doi.org/10.17226/26526

National Academies of Sciences, Engineering, and Medicine. (2022c). The nursing home workforce. In *The national imperative to improve nursing home quality: Honoring our commitment to residents, families, and staff* (pp. 221–302). The National Academies Press. https://www.ncbi.nlm.nih.gov/books/NBK584659/

Nolan, R. L. (1973). Managing the computer resource: A stage hypothesis. *Communications of the ACM, 16*(7), 399–405.

Office of the National Coordinator for Health Information Technology. (2015). *Electronic health records incentives and certification.* https://www.healthit.gov/providers-professionals/meaningful-use-definition-objectives.

Popejoy, L., Galambos, C., & Vogelsmeier, A. (2014). Hospital to nursing home transition challenges: Perceptions of nursing home staff. *Journal of Nursing Care Quality, 29*(2), 103–109.

Powell, K. R., & Alexander, G. L. (2021). Consequences of rapid telehealth expansion in nursing homes: Promise and pitfalls. *Applied Clinical Informatics, 12*(4), 933–943.

Powell, K. R., Winkler, A. E., Liu, J., & Alexander, G. L. (2022). A mixed-methods analysis of telehealth implementation in nursing homes amidst the COVID-19 pandemic. *Journal of the American Geriatric Society, 70*(12), 1–10. https://doi.org/10.1111/jgs.18020

Rantz, M. J., Scott-Cawiezell, J., Alexander, G. L., Conn, V., Madsen, R. W., Petroski, G. F., Hicks, L., Zwygart-Stauffacher, M., & RTI International. (2006). *Evaluation of the use of bedside technology to improve quality of care in nursing facilities.* https://www.cms.gov/research-statistics-data-and-systems/statistics-trends-and-reports/reports/downloads/rantz.pdf

Schoville, R. R. (2017). Discovery of implementation factors that lead to technology adoption in long-term care. *Journal of Gerontological Nursing, 43*(10), 21–26.

Shetty, K. D., Tolpadi, A. A., Robbins, M. W., Taylor, E. A., Campbell, K. N., & Damberg, C. L. (2020). Nursing home responses to performance-based accountability: Results of a national survey. *Journal of the American Geriatrics Society, 68*, 1979–1987.

Tate, K., Ma, R., Colin Reid, R., McLane, P., Waywitka, J., Cummings, G. E., & Cummings, G. G. (2023). A first look at consistency of documentation across care settings during emergency transitions of long-term care residents. *BMC Geriatrics, 23*(1), 17.

US Department of Health and Human Services. (2020). *21st century Cures Act: Interoperability, information blocking, and the ONC Health IT Certification Program*. https://www.federalregister.gov/documents/2020/05/01/2020-07419/21st-century-cures-act-interoperability-information-blocking-and-the-onc-health-it-certification

US Department of Health and Human Services. (2022). *Health IT legislation: 21st century Cures Act*. Office of the National Coordinator for Health Information Technology. https://www.healthit.gov/topic/laws-regulation-and-policy/health-it-legislation

Vogelsmeier, A. (2014). Identifying medication order discrepancies during medication reconciliation: Perceptions of nursing home leaders and staff. *Journal of Nursing Management, 22*(362), 372.

Vogelsmeier, A., Halbesleben, J. R. B., & Scott-Cawiezel, J. R. (2008). Technology implementation and workarounds in the nursing home. *Journal of the American Medical Informatics Association, 15*, 114–119.

Vogelsmeier, A., Popejoy, L., Canada, K., Galambos, C., Petroski, G., Crecelius, C., Alexander, G. L., & Rantz, M. (2021). Results of the Missouri Quality Initiative in Sustaining Changes in Nursing Home Care: Six-year trends of reducing hospitalizations of nursing home residents. *Journal of Nutritional Health and Aging, 25*(1), 5–12.

Walker, D., Mora, A., Demosthenidy, M. M., Menachemi, N., & Diana, M. L. (2016). Meaningful use of EHRs among hospitals ineligible for incentives lags behind that of other hospitals. *HealthAffairs, 35*(3), 495–501. https://doi.org/10.1377/hlthaff.2015.0924

INDEX

NOTE: Page references with an *f* are figures; page references with a *t* are tables.

4Ms (What Matters, Medication, Mentation, Mobility), 23, 23*f*, 28–29, 63, 64, 66, 309*t*–311*t*
24-hour presence of staff, 96
2567 Statement of Deficiencies, 264–265

A

AACN Essentials, 62–63
abbreviated standard survey, 257
abuse deficiencies, 267–268
academic-practice partnerships (APPs), 175, 176–178
academic reporting, competency-based education, 192–194
access
- to healthcare, 45, 47
- occupational therapists, 222

accountability, 33, 171
activities of daily living (ADLs), 77, 85, 186
- function-focused care (FFC), 78*t*
- occupational therapists, 221

acuity as indicator of education needs, 194–195
AD-8, 137
adaptive equipment, occupational therapists, 221–222
advance care planning, 236–237
advanced nursing
- practices, 168–170
- roles in long-term care, 190–191

advanced practice registered nurses (APRNs), 160
advancement for nursing assistants, 168
adverse events, preventing, 303. *See also* safety
age-friendly care, 21, 63–64
Age-Friendly Health Systems, 20, 22–35, 63, 64
- change in conditions, 26–28
- creating ecosystems, 25
- establishing baselines, 25
- 4Ms (What Matters, Medication, Mentation, Mobility), 23–24, 28–29
- leadership, 24
- Mentation, 26
- nursing home baselines, 24
- positive practice environments, 31–35
- resources and tools, 24–25
- shared governance, 31–35
- Teaching Nursing Homes, 29–30
- teamwork, 24

Agency for Healthcare Research and Quality (AHRQ), 149
almshouses, 2, 3
Alzheimer's Association, 65
Alzheimer's disease, 64, 65. *See also* cognitive impairment
American Association of Colleges of Nursing (AACN), 44, 62–63
American Hospital Association, 22, 63
ANCC Pathway to Excellence program, 20, 32*f*

appetite
  malnutrition, 141–143
  medication classes, 134*t*
assessments
  AACN Essentials, 62–63
  at-homeness, 67–70
  change in conditions, 26–28
  competency-based education, 192–194
  Confusion Assessment Method (CAM), 140
  deficiencies, 265*t*
  deficit-based model of, 65
  falls, 148–149
  4Ms (What Matters, Medication, Mentation, Mobility), 80*t*
  functional, 137
  function-focused care (FFC), 79–80
  Mentation, 26
  Minimum Data Set (MDS) 3.0, 136, 137, 142
  populations, 195
  preferences, 64–66, 75*t*
  questions, 68*t*–69*t*
  Simplified Nutritional Assessment Questionnaire, 142
  St. Louis University Rapid Geriatric Assessment, 133
  Tinetti Gait and Balance assessment, 138
  training materials, 71, 72
  urinary incontinence, 152
  well-being, 34
assignments, staff, 97
assistive technology, occupational therapists, 221–222
at-homeness, 67–70
attributes for information technology (IT) maturity, 323–324
avoiding burnout, 201–203

B

balancing safety and quality, 311–314
baselines
  Age-Friendly Health Systems, 25
  nursing homes, 24
bathing, 77
behavioral competency, 9
behaviors, 20. *See also* cultures
  dementia, 114
  expression of, 27
  management of, 28
belonging, 69
benefits of education, 196–197
billing services, 280–282
  Medicare consolidated billing, 283–285
biopsychosocial models, 8
Black older adults
  access to healthcare, 45
  inequities, 43–44
boarding homes, 3
Brief Inventory of Mental Status (BIMS), 137
Brigham and Women's Hospital (BWH), 21
burnout, avoiding, 201–203

C

capabilities of information technology (IT), 321
care
  age-friendly, 21
  competencies required for, 62–63
  Conceptual Model of Quality Nursing Home Care (NASEM, 2022), 307*f*
  creating culture of, 19 (*see also* culture of care)
  dementia, 65, 70, 113–123
  evaluation, 75–76
  Focused Dementia Care survey, 255
  function-focused care (FFC), 78*t*
  goals-of-care framework, 238
  good life model, 8–11, 9*f*
  hospice, 102–103
  models of, 6–11, 7*f*, 306–314
  nursing care-delivery models, 171–172
  palliative, 101
  patient-centered, 12
  person- and family-centered care, 61–62 (*see also* person- and family-centered care)
  person-centered, 12
  primary palliative, 104
  quality of, 248, 298 (*see also* quality)
  staff documentation, 285–293
  transitional, 106–107
Care Compare, 299

care-delivery models (CDLs), 95. *See also* delivery (of nursing care)
  dementia care model, 113–123
  engagement in care delivery, 200–201
  external palliative care consultations, 103
  hospice care, 102–103
  hospital readmissions, 107–108
  leadership and person-centered care, 99–101
  overview of, 96–101
  palliative care, 101
  poor transitions, 108–109
  primary palliative care, 104
  resources, 104–105
  transitional care interventions, 109–113
  used in modern nursing homes, 97–98
careers
  advancement for nursing assistants, 168
  opportunities in nursing homes, 175–180
  registered nurses (RNs), 165–166 (*see also* registered nurses [RNs])
  workforce, 159 (*see also* workforce)
Care Excellence, 77
caregiver training, 221–222
care partners, 165
care role models, 165
case studies, 30–31
  academic-practice partnerships (APPs), 176–178
  decision-making, 312–313
  dementia, 121–123
  diversity, equity, and inclusion (DEI), 52–54
  education, 203–204
  falls, 151
  frailty, 144–145
  geriatric syndromes, 146
  hospice care, 102–103
  interprofessional teams (IPCP), 238–242
  mealtimes, 269
  medications, 268
  preferences, 76
  quality, 308–309
  Quality Assurance and Performance Improvement (QAPI), 306
  speech-language pathologists, 224–228
  transitional care, 111–113
Catholic Health Association, 22, 63
Centers for Disease Control and Prevention (CDC), 41, 45
Centers for Medicare & Medicaid Services (CMS), 45, 160, 188, 195, 298
  deficiencies, 248
  information technology (IT), 320
  "Medicare and Medicaid Programs; Reform of Requirements for Long-Term Care Facilities" (2015), 250
  medication management, 213–214
  participation requirements, 252
  quality measures, 298
  State Operations Manual (SOM), 253
central pharmacies, 212–213
certification
  benefits of, 196–197
  nursing, 196
  recreation therapists, 230–231
certified nursing assistants (CNAs), 5, 12, 41, 186
  development, 35, 198
  inequities, 13–14
  medications, 188
  positive practice environments, 32
certified therapeutic recreation specialist (CTRS), 230
change in conditions, 26–28
charities, nursing homes and, 3
charting, clinical, 327–328
classification of payment models, 287
cleaning, 77
clinical charting, 327–328
clinical indicators, quality, 299. *See also* quality
clinical nurse specialists (CNSs), 160
CMS SOM Chapter 7, 258–260
coding, Minimum Data Sets (MDSs), 288*t*–289*t*
cognitive impairment, 135–141. *See also* delirium
  delirium, 138–140
  dementia, 136–138
  interventions, 140–141
  medication classes (geriatric syndromes), 134*t*
  physical therapist interventions, 217
collaborative practice, 209–210
comfort, 69

communication, 209, 312, 330*f*
- about preferences, 72–73
- case studies, 102–103
- dementia, 114 (*see also* dementia)

comparing nursing homes, 172
compensation, how nurses are paid, 276
competency-based education, 192–194
compliance, Medicare/Medicaid, 253
components of care-delivery models, 171*t*
computers, 329. *See also* information technology (IT)
Conceptual Model of Quality Nursing Home Care (NASEM, 2022), 307*f*
conditions, changes in, 26–28
Confusion Assessment Method (CAM), 140
consultant pharmacists, 213
consultations, external palliative care, 103
content (education) for older adults, 44
continence, 77
contracture management, occupational therapists, 222
convalescent homes, 3
cooking, 77
Council of State Governments, 249
COVID-19, 298
- inequities during, 43–44
- telehealth and, 211

Critical Element Pathways (CEPs), 260
Crossing the Quality Chasm (IOM, 2001), 62
culture of care
- Age-Friendly Health Systems, 22–35 (*see also* Age-Friendly Health Systems)
- creating, 19
- descriptions of organizational culture (OC), 20
- Just Culture, 21–22
- punitive cultures, 21–22

cultures
- changes in nursing homes, 11–12
- organizational culture (OC), 19–20
- of safety, 303–304

D

decision-making, 47, 171, 191. *See also* leadership
- case studies, 312–313
- sharing, 32–33, 302–303

deficiencies
- 2567 Statement of Deficiencies, 264–265
- abuse, 267–268
- assessments, 265*t*
- Centers for Medicare & Medicaid Services (CMS), 248
- CMS SOM Chapter 7, 258–260
- safety, 298 (*see also* safety)

deficit-based model of assessment, 65
delirium, 26–28, 115
- cognitive impairment, 138–140
- detection of, 28
- medication classes (geriatric syndromes), 134*t*
- risks, 139*t*
- types of, 139

Delirium Rating Scale, 140
delirium superimposed on dementia (DSD), 26
delivery (of nursing care), 95
- dementia care model, 113–123
- external palliative care consultations, 103
- hospice care, 102–103
- hospital readmissions, 107–108
- leadership and person-centered care, 99–101
- nursing care-delivery models, 171–172
- overview of, 96–101
- palliative care, 101
- poor transitions, 108–109
- primary palliative care, 104
- resources, 104–105
- transitional care, 106–107
- transitional care interventions, 109–113
- used in modern nursing homes, 97–98

delivery, engagement in, 200–201
dementia, 25, 64, 65
- care, 65, 70
- care model, 113–123
- case studies, 121–123
- cognitive impairment, 136–138
- definition of, 114

Focused Dementia Care survey, 255
Hogeweyk Dementia Village, 6
interventions, 115–118
key care essentials, 118–120
nonpharmacological interventions, 116*t*–117*t*
symptoms of, 120, 138
Department of Health and Human Services, 249, 303
depression, 214
Describe, Investigate, Create, and Evaluate (DICE), 117*t*
descriptions of organizational culture (OC), 20
design, roles of therapeutic, 69
detection of delirium, 28
development, 159–160
advanced nursing practice, 168–170
certified nursing assistants (CNAs), 198
information technology (IT), 324–325, 331
leadership, 191
licensed nursing staff, 164–168
licensed practical nurses (LPNs), 41, 167
nurse practice environments, 170–180
nursing assistants, 167–168
nursing positions, 160–170
performance evaluation, 192
professional, 35
Professional Nurse Practice model (PNP), 187–189
registered nurses (RNs), 164–166
staff, 185
Teaching Nursing Homes, 185–187
direct care staff, 12
director of nursing (DON), 33, 160–164
discharge planning, 235–236
disparities
health, 45, 48–54
information technology (IT), 325–326
diversity, definition of, 49–50
diversity, equity, and inclusion (DEI), 41–42
case studies, 52–54
inequities, 42, 43–44
nursing disparities/inequities, 48–54
nursing home resident populations, 44–54
documentation
eligibility, 290–293
staff, 285–293
dressing, 77
drugs, 133–134. *See also* medications
drumming, 29

E

Eden Alternative model, 12, 118
education
acuity as indicator of needs, 194–195
avoiding burnout, 201–203
benefits, 196–197
case studies, 203–204
competency-based, 192–194
content for older adults, 44
engagement in care delivery, 200–201
function-focused care (FFC), 83
long-term care, 188
methods of training, 199–200
nurse residency programs (NRPs), 178–180
nursing certification, 196
physical therapists, 215–216
Professional Nurse Practice model (PNP), 187–189
registered dietitian/nutritionists (RDNs), 228–229
role of educators, 198–199
Teaching Nursing Homes, 185–187
educators
responsibilities of, 199
role of, 198–199
electronic health records (EHRs), 333–334
eligibility
documentation, 290–293
Medicaid, 280
Elizabethan Poor Laws, 2
employment. *See also* careers; staff
opportunities in nursing homes, 175–180
selecting nursing home for, 173–175
empowerment, staff, 73–74
environmental approaches, function-focused care (FFC), 82

environments
information technology (IT), 323–333
nurse practice, 170–180
equity
definition of, 50
diversity, equity, and inclusion (DEI), 41–42 (*see also* diversity, equity, and inclusion [DEI])
equality and, 42*f*
evaluation
care, 75–76
performance, 192
everyday living inventories, 71, 72*t*
evolution of information technology (IT), 333–334
examples of competency-based education, 194
experience of transitions, 107*f*
expressions of unmet needs, 115
external palliative care consultations, 103

F

facility-level factors, 163
failure of adoption (IT), 320–323
falls, 115
assessments, 148–149
case studies, 151
definition of, 147
geriatric syndromes, 146–151
interventions, 149–151
medication classes (geriatric syndromes), 134*t*
occupational therapists, 222
physical therapist interventions, 217
risks, 147*t*–148*t*
families
function-focused care (FFC), 84–86
person- and family-centered care, 61–62 (*see also* person- and family-centered care)
training, 221–222
federal government intervention, 3–4
federal policies (IT), 320–323
Federal Register, 250
federal requirements, competency-based education, 193
feedback, competency-based education, 192–194
feeding, 77
Final Rule, 247, 250. *See also* regulatory processes
finances
billing services, 280–282
for-profit nursing homes, 293
hospice care, 282–283
how nurses are paid, 276
insurance plans, 279–280
long-term care (LTC), 275
Medicare consolidated billing, 283–285
Medicare long-stay residents, 280
nonprofit nursing homes, 293
nursing homes, 276–277
palliative care, 282–283
payors for nursing homes, 278–280
personal finance management, 77
private pay, 278–279
respite care, 282
short-stay residents, 279–280
staff documentation, 285–293
staff reimbursements, 285
systems (long-term care), 277–278
Five Star Rating system, 248, 266
Focused Dementia Care survey, 255
Focused Infection Control (FIC) survey, 256
focused surveys, 255–256. *See also* surveys
food service managers, 230
for-profit nursing homes, 293
for-profit status, 4–5
4Ms (What Matters, Medication, Mentation, Mobility), 23, 23*f*, 28–29, 63, 64, 66, 309*t*–311*t*
function-focused care (FFC), 80*t*
implementing, 23–24
organizational culture (OC), 30
frailty, 143–145
frameworks
4Ms (What Matters, Medication, Mentation, Mobility), 23*f* (*see also* 4Ms [What Matters, Medication, Mentation, Mobility])
goals-of-care, 238
information technology (IT), 323–333
occupational therapists, 219–221
SMART goal, 81–82
functional assessments, 137

functional nursing models, 97*t*, 98
functional urinary incontinence, 152, 217
function-focused care (FFC), 77–84
  assessments, 79–80
  barriers to, 79
  care activities, 78*t*
  education, 83
  environmental approaches, 82
  families, 84–86
  4Ms (What Matters, Medication, Mentation, Mobility), 80*t*
  interventions, 80–82
  planning, 80–82
  policies, 82–83
  risks, 83–84
function-focused care approach, 77–84

G

gathering information about preferences, 71–72
gender
  diversity, equity, and inclusion (DEI), 41
  inequities, 43–44
General Accounting Office (GAO), 249
geriatric syndromes, 131
  approaches to, 132–135
  case studies, 146
  characteristics of nursing home residents, 135
  cognitive impairment, 135–141
  falls, 146–151
  frailty, 143–144
  malnutrition, 141–143
  medications, 133–134
  presentation of illnesses, 134–135
  screening for, 133
  urinary incontinence, 151–153
gerontological nurses, 165
goals
  of nursing home care, 6, 7
  SMART goal framework, 81–82
goals-of-care framework, 238
Good Life model, 8–11, 9*f*
governance, sharing, 31–35
government
  federal government intervention, 3–4
  running almshouses, 2
Green House model, 13, 69, 118
groupers, 287

H

Harvard Business Review, 20
healthcare
  access to, 45, 47
  federal government intervention, 3–4
  for-profit status, 4–5
  geriatric syndromes (*see* geriatric syndromes)
  history of nursing homes, 2–3
  holistic, 6
  services, 45 (*see also* nursing homes)
health disparities, 45, 48–54
health information technology, 318. *See also* information technology (IT)
Health Insurance Prospective Payment System (HIPPS) codes, 207
Henry L. Hillman Foundation, 64
Hill-Burton Act (1946), 3
Hispanic older adults, health disparities, 45
history
  management of falls, 150*t*
  of nursing homes, 2–3
  of regulatory processes, 248–251
Hogeweyk Dementia Village, 6
holistic approaches to geriatric syndromes, 132–135
holistic healthcare, 6
home, searching for, 67. *See also* at-homeness; nursing homes
home safety, occupational therapists, 222
hospice care, 102–103
  case studies, 102–103
  finances, 282–283
  resources, 104–105
hospital readmissions, 107–108
hourly positions, 276
household model, 12
hyperactive delirium, 139
hypoactive delirium, 139

I

IHI Global Trigger Tool for Measuring Adverse Events, 303
illnesses, presentation of, 134–135
immediate jeopardy, 264
implementing
  4Ms (What Matters, Medication, Mentation, Mobility), 23–24
  information technology (IT), 321–322, 331
Improving Medicare Post-Acute Care Transformation Act of 2014, 331
improving nursing care, 1–2
  Continuous Quality Improvement (CQI) activities, 305
  federal government intervention, 3–4
  for-profit status, 4–5
  history of nursing homes, 2–3
  models of care, 6–11 (*see also* models)
  nursing home culture change, 11–12
  organizational culture (OC), 30
  Quality Assurance and Performance Improvement (QAPI), 305–306
  quality efforts, 5–6 (*see also* quality)
Improving the Quality of Nursing Home Care (IOM, 1986), 11, 298
inclusion
  definition of, 50–51
  diversity, equity, and inclusion (DEI), 41–42 (*see also* diversity, equity, and inclusion [DEI])
incontinence
  assessments, 152
  geriatric syndromes, 151–153
  interventions, 152–153
  medication classes (geriatric syndromes), 134*t*
Independence Foundation, 64
Individualized Positive Psychosocial Interaction (IPPI) program, 74
inequalities, 42
inequities, 42, 43–44
infections, Focused Infection Control (FIC) survey, 256
information technology (IT), 318
  capabilities, 321
  Centers for Medicare & Medicaid Services (CMS), 320
  current state of, 333–334
  development, 324–325, 331
  disparities, 325–326
  electronic health records (EHRs), 333–334
  environments, 323–333
  evolution of, 333–334
  failure of adoption, 320–323
  federal policies, 320–323
  implementing, 331
  maturity, 323–324
  quality, 320
  specialized technologies, 326–331
  telehealth, 334
  testing, 324–325
  use case interoperability, 331–333
infrastructure, information technology (IT), 321
instability, management of falls, 150*t*
Institute for Healthcare Improvement (IHI), 22, 61, 303, 309
Institute for Patient- and Family-Centered Care, 61
Institute of Medicine (IOM), 11, 45, 249
  Crossing the Quality Chasm (2001), 62
  Improving the Quality of Nursing Home Care (IOM, 1986), 298
instrumental activities of daily living (IADLs), 77
insurance plans, 279–280
integrating
  4Ms (What Matters, Medication, Mentation, Mobility), 30
  person-environment integration, 66
interactions, drug, 133–134
interoperability of use cases, 331–333
interprofessional teams (IPCP)
  case studies, 238–242
  collaborative practice, 209–210 (*see also* collaborative practice)
  definition of, 210
  introduction to nurses, 210–211
  nurses, 211–212

occupational therapists, 219–222
pharmacists, 212–214
physical therapists, 215–219
recreation therapists, 230–233
registered dietitian/nutritionists (RDNs), 228–230
rehabilitation services, 214–215
social workers, 233–238
speech therapists, 223–228
interventions
cognitive impairment, 140–141
dementia, 115–118
falls, 149–151
function-focused care (FFC), 80–82
incontinence, 152–153
malnutrition, 143
nonpharmacological, 116*t*–117*t*
physical therapists, 216–219
transitional care, 109–113
Interventions to Reduce Acute Care Transfers (INTERACT), 110
investigation processes, surveys, 262–263

J

JASON report, 320
Jewish Healthcare Foundation, 64
job satisfaction, staff, 85
John A. Hartford Foundation, 22
Just Culture, 21–22

K–L

key dementia care essentials, 118–120

Latino older adults
access to healthcare, 45
inequities, 43–44
laundry, 77
Lawton, M. Powell, 8
leadership, 33
acuity as indicator of education needs, 194–195
avoiding burnout, 201–203
benefits, 196–197
development, 191
engagement in care delivery, 200–201
methods of training, 199–200
nursing certification, 196
and person-centered care, 99–101
resources for, 100*t*
role of educators, 198–199
and teamwork, 24
legal requirements, medications, 213–214
legislation, 248. *See also* regulatory processes
Hill-Burton Act (1946), 3
Improving Medicare Post-Acute Care Transformation Act of 2014, 331
Omnibus Reconciliation Act of 1987, 298
Social Security Act (1935), 249
Lewy body dementia, 136
licensed nursing staff, 164–168
licensed practical nurses (LPNs), 41, 167
licensed practical/vocational nurses (LPNs/LVNs), 160
licensure, physical therapists, 215–216
life, quality of, 77
Life Safety Code (LSC) survey, 255, 304
long-stay residents, 280, 300–302
long-term care (LTC), 5. *See also* nursing homes
advanced nursing roles in, 190–191
development of nurses, 198
education, 188
finances, 275 (*see also* finances)
telehealth and, 211
long-term/post-acute care (LT/PAC) facilities, 248, 249, 250, 251, 252, 253
surveys, 260–261
love, 69

M

malnutrition, 141–143
interventions, 143
risks, 142
management
of behaviors, 28
contracture, 222
of falls, 150*t*
food service managers, 230
medications, 213–214, 329
personal finances, 77
use cases, 328*f*

Mandatory Medicaid Managed Care Programs for Long Term Services and Supports, 278
maturity, information technology (IT), 323–324
measurements
- IHI Global Trigger Tool for Measuring Adverse Events, 303
- performance, 47

measures
- quality, 298–303, 301*t*–302*t*
- safety, 303–306

Medicaid, 4, 45, 46, 250
- billing services, 280–282
- compliance, 253
- eligibility, 280
- regulatory processes, 247 (*see also* regulatory processes)

medical director (MD), 160
medical facilities, 6
medical records, 333. *See also* information technology (IT)
- electronic health records (EHRs), 333–334

Medicare, 45, 46, 250
- billing services, 280–282
- compliance, 253
- consolidated billing, 283–285
- long-stay residents, 280
- payments, 279–280
- regulatory processes, 247 (*see also* regulatory processes)
- reimbursements, 195, 279–280

Medicare Advantage Plan/Managed Care Plan, 279
Medicare Advantage plans, 278
medications
- certified nursing assistants (CNAs), 188
- classes (geriatric syndromes), 134*t*
- geriatric syndromes, 133–134
- management, 213–214, 329
- pharmacists, 212–214

memory, loss of, 114. *See also* dementia
- case studies, 121–123

Mentation, 26
mentors, 165
methods of training, 199–200
metrics, performance, 47
Mini-Cog, 137
Minimum Data Sets (MDSs), 25, 195, 279, 288
- 3.0, 136, 137, 142
- coding, 288*t*–289*t*
- Resident Assessment Instrument/Minimum Data Set (RAI/MDS), 299–300
- survey, 256

mixed delirium, 139
mobility, 25
- physical therapist interventions, 217–219

mock surveys, 261
models
- biopsychosocial, 8
- of care, 6–11, 7*f*
- components of care-delivery, 171*t*
- *Conceptual Model of Quality Nursing Home Care* (NASEM, 2022), 307*f*
- deficit-based model of assessment, 65
- dementia care, 113–123
- Eden Alternative, 12, 118
- functional nursing, 97*t*, 98
- Good Life, 8–11, 9*f*
- Green House, 13, 69, 118
- household, 12
- nursing care delivery, 95, 171–172 (*see also* delivery [of nursing care])
- Patient Driven Payment Model (PDPM), 195, 286–287
- payments, 96
- primary nursing, 97*t*, 98
- Professional Nurse Practice model (PNP), 187–189
- of quality care, 306–314
- quality-of-life, 8
- team nursing, 97*t*, 98
- total patient care, 97*t*, 98
- traditional medical, 7
- transitional care, 106–107
- Wellspring model, 13, 118

modernization of nursing homes, 4
Montreal Cognitive Assessment, 137
multifactorial approaches to geriatric syndromes, 132–135
music therapy, 116*t*

N

National Academies of Practice (NAP), 210
National Academies of Science, Engineering, and Medicine (NASEM), 298, 320
    Conceptual Model of Quality Nursing Home Care (NASEM, 2022), 307*f*
    The National Imperative to Improve Nursing Home Quality (NASEM, 2022), 298
National Association of Health Care Assistants, 44
National Citizens' Coalition for Nursing Home Reform (NCCNHR), 11
National Council for Therapeutic Recreation Certification (NCTRC), 230
National Fire Protection Association, 255
The National Imperative to Improve Nursing Home Quality (NASEM, 2022), 298
National Institute of CNA Excellence, 168
near misses, reporting, 21
neglect, 115
neurocognitive disorders, 136. *See also* cognitive impairment
nonpharmacological interventions, 116*t*–117*t*
nonprofit nursing homes, 293
nurse managers (NMs), 33
nurse practice environments, 170–180
nurse practitioners (NPs), 160, 169–170
nurse residency programs (NRPs), 175, 178–180
nursing. *See also* staff
    avoiding burnout, 201–203
    certification, 196
    disparities/inequities, 48–54
    how nurses are paid, 276
    interprofessional teams (IPCP), 211–212
    interventions (*see* interventions)
    long-term care education, 188
    staff reimbursements, 285
    staffs, 173 (*see also* staff)
    strengths-based, 65, 66
    workforce (*see* workforce)
nursing assistants, 167–168
    advancement for, 168
nursing care
    delivery, 95 (*see also* delivery [of nursing care])
    federal government intervention, 3–4
    for-profit status, 4–5
    history of nursing homes, 2–3
    improving, 1–2
    models of care, 6–11 (*see also* models)
    nursing home culture change, 11–12
    quality efforts, 5–6
nursing care-delivery models, 171–172
nursing home administrator (NHA), 160
Nursing Home Reform Act. *See* OBRA '89
nursing homes
    Age-Friendly Health Systems, 22–35 (*see also* Age-Friendly Health Systems)
    baselines, 24
    billing services, 280–282
    characteristics of residents, 135
    comparing, 172
    culture change, 11–12
    dementia care model, 113–123, 118*f*
    finances, 276–277
    for-profit status, 4–5, 293
    4Ms (What Matters, Medication, Mentation, Mobility), 309*t*–311*t*
    history of, 2–3
    inequities (workforce), 43–44
    information technology (IT), 318 (*see also* information technology [IT])
    Medicaid, 4
    models of care, 6–11 (*see also* models)
    modernization of, 4
    nonprofit, 293
    partnerships, 24–25
    payment structures, 286–289
    payors for, 278–280
    populations (*see* populations)
    presentation of illnesses, 134–135
    quality efforts to improve, 5–6
    regulatory processes (*see* regulatory processes)
    resident populations, 44–54
    resident wishes, 73–74
    resources, 24–25
    roles of, 297
    selecting for employment, 173–175
    specialized technologies, 326–331

teaching, 185–187
tools, 24–25
workforce, 41 (*see also* development)
nursing positions, 160–170
director of nursing (DON), 160–164

O

objective environment, 9
OBRA '89, 248–253
purpose/intent, 251–253
occupational therapists, 219–222
Office of Inspector General (OIG), 303
Office of the National Coordinator for Health Information Technology, 331, 333
older adults, health disparities, 45
Omnibus Reconciliation Act of 1987, 298
organizational culture (OC), 19–20, 30
overflow urinary incontinence, 152
ownership, 33

P

pain, 115
palliative care, 101
external palliative care consultations, 103
finances, 282–283
primary, 104
resources, 104–105
Parkinson's disease dementia, 136
participation requirements (CMS), 252
partnerships, nursing homes, 24–25
Pathway-LTC, 32
patient-centered care, 12
Patient Driven Payment Model (PDPM), 195, 286–287
patients
balancing quality and, 311–314
focus on needs of, 210
preferences, 311–314
scheduling, 327–328
payments
billing services, 280–282
insurance plans, 279–280
long-term care finance systems, 277–278 (*see also* finances)
Medicare, 45, 46, 279–280 (*see also* Medicaid)
Medicare Advantage plans, 278
Medicare consolidated billing, 283–285
Medicare long-stay residents, 280
models, 96
Patient Driven Payment Model (PDPM), 195, 286–287
private pay, 278–279
short-stay residents, 279–280
staff documentation, 285–293
staff reimbursements, 285
structures for nursing homes, 286–289
payors for nursing homes, 278–280
Pennsylvania Revisiting the Teaching Nursing Home program, 20
Pennsylvania State University College of Nursing, 64
perceived valuation, 9
performance
case studies, 306
evaluation, 192
measurements, 47
Quality Assurance and Performance Improvement (QAPI), 305–306
performance improvement (PI), 305
personal finance management, 77
personal power, 67
person- and family-centered care, 61–62
AACN Essentials, 62–63
age-friendly care, 63–64
approaches to, 70–76
assessing preferences for care, 64–66
at-homeness, 67–70
care evaluation, 75–76
case studies, 76
function-focused care approach, 77–84
staff empowerment, 73–74
person-centered care, 12
leadership and, 99–101
person-environment integration, 66
pharmacists, 212–214
pharmacy systems, 329*t*, 330*f*. *See also* information technology (IT)
physical activities, 79
Physical Capability Measure, 138

physical therapists, 215–219
  education, 215–216
  licensure, 215–216
Pioneer Network, 12
planning
  advance care, 236–237
  at-homeness, 67–70
  discharge, 235–236
  function-focused care (FFC), 80–82
  person- and family-centered care, 61–62 (*see also* person- and family-centered care)
point of care (POC) systems, 326, 327
policies
  function-focused care (FFC), 82–83
  information technology (IT), 320–323
  nursing disparities/inequities, 48–54
  nursing homes, 24
poorhouses, 2
populations
  assessments, 195
  nursing home resident, 44–54
positions. *See* nursing positions
positive practice environments, 31–35
post-acute and long-term care (PA-LTC) settings, 132, 133
poverty, 2
power, personal, 67
practices
  advanced nursing practice, 168–170
  collaborative (*see* collaborative practice)
  nurse practice environments, 170–180
  nursing disparities/inequities, 48–54
  nursing homes, 24
  Professional Nurse Practice model (PNP), 187–189
pre-assessments, 63. *See also* assessments
preferences
  assessments, 75*t*
  for care, 64–66
  case studies, 76
  communication about, 72–73
  everyday living inventories, 71, 72*t*
  gathering information, 71–72
  patient wishes, 73–74, 311–314
Preferences for Activities and Leisure (PAL) cards, 72, 73*f*
preparation
  Quality Review/Mock Survey, 261
  for surveys, 262
presentation of illnesses, 134–135
pressure ulcers, 115
primary nursing models, 97*t*, 98
primary palliative care, 104
private equity firms, 4
private pay, 278–279
processes
  Quality Assurance and Performance Improvement (QAPI), 253
  regulatory, 247–248 (*see also* regulatory processes)
  surveys, 260–269
professional development, 35
Professional Nurse Practice model (PNP), 187–189
profits, for-profit status, 4–5
protocols, safety, 304
psychological well-being, 9
punitive cultures, 21–22

Q

quality, 34
  balancing safety and, 311–314
  of care, 248
  case studies, 308–309
  Conceptual Model of Quality Nursing Home Care (NASEM, 2022), 307*f*
  Continuous Quality Improvement (CQI) activities, 305
  COVID-19, 298
  efforts to improve nursing homes, 5–6
  4Ms (What Matters, Medication, Mentation, Mobility), 309*t*–311*t*
  information technology (IT), 320
  of life, 77
  long-stay residents, 300–302
  measures, 298–303, 301*t*–302*t*
  models of quality care, 306–314

Resident Assessment Instrument/Minimum Data Set (RAI/MDS), 299–300
safety measures, 303–306
sharing decision-making, 302–303
short-stay residents, 300–302
Quality, Safety, and Oversight (QSO) memoranda, 253
quality assurance (QA), 305
Quality Assurance and Performance Improvement (QAPI), 253, 305–306
quality-of-life model, 8
questions, assessments, 68*t*–69*t*

R

race inequities, 43–44
rating methodologies, abuse deficiencies, 267–268
readmissions, hospital, 107–108
real estate investment trusts (REITS), 4, 5
re-authorization, 280
records, 333. *See also* information technology (IT)
electronic health records (EHRs), 333–334
recreation therapists, 230–233
refuge, 67
registered dietitian/nutritionists (RDNs), 228–230
registered nurses (RNs), 41, 160, 164–166. *See also* nursing
opportunities in nursing homes, 175–180
roles, 166*t*
regulatory processes, 247–248
for-profit nursing homes, 293
history of, 248–251
nonprofit nursing homes, 293
OBRA '89, 248–253
purpose/intent of OBRA '89, 251–253
Social Security Act (1935), 249
types of surveys, 253–258 (*see also* surveys)
rehabilitation services, 214–215
reimbursements. *See also* finances; payments
Medicare, 195, 279–280 (*see also* Medicaid)
Medicare Advantage plans, 278
staff, 285
relationships, 67
reporting
competency-based education, 192–194
JASON report, 320
near misses, 21
Office of the National Coordinator for Health Information Technology, 331
requirements
Centers for Medicare & Medicaid Services (CMS), 252
competency-based education, 193
information technology (IT), 321
medications, 213–214
regulatory processes (*see* regulatory processes)
Resident Assessment Instrument/Minimum Data Set (RAI/MDS), 299–300
residents
balancing quality and, 311–314
wishes, 73–74
resident rights, 234–235
resources
Age-Friendly Health Systems, 24–25
care-delivery models (CDLs), 104–105
delivery (of nursing care), 104–105
for leadership, 100*t*
respite care finances, 282
responsibilities
director of nursing (DON), 163–164
of educators, 199
rest homes, 3
restraints, 115
results, surveys, 264–268
Revisiting the Teaching Nursing Home (RTNH), 64, 185–187
rights, resident, 234–235
risks
communication, 312
delirium, 139*t*
falls, 147*t*–148*t*
function-focused care (FFC), 83–84
geriatric syndromes, 132
Just Culture, 21
malnutrition, 142
reducing, 6
Robert Wood Johnson Foundation, 61, 64

roles
advanced nursing roles in long-term care, 190–191
dementia interventions, 116
of director of nursing (DON), 163–164
of educators, 198–199
of nurse practitioners, 169–170
of nursing homes, 297
of registered dietitian/nutritionists (RDNs), 229–230
of registered nurses (RNs), 166*t*
of staff, 189*f*
of therapeutic design, 69

S

safety, 34
AHRQ Survey on Patient Safety Culture (SOPS), 304
balancing quality and, 311–314
COVID-19, 298
creating culture of, 303–304
measures, 303–306
protocols, 304
salaried positions, 276
scheduling patients, 327–328
scoring rules summaries, surveys, 266–267
screening for geriatric syndromes, 133, 137. *See also* assessments
selecting nursing home for employment, 173–175
self, maintaining sense of, 119–120
self-care, definition of, 202–203
self-reconciliation, 67
self-reflection, 192–194
Serial Trial Intervention (STI), 117*t*
services
billing, 280–282
healthcare, 45 (*see also* nursing homes)
sharing
decision-making, 32–33, 302–303
governance, 31–35
short-stay residents
finances, 279–280
quality, 300–302
Simplified Nutritional Assessment Questionnaire, 142
skilled nursing facilities (SNFs), 288
SMART goal framework, 81–82
Social Security Act (1935), 3, 4, 249
social workers, 49, 233–238
Special Committee on Aging, 249
Special Focus Facilities (SFF), 258
specialized technologies, 326–331
medication management, 329
pharmacy systems, 329*t*, 330*f*
use cases, 328*f*
speech-language pathologists, 224–228
speech therapists, 223–228
splinting, occupational therapists, 222
staff. *See also* workforce
24-hour presence of, 96
assignments, 97
certified nursing assistants (CNAs), 5, 12
compensation, 276
competency-based education, 192–194
development, 185
direct care, 12
director of nursing (DON), 160–164
diversity, equity, and inclusion (DEI), 47 (*see also* diversity, equity, and inclusion [DEI])
documentation, 285–293
empowerment, 73–74
engagement in care delivery, 200–201
job satisfaction, 85
leadership, 191 (*see also* leadership)
licensed nursing, 164–168
nursing, 173
nursing positions, 160–170
opportunities in nursing homes, 175–180
performance evaluation, 192
Professional Nurse Practice model (PNP), 187–189
registered nurses (RNs), 164–166
reimbursements, 285
roles, 189*f*
staffing mixes, 97
training, 185
turnover, 12

Staff Training in Assisted Living Residencies (STAR), 117*t*
Standard Health Care Facilities Code (HCFC) survey, 304
standards, surveys, 254
state, 248
statements, 2567 Statement of Deficiencies, 264–265
State Operations Manual (SOM), 253
  Appendix PP, 193
State Survey Agency (SSA), 252, 260
St. Louis University Mental Status Exam, 137
St. Louis University Rapid Geriatric Assessment, 133
strategies
  care delivery, 171
  culture change, 11–12
  family effectiveness, 84–86
strength-based approach to dementia care, 114
strengths-based nursing, 65, 66
stress urinary incontinence, 151
support, 171
  function-focused care (FFC), 82–83
Surveyor Minimum Qualifications Test (SMQT), 254
surveys
  abbreviated standard survey, 257
  abuse deficiencies, 267–268
  AHRQ Survey on Patient Safety Culture (SOPS), 304
  CMS SOM Chapter 7, 258
  compliance, 257–258
  Five Star Rating system, 266
  Focused Dementia Care survey, 255
  Focused Infection Control (FIC) survey, 256
  investigation processes, 262–263
  Life Safety Code (LSC), 255, 304
  long-term/post-acute care (LT/PAC) facilities, 260–261
  Minimum Data Set (MDS) survey, 256
  preparation for, 262
  processes, 260–269
  Quality Review/Mock Survey, 261
  regulatory, 247 (*see also* regulatory processes)
  results, 264–268
  scoring rules summaries, 266–267
  Special Focus Facilities (SFF), 258
  standard, 254
  Standard Health Care Facilities Code (HCFC) survey, 304
  State Survey Agency (SSA), 252, 260
  2567 Statement of Deficiencies, 264–265
  types of, 253–258
symptoms
  of dementia, 114, 120, 138
  geriatric syndromes (*see* geriatric syndromes)

T

Tailored Activity Program (TAP), 116*t*
Teaching Nursing Homes, 29–30, 64, 185–187
team nursing models, 97*t*, 98
teamwork
  4Ms (What Matters, Medication, Mentation, Mobility), 30
  function-focused care (FFC), 84–86
  leadership and, 24
technology. *See* information technology (IT)
telehealth, 210, 334
testing information technology (IT), 324–325
theories, occupational therapists, 219–221
therapeutic design, roles of, 69
Tinetti Gait and Balance assessment, 138
tools
  Age-Friendly Health Systems, 24–25
  IHI Global Trigger Tool for Measuring Adverse Events, 303
total patient care models, 97*t*
traditional medical models, 7
training
  caregivers, 221–222
  competency-based education, 192–194
  leadership, 181
  materials, 71, 72
  methods of, 199–200
  nurse residency programs (NRPs), 178–180
  occupational therapists, 221–222
  opportunities, 175
  performance evaluation, 192

Professional Nurse Practice model (PNP), 187–189
role of educators, 198–199
staff, 185
Staff Training in Assisted Living Residencies (STAR), 117*t*
Teaching Nursing Homes, 185–187
transferring, 77
transitional care, 106–107
case studies, 111–113
hospital readmissions, 107–108
interventions, 109–113
poor transitions, 108–109
transitions, experience of, 107*f*
transportation, 77
treatments
COVID-19, 298
depression, 214
geriatric syndromes, 133–134 (*see* geriatric syndromes)
turnover, 12
24-hour presence of staff, 96
2567 Statement of Deficiencies, 264–265
types of surveys, 253–258

U–V

University of Pennsylvania School of Nursing, 64
University of Pittsburgh School of Nursing, 186
unmet needs, expressions of, 115
urge urinary incontinence, 151
urinary incontinence
assessments, 152
geriatric syndromes, 151–153
interventions, 152–153
medication classes (geriatric syndromes), 134*t*
physical therapist interventions, 217
types of, 151–152
US Bureau of Labor Statistics (BLS), 41
use cases, 328*f*, 332*f*
interoperability, 331–333

W–Z

wages, how nurses are paid, 276
Watkins, Michael D., 20
weight loss
malnutrition, 141–143
medication classes (geriatric syndromes), 134*t*
well-being, 34–35
psychological, 9
Wellspring model, 13, 118
workforce
adopting information technology (IT), 322
development (workforce), 159–160 (*see also* development)
diversity, equity, and inclusion (DEI), 41 (*see also* diversity, equity, and inclusion [DEI])
inequities, 43–44
nursing homes, 41
World Health Organization (WHO), 202
wounds, physical therapist interventions, 217